Imaging

Radiotherapy in Practice

Series editor: Peter Hoskin

Radiotherapy in Practice: *Radioisotope Therapy*, edited by Peter Hoskin

Radiotherapy in Practice: *Brachytherapy*, edited by Peter Hoskin and Catherine Coyle

Radiotherapy in Practice: *External Beam Therapy*, edited by Peter Hoskin

Radiotherapy in Practice Imaging

Edited by

Peter Hoskin and
Vicky Goh

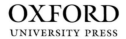

OXFORD

UNIVERSITY PRESS

Great Clarendon Street, Oxford OX2 6DP

Oxford University Press is a department of the University of Oxford.
It furthers the University's objective of excellence in research, scholarship,
and education by publishing worldwide in

Oxford New York

Auckland Cape Town Dar es Salaam Hong Kong Karachi
Kuala Lumpur Madrid Melbourne Mexico City Nairobi
New Delhi Shanghai Taipei Toronto

With offices in

Argentina Austria Brazil Chile Czech Republic France Greece
Guatemala Hungary Italy Japan Poland Portugal Singapore
South Korea Switzerland Thailand Turkey Ukraine Vietnam

Oxford is a registered trade mark of Oxford University Press
in the UK and in certain other countries

Published in the United States
by Oxford University Press Inc., New York

British Library Cataloguing in Publication Data

Data available

Library of Congress Cataloging-in-Publication Data

Radiotherapy in practice : imaging / edited by Peter Hoskin and Vicky Goh.
      p. ; cm.—(Radiotherapy in practice)
   Includes bibliographical references and index.
   ISBN 978–0–19–923132–4 (alk. paper) 1. Cancer—Diagnosis.
2. Cancer—Radiotherapy. 3. Tumors—Classification. I. Hoskin, Peter J.
II. Goh, Vicky. III. Title: Imaging. IV. Series: Radiotherapy in practice.
   [DNLM: 1. Neoplasms—diagnosis. 2. Neoplasms—radiotherapy.
3. Diagnostic Imaging. 4. Neoplasm Staging. 5. Radiotherapy Dosage.
QZ 269 R1323 2010]
   RC270.R33 2010
   616.99'40642—dc22   2009033187

Typeset in Minion by Glyph International, Bangalore, India
Printed in Great Britain
on acid-free paper by the
MPG Books Group, Bodmin and King's Lynn

ISBN 978–0–19–923132–4

10 9 8 7 6 5 4 3 2 1

Contents

Contributors

Dr Edwin Aird,
Mount Vernon Hospital,
Northwood

Dr Steve Allen,
Royal Marsden Hospital,
Sutton

Dr Jamshed Bomanji,
University College Hospital,
London

Dr Guy Burkill,
Royal Sussex County Hospital,
Brighton

Dr Anthony Chambers,
Northwick Park and
St Mark's Hospitals,
Harrow

Dr R. Jane Chambers,
Mount Vernon Hospital,
Northwood

Dr Yong Du,
Christie Hospital/University of
Manchester

Dr Sara C. Erridge,
Edinburgh Cancer Centre

Dr Charlotte Fowler,
Harefield Hospital,
Harefield

Dr Mark Gaze,
University College Hospital,
London

Dr Ian Geh,
Queen Elizabeth Hospital,
Birmingham

Dr Rod Gibson,
Western General Hospital,
Edinburgh

Dr Rob Glynne-Jones,
Mount Vernon Hospital,
Northwood

Dr Vicky Goh,
Mount Vernon Hospital,
Northwood

Professor Peter Hoskin,
Mount Vernon Hospital,
Northwood

Dr Paul Humphries,
University College Hospital,
London

Dr Steven James,
The Royal Orthopaedic
NHS Foundation Trust,
Birmingham

Dr Julian Kabala,
Bristol Royal Infirmary,
Bristol

Dr Vincent Khoo,
Royal Marsden Hospital,
Sutton

Dr Kate Lankester,
Royal Sussex County Hospital,
Brighton

Dr Jonathan Liaw,
Memorial Hermann Hospital,
Houston, USA

Dr Brinder Mahon,
Queen Elizabeth Hospital,
Birmingham

Dr Ben Miller,
Birmingham Heartlands Hospital,
Birmingham

Dr Eleanor Moskovic,
Royal Marsden NHS Foundation Trust,
London

Dr Noelle O'Rourke,
The Western Infirmary,
Glasgow

Dr Francesca Peters,
University College Hospital,
London

Dr Shuvro Roy-Choudhury,
Birmingham Heartlands Hospital,
Birmingham

Dr Bal Sanghera,
Mount Vernon Hospital,
Northwood

Dr Frank Saran,
Royal Marsden NHS Foundation Trust,
London

Professor Michele Saunders,
University College Hospital,
London

Dr Beatrice Seddon,
University College Hospital,
London

Ms Jane Shekhdar,
Mount Vernon Hospital,
Northwood

Dr S. Aslam Sohaib,
Royal Marsden Hospital,
Sutton

Dr David Spooner,
Queen Elizabeth Hospital,
Birmingham

Dr Michael Sproule,
The Western Infirmary,
Glasgow

Dr David Summers,
Western General Hospital,
Edinburgh

Dr Derek Svasti-Salee,
Royal Marsden NHS Foundation Trust,
London

Dr Jane Taylor,
Mount Vernon Hospital,
Northwood

Dr Charlotte Whittaker,
St Mary's Hospital,
London

Dr Oliver Wignall,
Royal Marsden Hospital,
Sutton

Dr Wai-Lup Wong,
Mount Vernon Hospital,
Northwood

Chapter 1

Introduction

Peter Hoskin and Vicky Goh

Imaging is an essential component in the management of any patient with cancer. With perhaps the exception of a small superficial basal cell carcinoma all patients will require imaging evaluation of their malignancy. Therefore it is essential that the principles of imaging and the specific requirements for each tumour site are clearly understood by those involved in the management of patients with malignant disease to enable optimum use of this essential modality.

1.1 The role of imaging

The role of imaging is extensive and integral to management at any point in the patient's journey. At a patient's initial presentation imaging may have led to the discovery of a tumour, resulting in the image-guided or surgical procedure to confirm its malignant nature. It will then be essential for assessing the full extent of that tumour and defining the tumour stage by evaluating pathways of direct, lymphatic, and blood-borne spread. The tumour stage is critical to subsequent management and it is therefore vital that appropriate imaging is undertaken at this point.

For the patient having radiotherapy, an accurate assessment of the tumour to be treated and of the surrounding organs at risk is critical to the planning of the radiotherapy. Detailed evaluation through diagnostic imaging is essential for delivering optimal radiotherapy. The most important step in radiotherapy planning is tumour localization and, with the few exceptions of readily palpable and visible skin tumours, a full appreciation of the anatomical localization, involvement of surrounding structures, and proximity to critical organs is essential, and can only be provided through appropriate radiological investigations.

Following treatment, further management is based on response assessment and continued surveillance in which imaging will play a major part. It is essential to have an understanding of the positive and negative predictive value of a test and the level of reliance that can be placed upon it. This is particularly the case in the response assessment scenario when patients may be subjected to major salvage procedures on the basis of failure to achieve a radiological complete response.

1.2 Imaging modalities

X-ray imaging was available soon after the discovery of X-rays by Roentgen in 1895. It is remarkable that despite technical improvements in the production of plain X-ray images and increased understanding of the use of contrast materials it took almost 80 years for the next revolution in imaging to appear in the clinical setting with the introduction of computed tomography (CT). Over the subsequent 30 years there has, however, been a major revolution in the imaging world with ever more sophisticated and rapid CT imaging, the advent of clinical magnetic resonance (MR), and in the last decade the development of functional imaging techniques harnessing not only CT and MR but also positron emission tomography (PET). The result of this dramatic technological change is that a modern cancer centre has a sophisticated range of imaging modalities available for each patient to provide detailed information on both the anatomical distribution and physiological characteristics of the tumour in question. The challenge in this setting is to optimize the use of each modality in order to obtain the most accurate and reliable information possible with the technology available.

1.3 Integration into the radiotherapy department

Modern radiotherapy is a complex multistep process, optimizing the many features of a modern linear accelerator in order to deliver a high dose of radiation to the tumour yet minimizing exposure to surrounding organs at risk, thus ensuring that patients receive accurate reproducible treatment. Imaging is an integral component of many of the stages through which a patient will pass in the radiotherapy department. The technological developments in imaging in recent years have also driven important changes in the radiotherapy department.

For many years imaging information and radiotherapy planning was undertaken in parallel rather than in an integrated fashion. Information from plain radiology film and later CT images would be manually and visually transferred to orthogonal X-ray films taken in the radiotherapy treatment simulator. Dosimetric planning would be undertaken with a manual outline of the patient's shape and size, which would be obtained using a piece of bendy wire or plaster of Paris transferred by hand to a sheet of paper and then the radiotherapist using co-ordinates would measure from the orthogonal X-ray films to derive the position and size of the treatment volume and any organs at risk which were important. This was a laborious and relatively inaccurate process. This has now been largely set aside with all modern radiotherapy departments using CT-based planning systems in which a CT scanning sequence is imported into a radiotherapy planning computer system and the treatment volume, together with the organs at risk, are defined on screen on sequential CT images so that an accurate three-dimensional reconstruction is obtained. This is then used by radiation physicists to define the beam sizes, shapes, and contributions to achieve a homogeneous dose distribution within the planning target volume whilst minimizing dose to organs at risk. It also provides information on tissue inhomogeneities for X-ray absorption corrections. For example, lungs will absorb far less energy, having lower electron density than other soft tissue such as skin and muscle. This enables a highly accurate dosimetric plan to be achieved based on the detailed anatomical information provided.

Critical to the successful treatment of a patient using this information is that the scanning for dosimetry purposes (the planning scan) is obtained in identical positions and circumstances to those that will be encountered on the linear accelerator during treatment. This will often be different to those used for optimal imaging sequences, for example the treatment couch is flat rather than scalloped, the patient may need to have their arms raised above their head out of the path of an X-ray beam, and there will be constraints on bladder filling and other physiological parameters. The use of intravenous contrast can be useful in radiotherapy planning as in diagnostic imaging to distinguish vessels from other soft tissue structures such as lymph nodes. Large volumes of oral contrast to outline bowel are not used because large volumes of contrast can alter the absorption characteristics of the dosimetric calculations. In the early years of using CT imaging it was usual for these to be performed on the imaging scanner, often allocating a half-day session to radiotherapy planning scans so that the altered scanning conditions could be accommodated without disruption of the imaging processes. In most modern departments now however, there are dedicated radiotherapy CT simulators designed for the acquisition of radiotherapy planning scans with appropriate couch tops and larger apertures to enable radiotherapy treatment positions, for example with the arms raised, to be accommodated in the scanner. These may produce images which have slightly lower resolution to the diagnostic images and thus not necessarily interchangeable with diagnostic images. Diagnostic scans will still be required to supplement information from the planning scan during tumour demarcation.

There are certain sites where MR is superior to CT in demarcating tumour and normal tissue structures: particular examples would include the brain and pelvis for prostate, bladder, and uterine tumours. At present however, MR cannot be used in radiotherapy dosimetry. This is related to the distortion characteristics at the edge of the MR field so that the patient outline is less accurate and also the fact that the information on X-ray absorption heterogeneities is not obtained in the process of MR scanning. This has been overcome in many departments by the use of MR/CT registration, so that the CT remains the platform for radiotherapy planning but the superior MR diagnostic information is available on the same screen overlaid on the CT template.

The next phase of development will undoubtedly be integration of information from PET/CT with both MR and diagnostic CT data. It is feasible that PET/CT could be used as a radiotherapy planning image incorporating the functional information from PET with the anatomical and X-ray absorption heterogeneity data in the CT images. This remains an investigational area at present and in most cases the diagnostic information from PET will be used alongside the diagnostic CT information during radiotherapy planning rather than integrated into the planning images.

1.4 **Summary**

- Imaging is an integral component of patient care throughout the cancer journey, being required for diagnosis and staging, treatment planning, and subsequent response evaluation and follow-up.

- The dramatic evolution of imaging modalities in recent years with widespread availability of high speed CT, MR, and functional imaging has driven major changes in radiotherapy practice, with most patients' treatment being planned using information from CT-based datasets, enabling three-dimensional reconstruction of treatment volumes and organs at risk and more accurate dosimetry.

- The precise requirements for individual tumours and tumour sites vary and a clear appreciation of the relative strengths and weaknesses of different imaging modalities for a given patient is essential. Alongside this it is critical to bear in mind that increased availability and use of imaging exposes the patient to a higher concomitant radiation dose, the long-term sequelae of which are as yet to be fully evaluated.

- Clear justification based on sound evidence is essential in this setting for each diagnostic radiation exposure to ensure that the imaging tools are used optimally for each patient.

Chapter 2

Principles of imaging

Jonathan Liaw, Jane Taylor,
Anthony Chambers, Bal Sanghera, and
Vicky Goh

Introduction

Imaging is fundamentally important to the management of the cancer patient. Anatomical imaging is the mainstay for patient evaluation; however, functional and hybrid (combined functional–anatomical) imaging have acquired an increasing role.

To obtain the most accurate and reliable information possible with the most appropriate imaging modality the relative performance of the imaging test has to be defined. Commonly used measures of test performance include:

- *Sensitivity*: how good the test is at picking up disease (true positive (TP)/TP + false negative (FN)), expressed as a percentage.
- *Specificity*: how good the test is at excluding disease (true negative (TN)/TN + false positive (FP)), expressed as a percentage.
- *Accuracy*: how good a test is at picking up and excluding disease (TP + TN/TP + FP + TN + FN), expressed as a percentage.

Test performance is also affected by the prevalence of disease in the population: test performance will be lower if disease prevalence in the population is low i.e. the *positive predictive value* (TP/TP + FP) will be lower (Table 2.1). Other parameters that have been used include receiver operator curve (ROC) analysis, frequency of management change, and cost–benefit analysis.

2.1 Plain X-ray

The traditional X-ray remains an important part of cancer management, and is still the first imaging used at presentation, e.g. patients with suspected lung cancer. Although it has poor sensitivity and specificity, it is widely available and cheap. Digital radiography systems which have replaced conventional films have the advantage that images can be viewed and distributed with a higher patient throughput. Digital detectors also demonstrate increased dose efficiency and a greater dynamic range, potentially reducing radiation exposure to the patient.

Table 2.1 Effect of disease prevalence on the performance of a test with 90% sensitivity and 90% specificity in the population imaged (1000 independent tests)

Disease prevalence (%)	True positives	False positives	Positive predictive value (%)
75	675	25	96
50	450	50	90
10	90	90	50

2.1.1 Production of X-rays

X-rays are produced from an X-ray tube, a glass envelope vacuum with a wire element at one end forming the cathode, and a heavy metal target (e.g. tungsten or copper) at the other end forming the anode. Application of a high voltage at the cathode results in the formation of electrons which are drawn towards the anode. On collision with the heavy metal target X-rays are produced. This is an inefficient process with >99% of the kinetic energy of electrons converted to heat, leaving <1% available for the production of X-rays.

2.1.2 X-ray quality and intensity

Quality describes the penetrating power of an X-ray beam. *Intensity* describes the quantity of radiation energy flowing in unit time. In practice an X-ray beam consists of a continuous spectrum of energies up to a maximum determined by the voltage applied between the cathode and the anode, e.g. a voltage setting of 120kV will produce a range of X-ray energies up to a maximum of 120keV.

Factors affecting X-ray tube output include:

- *Tube kilovoltage*: this affects both beam quality and intensity. The higher the kV, the greater the beam penetration: settings ranging from 28–30kV are used for mammography, and 70–90kV for body imaging.
- *Tube current*: this affects beam intensity only. In general, beam intensity is directly proportional to tube current.
- *Beam filtration*: filters are placed into the X-ray beam to improve beam quality by absorbing lower energy radiation, yet transmitting higher energy X-rays. Typical filters include aluminium, copper, molybdenum, or palladium.
- *Distance from source*: an X-ray tube produces a diverging beam, subject to a reduction in intensity with distance obeying the inverse square law.
- *Tube target material*: the proton number of the target affects the intensity of the beam produced. Beam quality is not affected.

2.1.3 Interaction of X-ray with matter

There are two main types of interaction between X-ray and matter at the photon energies produced for diagnostic radiology:

- *Photoelectric effect*: the interaction of X-ray photons with tightly bound electrons which absorb all the energy of the X-ray photon. The electrons are then ejected from the atom, a 'photoelectron'. Photoelectric interactions occur at lower energies

(<1MeV) and predominate in the diagnostic energy range. The degree of absorption is highly dependent upon the atomic number of the tissue.

♦ *Compton scattering*: the interaction of X-ray photons with loosely bound orbital electrons. The X-ray photons lose some energy and are deflected or scattered; this interaction predominates in the megavoltage energy ranges used for therapeutic radiation beams. The probability of interaction is independent of atomic number and varies with tissue electron density.

2.1.4 Tissue differentiation in the radiographic image

Different tissues in the body attenuate X-ray beams differently. Tube voltages between 20–65kV provide the best contrast for body imaging with excellent differentiation between soft tissue and bone as the photoelectric effect is dominant. At higher energies, when the Compton effect dominates, image contrast is predominantly due to tissue density. This is useful for high kV (150kV) chest radiography for example.

2.1.5 Image generation

Digital radiography has now replaced screen-film radiography. Digital images consist of picture elements or *pixels*; the two-dimensional (2D) representation of pixels in an image is called the *matrix*. Digital radiography consists of four separate steps:

♦ Image generation.

♦ Image processing.

♦ Image archiving.

♦ Image presentation.

Following exposure of digital detectors to X-rays, the energy absorbed is transformed into electric charges, which are then processed into a greyscale clinical image representing the amount of energy deposited. A digital header file containing patient information is added to the image generated.

The following factors influence image quality:

♦ *Spatial resolution*: in digital radiography, spatial resolution (the minimal resolvable separation of two high-contrast objects) is defined by minimum pixel size. This is in the order of 100–200 microns. The use of direct conversion detectors increases spatial resolution as the scatter of X-ray quanta and light photons within the detector influences spatial resolution.

♦ *Dynamic range*: this refers to the range of X-ray exposures over which a meaningful image can be obtained. Digital detectors have a wide and linear dynamic range in comparison to previously used screen-film combinations so that differences in specific tissue absorption (e.g. bone versus soft tissue) can be displayed in a single image without the need for additional imaging.

♦ *Detective quantum efficiency*: this refers to the efficiency of a detector in converting X-ray energy into an image signal. It is dependent on radiation exposure, radiation quality, spatial frequency, modulation transfer function (the capacity of the detector to transfer the modulation of input signal at a given spatial frequency to its output), and detector material.

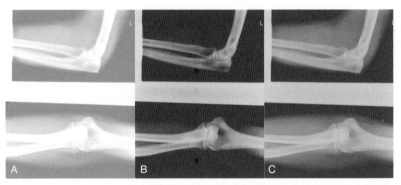

Fig. 2.1 Digital radiographs: Images can be digitally processed to alter image quality. The effect of contrast enhancement (A), contrast reduction (B), and edge enhancement is shown (C).

2.1.6 **Image processing**

Post-processing is performed following exposure and readout to ensure images are optimized for viewing (Fig. 2.1). Spatial resolution is dependent on the detector and cannot be altered by post-processing; however, manoeuvres including contrast optimization, noise reduction, and artefact removal can compensate for poorer spatial resolution. Different algorithms are generally applied to different anatomic regions in order to prevent inadvertent suppression of useful information.

2.2 **Computed tomography (CT)**

CT is currently the most widely used imaging modality for cancer imaging. Since its introduction in 1971, CT technology has evolved rapidly. In general it is a sensitive and specific test, though values vary depending on the body part examined.

2.2.1 **Basic principles**

CT is an *X-ray tomographic technique* that provides non-superimposed cross-sectional images of the body. As the X-ray tube rotates around the patient, the X-ray beam passes through an axial section of the patient's body from different directions. Detectors around the patient measure the intensity of the attenuated radiation beam as it emerges from the body. Detectors convert the X-ray intensity into electric signals which are amplified and processed to compensate for inhomogeneities in the detector system and to correct for beam hardening effects. Data is then transformed into X-ray attenuation values producing the CT raw data. This is then filtered and reconstructed mathematically to yield the image dataset, for example, using *filtered back projection*. Different *convolution kernels* can be applied for filtered back projections thus enabling different types of images to be obtained (e.g. soft, smooth, sharp, edge enhanced).

During image reconstruction a *CT number* (Hounsfeld unit) is assigned according to the degree of attenuation. This is defined as

$$CT = 1000 \times (\mu - \mu_{\text{water}})/\mu_{\text{water}}$$

A CT number of −1000 represents air, 0 represents water, around 50 represents soft tissue, and >1000 represents cortical bone. There is no upper limit. Images are displayed as a greyscale image. The resulting CT image is composed of a square matrix ranging in size from 256×256 to 1024×1024 pixel elements. Each pixel represents a scanned voxel, each with its own CT number. Axial CT images can be manipulated further to produce reformatted images in any secondary plane and three-dimensional (3D) images.

2.2.2 **CT acquisition**

CT is currently based on helical CT, which was made possible by the introduction of slip ring technology allowing for a continuously rotating CT gantry. Images are acquired using the continuously rotating X-ray tube by moving the table top on which the patient lies through the scan plane. This results in a helical scan pattern and acquisition of a data volume. Because of the helical acquisition, *interpolation* has to be performed during image reconstruction to generate a planar dataset for each table position and to produce artefact-free images. Images can be generated from any segment within the scanned volume by overlapping reconstructions as often as required. Different reconstruction intervals (spacing between sections) and section collimations (section thickness) can be used.

Multidetector helical CT, introduced in 1998, has resulted in a large gain in CT performance including a shorter acquisition duration, longer scan ranges, and thinner sections with near isotropic resolution. Multidetector helical CT uses the radiation delivered more efficiently. The number of detector rows currently stands at 320 for state-of-the-art scanners. Dual-source CT with two X-ray tubes and two corresponding multidetector arrays has also been developed. The acquisition systems are mounted on a rotating gantry with a 90-degree angular offset. The gantry rotation time is 0.33s, and dual-source CT can provide temporal resolutions one-quarter of the gantry rotation time.

Typical acquisition parameters for general imaging of the thorax, abdomen, and pelvis are summarized in Table 2.2.

◆ *Kilovoltage (kV)*: typically 120kV is applied for diagnostic body imaging. Dual-energy imaging is performed on a dual-source CT using 140kV and 80kV, while 80kV is applied for perfusion CT imaging as this is closer to the absorption point of iodine.

◆ *Milliampere second (mAs)*: this is the product of the tube current (e.g. 200mA) and rotation time of the scanner (e.g. 0.6s). In multidetector CT this is often quoted as *effective mAs* which is the product of the tube current and exposure time of one slice (rotation × collimation/feed per rotation). The mAs applied will depend on the body part examined. A higher mAs generally reduces image noise thus improving the detectability of low-contrast structures but has to be tempered by patient dose considerations. Current scanners use dose modulation techniques to reduce patient radiation exposure: the dose during each tube rotation is measured and altered depending on the attenuation level making it possible to reduce the dose by as much as 56%.

◆ *Collimation*: the radiation beam emitted by the X-ray tube can be shaped using special diaphragms or 'collimators' positioned either directly in front of the X-ray source (to shape the emitted beam) or directly in front of the detectors (to reduce the effect of scattered radiation). The collimation and focal spot size determines the quality of the slice profile. Images can be reconstructed with slice thicknesses equal to or greater than the detector collimation.

♦ *Increment*: the distance between images reconstructed from a data volume. This should be selected as an overlapping increment to lower noise and improve image quality. An overlap of up to 90% can be achieved but an overlap of 30–50% is generally used in clinical practice. For example, if slice thicknesses of 10mm are reconstructed with a 5mm increment, slices will overlap by 50%.

♦ *Pitch*: this traditionally refers to table feed per rotation/collimation for single-slice CT. For multidetector CT, pitch is more complicated. Its value will depend on whether a single section collimation or total collimation of the detector array is used. Good image quality is obtained with a pitch between 1–2, defined as table feed per rotation/single section collimation.

2.2.3 Image processing and display

Multidetector helical CT has had a major impact on 2D and 3D imaging. Multiplanar reformations (MPRs) are 2D reformatted images that are reconstructed secondarily from a stack of axial images, e.g. in the sagittal or coronal plane. Oblique and curved reformations can also be obtained but require interpolation between adjacent voxels. Curved reformations are needed for structures that pass through multiple axial planes, e.g. blood vessels and bronchi. Thin collimation axial images (<2mm) are required to produce MPRs of good image quality. MPRs are generally the width of 1 voxel but can be produced with a greater section thickness to reduce image noise and further improve image quality. An example is shown in Fig. 2.2.

Maximum (MIP) and minimum intensity projections (MinIP) are volume rendering techniques. Images are generated by displaying the maximum or minimum CT numbers encountered along the direction of the projection, known as the viewing angle. This ensures that contrast is optimized between high-contrast structures and surrounding tissue.

Table 2.2 Typical CT acquisition parameters for multidetector CT (64 rows and above)

	Thorax	Abdomen	Pelvis
Positioning	Thoracic inlet to below diaphragm	Above diaphragm to iliac crest	Iliac crest to symphysis pubis
kV	120	120	120
Effective mAs	200	280	300
Pitch	0.75	0.75	0.75
Detector collimation (mm)	0.6	0.6	0.6
Reconstruction increment (mm)	3–5	3–5	3–5
Reconstruction kernel	B30f medium smooth and B80f ultra sharp	B30f medium smooth	B30f medium smooth
Effective slice collimation (mm)	3–5	3–5	3–5

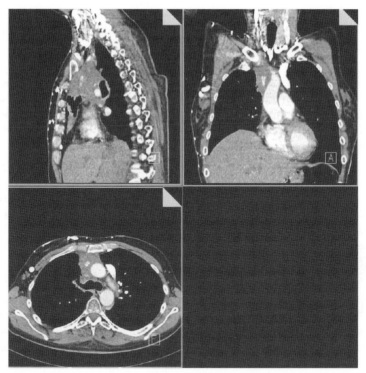

Fig. 2.2 CT Images of the thorax: multiplanar reformats can be obtained from manipulating the original dataset, in this case demonstrating a lung tumour causing superior vena cava obstruction.

MIP views are generally used for CT angiography and for specialized pulmonary studies. MinIP images are used mainly for visualizing the central tracheobronchial system. Volume rendering techniques have become the standard technique for CT angiography and for musculoskeletal imaging. Virtual endoscopy is a special type of volume rendered dataset giving a perspective view and the impression of 'flying through' the structure, e.g. colon.

2.2.4 Radiation dose

The radiation exposure in CT is dependent on scan parameters, scanner, and patient characteristics. Radiation dose with CT is generally 5–10 × higher than corresponding conventional radiography, hence the importance of the ALARA (As Low As Reasonably Achievable) principle in ensuring that the patient receives the lowest possible radiation dose without compromising diagnostic scan quality.

Parameters that are commonly used to describe dose are the volume CT dose index ($CTDI_{vol}$), the total scan dose (dose length product, DLP), and radiation risk (effective dose).

◆ *$CTDI_{vol}$*: this is the average local dose delivered to a phantom cross-section (in milliGray, mGy) and indicates the average local dose delivered to the patient. CTDI will underestimate the dose for children and slim patients, and overestimate this for obese patients.

- *DLP*: this is a measure of the cumulative dose delivered to the patient (in mGy.cm). It takes into account the average dose in the scan volume and the scan length (L).

$$DLP = CTDI_{vol} \times L$$

- *Effective dose*: this is an estimate of the radiation risk to patients (in millisieverts, mSv). Mathematical modelling is used to calculate effective dose appropriately weighted for individual organs for a standard male or female (of 70kg). Again such estimates of E will underestimate the dose for children and slim patients, and over-estimate it for obese patients.

The European guidelines for quality in CT[1] and UK national reference doses for CT (2003)[1] provide reference doses for CT indicating the CTDI$_{vol}$ and DLP that should not be exceeded (Table 2.3). The risk of death from radiation-induced cancer has been calculated from BEIR V and IRCP 60 data which extrapolate the risk estimates from accidentally or occupationally exposed groups. therefore reflecting high doses. The risk from diagnostic radiology (much lower doses) has to be extrapolated. The radiation-induced risk of death is approximately 0.5/10,000 persons, while the risk of fatal cancer is 3000/10,000 persons. The radiation-induced risk is age dependent (Table 2.4).

2.3 **Ultrasound (US)**

US has its origins in sonar technology and has been applied to medical imaging for over half a century. US remains one of the most widely used imaging modalities worldwide as it offers real-time imaging, is relatively inexpensive, safe, and portable. In general it has moderate sensitivity and specificity, e.g. in the order of 60–70% in the assessment of hepatic metastases[2]. High-frequency sound beams (usually >20kHz) are used to generate high-resolution anatomical imaging. Modern US equipment still uses a pulse echo approach with a brightness mode (B-mode) display but performance has been improved by the introduction of tissue harmonic imaging, extended field of view imaging, coded pulse excitation, and electronic section focusing; 3D and 4D imaging is also possible. In addition to anatomical information, US can also provide functional information, e.g. assessment of tissue regional perfusion using Doppler or contrast-enhanced US.

2.3.1 **Basic principles**

US pulses are generated by an US transducer made from piezoelectric crystals. As an alternating electric voltage is applied, the crystal changes thickness and vibrates,

Table 2.3 National reference dose levels for multislice CT as indicated by UK 2003 national dose review

Body part	CTDI$_{vol}$ (mGy)	DLP (mGy/cm)
Brain	65	930
Chest	13	580
Abdomen	14	470
Abdomen and pelvis	14	560

Table 2.4 Calculated radiation-induced risk of dying from cancer (ICRP 60)

Age (years)	Risk (death per mSv)
0–10	14/100,000
10–20	18/100,000
20–30	7.5/100,000
30–40	3.5/100,000
60	2.0/100,000
80	1.0/100,000

generating a *mechanical wave*. These mechanical waves range in frequency from 2–15MHz, travelling through biologic tissue at a velocity dependent upon the medium through which it is travelling. Sound travels more rapidly through tissues which demonstrate medium density and elasticity.

US wavelength (length of a single sine-wave cycle in a medium) is related to frequency and speed of sound as follows:

$$c = f\lambda$$

where c = speed of sound; f = frequency; and λ = wavelength.

As an US beam passes through tissue, it loses energy and amplitude. The following contribute to the attenuation of the US beam:

◆ Transfer of energy to tissue resulting in heating (*absorption*).

◆ Removal of energy by reflection and scattering.

The *attenuation*—measured in decibels per centimetre (dB/cm)—is proportional to path length and frequency. Longer path lengths and higher frequencies produce greater attenuation. Thus the depth of the field available when imaging at higher frequency is shorter than at a lower frequency: higher frequencies (>10MHz) are used to image objects near to the skin surface, while lower frequencies (3–5MHz) are used for tissue deeper within the body.

Echoes are produced from boundaries between tissues with different mechanical properties. The amount reflected from an interface between two tissues depends on the difference in *acoustic impedance* (Table 2.5), a measure of the tissue's resistance to distortion by US, in turn determined by the density and elasticity of the tissue. The intensity of the echo is proportional to the difference in acoustic impedance between the two tissues. For example, strong echoes are generated at a muscle:fat interface (intensity reflection coefficient = 1.5%). In most soft tissues, acoustic impedances are fairly similar, so the proportion of a sound pulse reflected at each interface is relatively small and most of the US energy is transmitted further into the body. If a US pulse encounters reflectors that has dimensions smaller than its wavelength (i.e. d <λ), then *scattering* occurs with echoes reflected through a wide range of angles. For example, the *speckled* texture of organs like the liver is the result of interference between multiple scattered echoes. The depth of any structure giving rise to an echo can be

Table 2.5 Acoustic impedance values of various tissues

Tissue	Acoustic impedance (g/cm^{-1}/s^{-1})
Air	0.0004×10
Fat	1.38×10
Water	1.48×10
Liver	1.65×10
Bone	7.80×10

determined from the time taken for the sound pulse to reach it and the time for the echo to return to the surface, because the velocity of sound is very similar in all soft tissue. Echoes returning from greater depths must be amplified to compensate for the attenuation.

2.3.2 US transducers

US pulses required for image generation are produced by transducers consisting of piezoelectric elements which also receive the reflected US pulse producing real-time images. Transducers may be linear, curvilinear, or radial. Most modern US machines use transducers consisting of multiple arrays with as many as 196 elements.

2.3.3 The US beam

The US beam is not uniform, altering in configuration as it moves away from the transducer. Initially the beam converges after leaving the transducer. This corresponds to the near field and is narrowest at its focal distance; it then diverges. The US beam diameter is affected by:

- *US frequency*: higher frequency US provides better image resolution as the near field is longer than at lower frequencies, but it is more heavily absorbed.
- *Distance from the transducer.*
- *Transducer diameter*: the near field is longer with larger diameter transducers thus image resolution is better.
- *Use of mechanical or electronic focusing*: focusing can only be achieved within the near field.

2.3.4 Image generation

Amplification of received echoes is necessary for image generation. Immediately after echoes are received by the transducer, echoes are pre-amplified uniformly. Noise and clutter are reduced by removal of small signals and demodulation.

2.3.5 US approaches

Modern US scanners are based on B-mode imaging where echoes of differing magnitudes are displayed as a greyscale. However, different methods can be applied to further improve imaging or obtain functional information.

2.3.5.1 Tissue harmonic imaging

Tissue harmonic imaging is based on frequencies that are multiples of the frequency of the transmitted pulse (fundamental frequency). The second harmonic (twice the fundamental frequency) is most commonly used to generate an image. Artefacts and clutter from multiple pulse reflections in surface tissues are also rejected, thus tissue harmonic imaging is ideal for patients with thick body walls who would normally be challenging and sub-optimally imaged.

2.3.5.2 Spatial compound imaging

Spatial compound imaging is a method to reduce speckle. Electronic steering of the US beam is used to image the same tissue multiple times using parallel beams oriented along different directions. Echoes from these multiple acquisitions are then averaged into a single composite image with the effect of reducing speckle and improving contrast and margin definition.

2.3.5.3 Extended field of view imaging

This allows a single composite image with a large field of view to be obtained. By slowly translating the transducer laterally across the region of interest, multiple images are acquired which are registered relative to each other to generate a single composite image. This is useful to assess vessels, e.g. for deep venous thrombosis or stenotic disease.

2.3.5.4 Doppler US

The Doppler principle states that there is a shift in frequency of a sound wave as the source of the sound moves relative to an observer. This change in frequency is called the Doppler frequency shift (DFS) which can be depicted by:

$$DFS = (2 \times IF \times BF/c) \times cosine\ \theta$$

where BF = blood flow; IF = incident frequency; c = speed of sound; θ = angle between the US beam and vascular flow

This can be exploited to demonstrate tissue or organ vascularity. Doppler techniques include:

- *Continuous wave (CW) Doppler*: velocity is portrayed as a function of time. The blood flow patterns in the arteries can be shown by a simple CW Doppler device with two transducers, one for transmitting and one for receiving.
- *Pulsed Doppler*: the spatial distribution of blood flow can be obtained from Doppler analysis of US pulses. Different velocities are portrayed in a range of colour in a 2D image. By convention, red represents flow towards and blue away from the transducer. Different intensities of colour represent velocity and turbulence.
- *Colour Doppler*: B-mode images with superimposed Doppler information in colour.

2.3.5.5 Imaging with US contrast agents

US contrast agents consist of gas microbubbles, stabilized by a shell of albumin or lipid that have very different acoustic impedances from soft tissue. The US contrast medium is injected into a vein and as it passes through the tissues the microbubbles are broken up by the US waves. The large number of small bubbles increases scatter, producing

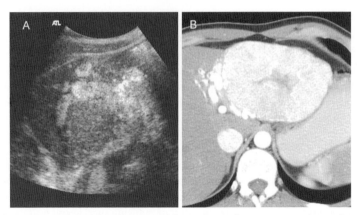

Fig. 2.3 Contrast-enhanced US images, with corresponding contrast-enhanced CT showing a benign focal nodular hyperplasia.

more echoes, enabling areas that are well perfused to be identified. Microbubbles enable abnormalities within the liver to be characterized, e.g. differentiation of a benign lesion such as haemangioma or focal nodular hyperplasia from a metastasis (Fig. 2.3).

2.4 **Magnetic resonance imaging (MRI)**

MRI is a versatile technique, capable of multiplanar acquisition, true 3D, and high-definition imaging of soft tissues with a good sensitivity and specificity generally. It is not suitable for investigating bony deformities, as solid bone appears dark on all images and certain body locations that are prone to motion and air/tissue boundaries (such as the lungs) provide a challenge. Despite this, its superior tissue resolution is invaluable. Whilst it does not carry the same risks of ionizing radiation exposure, special precautions to remove all ferromagnetic materials from the patient and to carefully assess prosthetic implants are required. Online databases exist for checking implant suitability. Most heart pacemakers are currently contraindicated and it is important to relate risk to magnetic field strength since an implant safe at one field strength may not be safe at another.

2.4.1 **MR principles**

The main part of the MR scanner is a large magnet. Three main types of magnet are used in clinical MRI installations: permanent ferromagnets, and resistive and super-conducting electromagnets. The most commonly used superconducting MRI scanners work at a field strength of 1.5 tesla. Lower field strengths may be preferred for specialist applications such as extremity imaging and higher field strengths confer advantages in image signal-to-noise, speed of acquisition or resolution.

   MR imaging is based on the principle that positively-charged protons in the body water line up with or against the magnetic field B_0, depending on their energy. A relatively small number of them line up predominantly with the field, and are termed the net magnetization, M_0. For most applications, this is taken to lie along the main (Z) axis of the scanner, and therefore along the patient. The individual protons do not actually line up: they rotate or spin around the Z axis with a frequency directly proportional to the field strength: this is termed the *Larmor frequency* and is given by the *Larmor equation*:

$$\omega_o = \gamma B_o$$

where ω_o is the angular frequency of rotation, γ is the gyromagnetic ratio (constant of proportionality: fixed for a given nucleus) and B_o the magnetic field strength in tesla (T). Bold italic text indicates a vector quantity, i.e. there is implied direction as well as magnitude. The nuclei are usually referred to as *spins*.

To acquire an image, a radiofrequency (RF) energy pulse with a bandwidth of frequencies centred around the Larmor frequency is produced using an RF power amplifier. It feeds currents to the RF transmit coil (usually the *body coil*), producing a circularly polarized magnetic field. This so-called B_1 field locally overcomes the main field B_o and so the spins in the body tip to rotate around the B_1 field direction instead, gaining energy as they do so. The RF pulses can either be given enough energy to flip the spins exactly orthogonal to their starting position (the RF pulse is then termed a 90° pulse), antiparallel to it (180° pulse), or any intermediate angle.

At the end of the RF pulse, the orientation of the spins returns to its base position giving off the energy they gained in an exponential decay, characterized by *relaxation times*, termed *T*1 and *T*2. The energy release is detected either by the same coil used to transmit the RF pulse, or a smaller, more sensitive *surface coil* which is much closer to the tissue of interest and can acquire higher resolution data. Most data are acquired via surface coils.

2.4.2 Image formation

A 'slice' of the patient is selected by applying a gradient, which changes the Larmor frequencies of spins along itself. This can be in any orientation, as the XYZ gradients can be used singly or in combination. An RF pulse with a given bandwidth of frequencies is applied, and only those spins in the patient with corresponding Larmor frequencies will be excited. The spins in the slice are then encoded using an orthogonal combination of gradients in Z (transverse, or axial), X (sagittal), and Y (coronal) orientations. For a typical axial image, X will be termed the 'frequency encoding' direction and Y the 'phase encoding' direction. However this encoding takes time, and the *free induction decay* (FID- the exponential decay of the signal as the protons return to their original position), is usually much faster than the time it takes to perform the encoding. To compensate for this, more gradients and/or (usually) 180° RF pulses are used to form an *echo* of the initial signal, which is detected after the encoding. If the echo is formed by an RF pulse, it is termed a *spin echo*; if a gradient is used, it is a *gradient echo*. A diagram of spin echo formation (and associated T2* decay) is given in Fig. 2.4.

Images are built up line-by-line using multiple *repetitions* of pulse + gradient sequences and the signal amplitudes of each line recorded by the computers in the scanner. At the end of a sequence, the images are reconstructed using a mathematical transformation called a *Fourier transform*. Usually, sequences can be designed to collect many image slices at once, in order to save time.

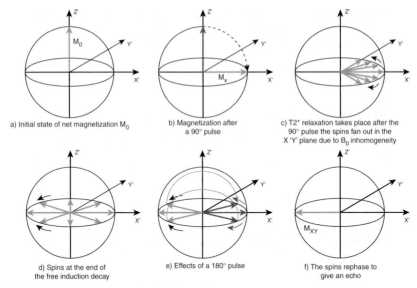

a) Initial state of net magnetization M_0

b) Magnetization after a 90° pulse

c) T2* relaxation takes place after the 90° pulse the spins fan out in the X 'Y' plane due to B_0 inhomogeneity

d) Spins at the end of the free induction decay

e) Effects of a 180° pulse

f) The spins rephase to give an echo

Fig. 2.4 Diagram showing spin echo formation.

Variables which can be changed by the scanner operator include the echo time TE, repetition time TR, and flip angle, α. These cause the amount of relaxation in the spins to vary before signal readout, and a knowledge of the intrinsic relaxation times T1 and T2 for a given tissue allows the changing of image contrast between imaging sequences, allowing different physiological characteristics to be assessed. Most basic images are therefore termed *T1-weighted* or *T2-weighted* (Fig. 2.5).

T1-weighted scans have short TE and short TR, and show long T1 tissues as dark and short T1 tissues as bright. Contrast agents such as gadolinium, which tend to shorten T1, therefore highlight tissues where it is taken up. Water, which has a long T1, appears relatively dark, and fat, with a short T1 is bright. T2-weighted scans have long TE and long TR. They show tissues with longer T2 as bright, as the shorter T2 tissues' signal will have decayed away at the long echo times used. This is very useful for showing fluid around tumours, e.g. gliomas, or tumours in prostate peripheral zones, which appear dark. Fat is less bright than water. Another common sequence used is termed *proton-density* (Fig. 2.5) as it shows the relative proton densities within the slice. Gradient echo sequences bring in another relaxation time weighting called *T2**, which allows magnetic field variations to be assessed.

In Fig. 2.4, T2* is the decay constant of the free induction decay. This can be refocused by a spin echo but not a gradient echo sequence, thus is only a significant contrast mechanism in the latter. A combination of T2* and T1-weighting is useful for looking at contrast agents such as ferromagnetic or gadolinium particles, which work by changing the local field around them, and therefore the tissue relaxation times. A post-contrast T1-weighted gradient echo image is shown in comparison with the pre-contrast (Fig. 2.5).

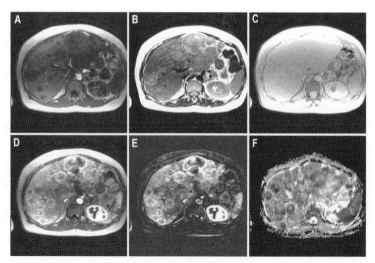

Fig. 2.5 MR images acquired at 1.5T showing colorectal liver metastases: T1-weighted pre-contrast (A), T2-weighted (B), PD-weighted (C), T1-weighted postcontrast (D), T1 subtraction (E), and ADC map (F).

2.4.3 Modern scanners and advanced imaging

Modern scanners permit much more flexible scanning than just the basic spin and gradient echo sequences. This stems from technological developments, for instance those which have made *parallel imaging* a clinical tool. This permits a speeding-up of image acquisition increasing resolution and reducing scan time.

Another development has been the development of *echo-planar imaging* (EPI) for routine use. This technique requires very fast gradient switching, but can acquire an entire image in <1s. It enables measurement of physiological factors such as *water diffusion* in tissues: depending on the cellular organization and density, this can be predominantly in one direction (isotropic) or all (anisotropic), restricted (dense cellular structure) or unrestricted (loose structure) (Fig. 2.5).

Dynamic contrast-enhanced (DCE) MRI (Fig. 2.6) consists of injecting contrast, usually gadolinium-based, while rapid T1-weighted gradient echo or EPI scanning takes place. Permeability of the vasculature can be assessed both semi-quantitatively evaluating the initial area under the gadolinium concentration-time curve in the first minute ($IAUGC_{60}$) or by generating fully-quantitative data such as K^{trans} (the rate at which the contrast passes into the extracellular space), the extracellular space volume, v_e, the onset time at which the contrast arrives at a given region, and the rate at which it passes back out to the plasma again, k_{ep}.

2.5 Nuclear medicine (radionuclide radiology)

This section deals with common investigative techniques that utilize the administration of a radiopharmaceutical, which is then imaged (or counted) with a gamma camera, concentrating on the management of patients with malignant conditions.

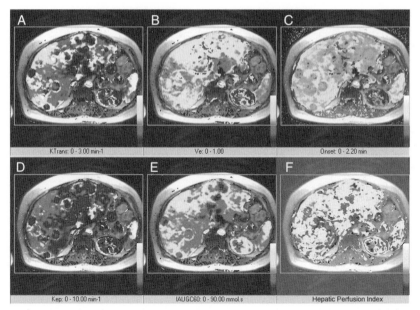

Fig. 2.6 Parametric images, all calculated from one DCE-MRI data set of 40 images: K^{trans}, (A), v_e, (B), onset time (C), k_{ep} (D), $IAUGC_{60}$ (E), and Hepatic Perfusion Index (F). See colour section.

2.5.1 The radiopharmaceutical (radiotracer)

A radiopharmaceutical consists of a radionuclide bound to a pharmaceutical. The radionuclide provides the gamma radiation which forms the image and is chosen for its physical properties of half-life, gamma energy emitted (i.e. in the range of 100–250keV which is best captured by a gamma camera), 'purity' of emission (i.e. no undesirable alpha or beta particles), and simplicity of production. It should also bind well to the bioactive compound/molecule, not dissociating under physiological conditions. The pharmaceutical enables the targeting of the particular physiological process of interest to the investigator. This can range from osteoblastic activity to left ventricular ejection fraction to specific peptide receptor expression.

Some physiological processes can be targeted by the radionuclide without a pharmaceutical. Iodine transport in the thyroid via the sodium iodine symporter can be imaged with radioisotopes of iodine, ^{123}I and [131]I. For imaging ^{123}I is preferred as it is a pure gamma emitter, whereas ^{131}I is also a beta emitter and therefore can be used for therapy. [123]I can only be produced in a cyclotron, limiting its availability and so benign thyroid disease is imaged with ^{99m}Tc-pertechnetate which follows a similar physiological pathway.

[99m]Tc (an isomer of technetium) is the workhorse of the nuclear medicine department due to its ideal imaging properties. It emits a 140keV gamma ray, giving good penetration of soft tissue while causing minimal damage. This energy is ideal for imaging by the gamma camera crystal. Its half-life of 6.03 hours is convenient for the logistics of production, administration, and imaging over a few hours—and short enough to allow acceptable outpatient use (it doesn't linger, giving the patient and surroundings

ongoing radiation exposure). The daughter isotope ^{99}Tc (a beta emitter) has a long half-life and is excreted in the urine before it decays. It is generated from molybdenum-99 which has a long half-life of 66 hours allowing a generator to last a working week. It readily binds to a variety of pharmaceuticals.

2.5.2 The gamma camera

2.5.2.1 The crystal

The crystal captures the gamma photons emitted from the patient. This is a flat crystal of sodium iodide with added thallium. The crystal's average atomic number is high enough to stop incident gamma photons. The photon releases its energy to an electron, exciting it. The electron then falls back to a lower energy state and a light photon is emitted. The crystal is linked to a close fitting array of photomultiplier tubes (PMTs).

2.5.2.2 The photomultiplier tube (PMT)

The PMT amplifies and locates the signal. The incident light photons from the crystal hit the entry window which is a photocathode. They liberate electrons—the photoelectric effect. These are accelerated and amplified via a series of dynodes through the tube to reach the end anode. This produces a current which gives a voltage which varies over time depending on the energy of the original gamma photon. Every incident gamma photon on the crystal will produce a scatter of light from the crystal into a group of PMTs at varying distances from the collision. The relative intensity of the signal from each neighbouring tube can be compared to give the location of each collision event.

2.5.2.3 The collimator

This is placed between the patient and crystal to exclude radiation that is not useful in forming the image, thus brings the image into 'focus'. Gamma photons leave the patient in random directions. Gamma radiation is too energetic to be focused with a lens, and has no charge and so is not deflected by electromagnetic fields. A filter (the collimator) is used to exclude radiation with an oblique incident angle (by absorption and scatter)—only allowing through gamma photons at a narrow angle useful in forming the image. The choice of collimator depends on the gamma energies involved and the particular examination. The most commonly used is a lead collimator with a series of parallel holes. A pinhole collimator is a cone which works like a camera obscura, giving a sharp image but with a small field of view and longer imaging time.

2.5.2.4 The gamma camera head

The three parts are assembled to form the 'head' which is mounted on a gantry. The computer system controls the operation of the camera, acquisition, and storage of acquired images. It is important for image quality to have the head as close as possible to the patient. A simple gamma camera has a single head and is static. A dual-headed camera can image a patient from two different angles simultaneously. Either can be used with a moving table. The heads can be positioned manually or automatically. Some have software and infrared sensors to adjust the position of the head according to the contours of the patient's body as it moves past. Pressure sensors stop the movement of the table if the gamma camera head is touched.

2.5.2.5 Single photon emission computed tomography (SPECT)

A SPECT camera is a type of gamma camera. It can acquire images tomographically. SPECT imaging is analogous to X-ray CT in that the image is acquired by rotating detectors around the patient, i.e. gamma camera heads (usually two) then reconstructing an image in three planes. This localizes the focus of activity in 3D and improves the visualization of faint foci of activity. Very intense concentrations of activity (e.g. the bladder in a bone scan) will produce artefacts, obscuring activity in adjacent structures. SPECT acquisitions can be gated to an electrocardiogram (ECG) allowing imaging of the myocardium and definition of the left ventricular volume. Gamma camera images can also be co-registered with radiographs and CT images to further localize the physiological process to the anatomy.

2.5.3 Imaging

Once the radiopharmaceutical is administered then, depending upon the half-life, multiple subsequent images can be obtained with no further patient dose (unlike X-rays). This allows images of different phases of the radiopharmaceutical's progress through the patient, e.g. the perfusion, blood pool, and delayed skeletal images of a bone scan, or several views of the same body part from various projections.

Data can be acquired in dynamic or 'spot' modes. The dynamic mode measures activity level as it changes over time. It is used for physiological processes which operate in the time period of the scan, e.g. the passage of tracer through the kidneys in a MAG3 (mercaptoacetyltriglycine) renogram. The data can be displayed as a series of images or as a time-activity graph. The spot mode records the sum of all activity in a given time. It is used for activity which is more or less constant during the scan, e.g. renal cortical activity in a DMSA (dimercaptosuccinic acid) scan. The data can also be used to produce an image or as a number of total counts giving the relative function in various defined regions of interest.

Thus the image produced is not directly of an organ or patient, but a map of the amount of the physiological process under study within the organ or patient. Therefore, on a DMSA study, an image of a fully functioning kidney will be kidney shaped but a damaged kidney will produce an irregular image indicating the level of function within different parts of the kidney. Gamma camera images can be co-registered with radiographs and CT images to further localize the physiological process to the anatomy. In cardiac imaging, acquisitions can be gated to an ECG, allowing imaging of the myocardium or left ventricular volume.

The great strength of these techniques is that they complement the anatomical detail of radiological examinations with functional information. The target physiology can be highly specific, e.g. iodine uptake in a deposit of papillary thyroid carcinoma. Often, however, the physiological process targeted is a surrogate marker for malignancy. This can reduce the specificity, e.g. gallium uptake as a marker for metabolic activity and transferrin receptor status is increased in lymphoma, but also sarcoidosis.

An isotope bone scan uses osteoblastic activity as a marker for the presence of metastases and so produces false negatives if there are lytic deposits with a poor osteoblastic reaction and false positives due to osteoblastic reactions to other processes such as fractures or infection. This makes it essential to interpret results in conjunction with the complete clinical picture, particularly correlating functional and anatomical investigations.

The following are examples of the way in which radionuclide imaging contributes to the management of patients with malignancy.

2.5.3.1 The isotope bone scan

The radiopharmaceutical ^{99m}Tc MDP (methylene-diphosphonate) is taken up by active osteoblasts. Osteoblastic activity may be a marker for the presence of metastases but will produce false positives due to osteoblastic reactions in other processes such as fractures or infection and false negatives with lytic deposits with a poor osteoblastic reaction. Causes of apparent increased activity on a ^{99m}Tc MDP bone scan include:

- True increased osteoblastic activity.
- Increased arterial supply to a body part, e.g. inflammation.
- Impaired venous drainage of a body part, e.g. deep vein thrombosis.
- Excretion of radiopharmaceutical, e.g. in urine.
- Distance from gamma camera head, e.g. iliac crests appear more active on anterior images, sacroiliac joints appear more active on posterior images.
- Lack of intervening soft tissue, e.g. the sternum.
- Thickness of bone, e.g. the distal humerus.

True osteoblastic activity can be in response to many processes from malignancy to infection, Paget disease to fractures. Thus the art of interpretation is to pay attention to the pattern of activity and correlation with the clinical picture and other imaging techniques (Fig. 2.7). Lytic deposits without osteoblastic reactions will produce photopenic 'holes' in the normal bone activity. The isotope bone scan can also demonstrate paraneoplastic processes such as hypertrophic osteoarthropathy (Fig. 2.8).

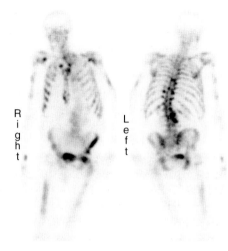

Fig. 2.7 ^{99m}Tc MDP bone scan: patchy diffuse foci of increased activity throughout the central axial skeleton and proximal long bones with low background and renal activity indicates a metastatic 'superscan'. This results from the osteoblastic response to the widespread skeletal malignant deposits typical of prostate carcinoma metastases.

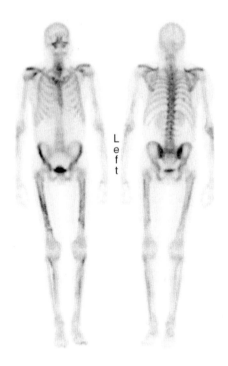

Fig. 2.8 Irregular increased cortical activity in both femora in a patient with lung cancer, typical of HOA.

2.5.3.2 The MUGA scan

Multi-gated acquisition (some companies use analysis). This technique is used as a method of measuring left ventricular ejection fraction in a reproducible manner. This is important in oncology for monitoring patients undergoing therapies with cardio-toxic side effects such as trastuzumab (Herceptin®).

To assess the left ventricular luminal volume the radiotracer must stay within the intravascular space, thus red blood cells are the ideal 'tracer'. In order to label the red cells with the radionuclide (^{99m}Tc), the patient is injected with a stannous (tin) salt. Later the pertechnetate is injected, enters the red cell, is reduced by the stannous salt, and then cannot diffuse back out again. A more laborious *in vitro* labelling method is not often used in clinical departments.

The camera head is put in an oblique position to throw the left ventricle into relief, free of overlapping structures, and the number of radioactive counts obtained over about 10–15min. This data acquisition is gated to an ECG—so the software can divide the counts into those acquired during different phases of the cardiac cycle, plotting a graph of activity versus phase of cardiac cycle. The total activity in all the time points in end systole is compared to those in end diastole. This activity is proportional to the volume of the ventricle and so an ejection fraction can be calculated.

The final report includes a summated image acquired in end systole and end diastole to demonstrate the regions of interest have been accurately sited over the left ventricle and area of lung for background correction and that there is no overlapping activity from adjacent structures, such as the spleen. There is also a diagram showing the wall motion divided into segments, but the oncologist will generally be interested in the overall percentage figure and any change in the value over the course of treatment.

2.6 **Positron emission tomography (PET)**

PET is used for detecting and localizing cancers, distinguishing benign from malignant tumours, staging, and monitoring response to treatment. It is generally more sensitive than anatomical imaging for cancer detection, and may be more specific.

2.6.1 **Basic principles**

PET relies upon the administration of positron-emitting radio pharmaceuticals of which the most common in routine use is the glucose analogue ^{18}F-fluorodeoxyglucose (FDG). The ^{18}F molecule is unstable and decays via emission of a positron and neutrino to form stable non-toxic ^{18}O. Energetic emitted positrons scatter with electrons in tissue before combining to annihilate, creating two 511keV photons emitted ~180° apart that are detected in PET scanners.

These two emitted 511keV photons travel through tissue before being recorded in rings of detectors surrounding the patient. The detectors consist of scintillator crystals coupled to photo multiplier tubes where interacting photons create pulses of light that are converted to electrical signals. If two signals are recorded within a small time window (nanoseconds) in the detection circuitry then a coincidence event has potentially occurred, creating a line-of-response (LOR) that defines the relative position of the event for use in image reconstruction.

Typical crystal scintillators employed today are based on bismuth germanate (BGO), lutetium oxyorthosilicate (LSO), and gadolinium oxyorthosilicate (GSO). Required characteristics for PET crystals are high detection efficiency for good sensitivity, fast speed to reduce random noise, and good energy resolution to reduce scatter. Some scanners can be operated in 2D or 3D acquisition mode. In 2D scanning, physical septa are placed between detector rings to accept relatively parallel LOR in order to reduce interplane scatter (~20%) and enable simple and speedy image reconstruction at the expense of detection sensitivity. In 3D scanning, septa are retracted and all LOR are accepted resulting in approximately five times the sensitivity compared with 2D. However, scatter increases by up to 50% as do random events thus requiring superior timing and scatter compensation in hardware and software compared with 2D. In 3D more bed positions are also scanned due to the non-uniform axial sensitivity encountered. Modern scanners utilize 3D-list mode data acquisition for increased versatility with iterative image reconstruction and recent fast time-of-flight systems offer superior signal-to-noise ratio.

2.6.2 **Fundamental limitations**

Positron range depends upon its kinetic energy and Table 2.6 illustrates this for different radiopharmaceuticals and tissues. The residual kinetic energy of the positron before annihilation translates into an angular variation of ~0.5° for photons created post annihilation. FDG positron range and photon non-colinearity are limitations to image resolution.

Table 2.6 The effect of energy on positron range in different tissues

Radioisotope	Max energy (KeV)	Cortical bone FWHM (mm)	Soft tissue FWHM (mm)	Lung tissue FWHM (mm)
^{18}F	633	0.18	0.19	0.37
^{11}C	959	0.22	0.28	0.52
^{13}N	1197	0.26	0.33	0.62
^{15}O	1738	0.33	0.41	0.86
^{68}Ga	1900	0.36	0.49	0.98
^{82}Rb	3350	0.56	0.76	1.43

FWHM, full width at half-maximum.

2.6.3 Imaging

FDG is phosphorylated intracellularly into FDG-6-phosphate and trapped, taking no further part in the glycolytic pathway, and the image therefore represents a map of glucose utilization in the scanned area. Typically scanning is performed at least 1 hour after intravenous injection which allows for sufficient FDG uptake to achieve good signal-to-noise ratio for imaging lesions.

Modern imaging combines PET with CT to give added topographical information on the distribution of FDG. Initially a full helical CT image set is acquired, then the couch moves into the PET component where individual bed positions, typically about 16cm in length, are scanned to cover the entire body length required; this may take up to 30min (Fig. 2.9). In fused images the registration accuracy of ~1mm arises from precise mechanical alignment in scanners. Artefacts arising from respiratory motion

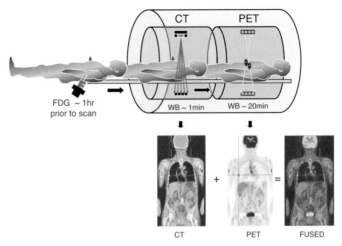

Fig. 2.9 Clinical PET/CT depicting transmission scanning in CT and emission scanning in PET leading to fused whole body images. See colour section.

and attenuation correction are known pitfalls and can be minimized with experience and by using gating techniques.

Malignant cells typically have a higher glucose metabolism compared with normal cells and hence may be identified on PET; however, increased glucose metabolism is not unique to malignancy and hence false positive scans may occur in areas of infection and inflammation. Additional functional information is available by performing kinetic investigations in PET with dynamic scanning techniques.

References

1. Shrimpton PC, Hillier MC, Lewis MA, *et al. Doses from computed tomography (CT) examinations in the UK-2003 review. NRPB-W67.* Chiltern: National Radiation Protection Board, UK, 2003.
2. European Commission. *European guidelines on quality criteria for computed tomography. EUR 16262 EN.* Luxembourg: Office for Official Publications for the European Communities, 1999.

Additional resource

Information on specific CT scanning protocols can be found on websites such as http://www.CTisus.org.

Chapter 3

Breast

Steve Allen

3.1 Clinical background

3.1.1 Incidence

Breast cancer is the commonest cancer in women in the Western world, and prior to 1999 was the most common cause of cancer death in women until it was overtaken by lung cancer[1]. Breast cancer mortality rates in the UK have fallen dramatically since 1989 when 15,625 women died from the disease compared with 12,417 in 2005[3]. The reduction in breast cancer mortality rates is likely to have several different causes including screening, increasing standardization and specialization of care, and the widespread adoption of tamoxifen treatment since 1992[2].

3.1.2 Screening

The UK NHS breast screening programme (NHSBSP) invites each year more than 2 million women aged 50–70 years for mammography. In 2005, 4.8% of women screened were recalled for further tests, and nearly 14,000 cancers were detected—17% of those underwent further tests, 0.8% of all women screened. The latest research shows that the NHSBSP is now saving 1400 lives every year in England[3].

Ductal carcinoma in situ (DCIS) registrations have increased markedly since the introduction of breast screening, because it is a condition that is usually not palpable and therefore is mostly diagnosed by mammography. DCIS accounts for approximately 20% of screen-detected cancers. Critics of the breast screening programme have voiced concerns that identifying DCIS is overdiagnosis of breast cancer, as these lesions may never progress or threaten the woman's life. However, the majority of screen-detected DCIS is high grade (69%) and necrotic (87%), and there is growing and convincing evidence that the detection of high-grade and necrotic DCIS by screening and its subsequent treatment prevents the development of high-grade invasive cancer with poor prognosis[4–7]. Some debate has centred around the age of women screened. A recent large UK randomized control trial assessing the mortality benefit of screening women annually from 40–49 years, suggests that accounting for the necessity to perform annual mammography due to a more aggressive tumour biology and generally denser mammographic pattern, there is no statistical survival benefit in screening women of this age group[8]. The screening interval in the vast majority of trials has been 2 years rather than the 3 years implemented by the NHSBSP, so the effectiveness of this programme is somewhat reduced as evidenced by the increased interval cancer rate in the third year after screening compared to the first 2 years[9]. However, optimum mammographic technique including two-view mammography, double reading of mammograms, and regular quality assurance and audit both locally and nationally within the NHSBSP has led to improved standardized detection rates.

3.2 Diagnosis and staging

3.2.1 Radiological diagnosis

Despite advances in many imaging techniques over the last two decades, in particular MRI, the main diagnostic tools used radiologically in the diagnosis of breast cancer remain mammography and ultrasound. In women younger than 35 years of age mammography is not routinely performed in the assessment of a breast lesion, as the breasts are radiosensitive, dense, and therefore difficult to interpret mammographically. Ultrasound will usually be sufficient. In women of 35 years and over, a mammogram is the first-line investigation, often accompanied by a focused ultrasound of the area of clinical concern[10]. Mammography is now increasingly performed using full-field digital mammogram machines, and these are now being gradually rolled out in the NHSBSP. This technology, although expensive, shows an equivalent cancer detection rate, though with an improved specificity, in part because the reader has much more capability to manipulate the images using a dedicated mammographic workstation[11]. The advantage of being filmless also confers seamless transfer of images into the patient's electronic imaging file in departments equipped with picture archive communication systems (PACS)[12].

The most common mammographic feature of breast cancer is a dense mass with an ill-defined border, though a spiculate irregular mass has a pathognomic appearance (Fig. 3.1). Usually a well-defined non-dense mass on a mammogram represents a benign entity such as a simple cyst, a fibroadenoma, or an intramammary node, though often an ultrasound and even a tissue sample is needed to confirm this. The less aggressive ductal carcinoma pathologies—such as medullary carcinoma—can appear very similar radiologically to a fibroadenoma, so usual practice is to biopsy/fine needle aspiration (FNA) any solid breast lesion in women locally considered to be of sufficient risk by age (usually at least 25 years). Another mammographic sign of cancer is a distortion of the breast tissue. This is commonly only seen on one mammographic view, and can be a very subtle mammographic finding. Post-surgical scarring, fat necrosis, radial scar, and sclerosing adenosis are all benign entities that show distortion or sometimes even a spiculate mass and hence can be indistinguishable radiologically from cancer[13]. Other mammographic features of cancer include asymmetric soft tissue, which although most commonly represents normal parenchymal breast tissue, can be a subtle appearance of invasive lobular cancer. Calcification is a common mammographic finding and when rounded, coarse, and scattered have features in keeping with benignity. Pleomorphism, linear and branching patterns, and fine clusters may all be features of malignant disease, though quite often calcifications are indeterminate[14]. When such clusters are considered suspicious or indeterminate, a tissue biopsy is indicated to exclude DCIS.

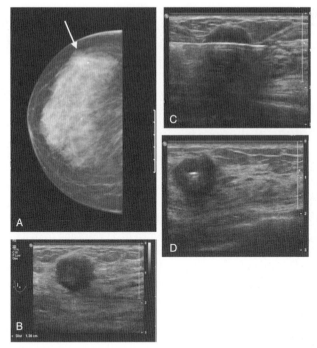

Fig. 3.1 Primary diagnostic images in a 57-year-old woman with breast cancer. (A) Right craniocaudal mammogram shows an ill-defined mass in the outer breast (arrow). (B) Focused US shows a heterogeneous mass with an irregular border suspicious for a carcinoma. (C) and (D) US images showing a core biopsy needle within the lesion which was used to histopathologically confirm the diagnosis.

On ultrasound, cancers are typically solid rather than cystic, have an irregular margin, and cast acoustic shadowing distantly. Both fast growing high-grade tumours as well as low-grade medullary carcinomas may be well defined and cast minimal acoustic shadowing, but will be solid. It is for this reason that any solid lesion, however innocent otherwise in appearance, will routinely be subjected to biopsy such that benignity can be confirmed. Doppler ultrasound has been employed in further assessing solid lesions, though tumour vascularity is quite variable, and benign lesions themselves may be very vascular[15].

Breast MRI has been shown to have a high sensitivity for the detection of breast cancer, but traditionally at the expense of a variable specificity[16]. The high detection rate is underpinned by the tendency of breast cancer (like other malignant tumours) to develop malignant angiogenesis. When gadolinium-DTPA contrast is administered dynamically intravenously, on T1-weighted images, there is an intense peak with subsequent washout (reflecting leaking capillaries). MRI false positives include fibroadenomas and papillomas, which also may focally avidly enhance. DCIS has been detected with low sensitivity, partly due to the inability of MRI to detect microcalcifications, though a recent study suggests that MRI may detect high-grade necrotic DCIS, which is non-calcified and therefore mammographically invisible (Fig. 3.2)[17].

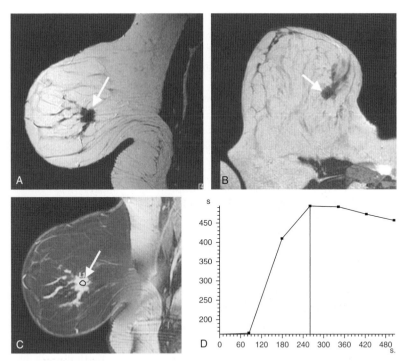

Fig. 3.2 MR images of a 63-year-old woman with right-sided breast cancer. (A) and (B) sagittal and axial T2-weighted images showing a low signal irregular mass (arrow) consistent with a carcinoma. Ductal prominence radiating from the mass anteriorly is suspicious for associated carcinoma in situ. (C) Dynamically enhanced sagittal fat-saturated T1-weighted image showing marked enhancement of the mass and associated anterior ducts confirming DCIS. The circle overlying the mass is a region of interest for which an enhancement-time curve may be displayed. (D) The enhancement curve shows rapid enhancement with slow washout, in keeping with a carcinoma.

Breast MRI was officially incorporated into the diagnostic armoury of the breast radiologist when the National Institute for Health and Clinical Excellence (NICE) published guidelines for screening women at high risk for familial breast cancer in July 2006. They appraised the evidence of a number of multicentre randomized control trials assessing the efficacy of MRI in breast cancer detection[18–20] including the UK trial, MARIBS[21]. The recommendations include annual contrast-enhanced breast MRI studies to supplement annual mammography in the very highest risk women (BRCA-1, -2, Tp53 carriers). This is currently being implemented in centres with family history breast clinics, but is in its early stages.

Other newer technologies include computer aided detection (CAD), a computer software package applied either to a digital mammography unit (or an MRI worksta-tion), which can flag abnormal areas on the mammogram (or MRI) by producing electronic markers on the image at the touch of a button. It aims to improve cancer detection, and reduce the false negative rate. Various mammographic software packages have been trialed in the USA and UK but to date have consistently suffered from very poor specificity and have not been diagnostically helpful[22]. This is a continuing area of research. Tomosynthesis is another developing technology. This essentially acquires sequential mammographic images using an X-ray source that is moved in an arc above a stationary breast and digital detector[23]. A number of prototypes are being tested, mainly in the USA, but as yet it has not been adopted into routine clinical practice.

[18]F-fluorodeoxyglucose positron emission tomography (FDG PET) has been shown to be able to detect primary breast carcinoma. However, this technique, which is now increasingly fused with computed tomography (PET/CT), has a better utility in disease staging, and so is discussed in section 3.2.2. In detection of small breast cancers it is insufficiently sensitive, and so is not used in the primary diagnostic setting[24].

3.2.2 Radiological staging

The TNM (tumour, node, metastasis) system has been widely adopted (Table 3.1), and although a largely clinical classification, is being increasingly influenced by imaging techniques. Primary disease radiological staging continues to be performed routinely by mammography and ultrasound, which although reasonable in accuracy when correlated to final pathology are not perfect (Table 3.2). On mammography surrounding tissue distortion spreading around a mass due to breast compression can make disease appear far more extensive than it actually is. On ultrasound, although well-defined lesions can be measured accurately, some cancers can be difficult to measure as these appear as ill-defined acoustic shadowing. Lobular carcinoma is classically very difficult to measure as it often grows by infiltrating along normal tissue planes without forming a mass[25].

MRI may be more accurate at primary disease staging, especially with contrast enhancement, as abnormal tissue that is difficult to distinguish from dense parenchymal tissue, can be assessed more accurately by its enhancement characteristics. It has been shown to be more accurate at detecting multifocal and multicentric disease than the other imaging modalities currently used in primary disease staging, though there have been only small studies to date[26]. MRI and mammography are believed to be superior to ultrasound in detecting associated *in situ* disease although their real accuracy in this regard is still not known. Lobular carcinoma may still be understaged by MRI, again due to its infiltrative growth pattern. As yet there is no published evidence to suggest a high accuracy in quantification of disease in this pathological subtype. In fact many clinical indications for breast MRI are not based on a high level of evidence, with studies being mainly retrospective and including only small patient numbers[27]. Many units are performing MRI on patients in order to better clarify disease extent prior to surgery, in particular where there is invasive lobular cancer. There has also been an interest in its utility in assessing disease response to chemotherapy preoperatively. For full utilization of this technique, specificity needs to be improved, as does availability of a compatible biopsy system. There would also need to be more standardization in terms of imaging protocols and reporting terminology, though this is currently under development.

Axillary lymph nodes metastatically involved by tumour usually lose their normal architecture such that an echogenic fatty hilum diminishes and an irregularly thickened low echogenic cortex predominates on ultrasound. Although reactive nodes can

Table 3.1 TNM classification of breast cancer

Primary tumour (T)	
TX	Primary tumour cannot be assessed
T0	No evidence of primary tumour
Tis	Intraductal carcinoma, lobular carcinoma *in situ*, or Paget disease of the nipple with no associated invasion of normal breast tissue: ♦ Tis (DCIS): ductal carcinoma *in situ* ♦ Tis (LCIS): lobular carcinoma *in situ* ♦ Tis (Paget): Paget disease of the nipple with no tumour. [Note: Paget disease associated with a tumour is classified according to the size of the tumour]
T1	Tumour not >2.0cm in greatest dimension: ♦ T1mic: microinvasion ≤0.1cm in greatest dimension ♦ T1a: tumour >0.1cm but ≤0.5cm in greatest dimension ♦ T1b: tumour >0.5cm but ≤1.0cm in greatest dimension ♦ T1c: tumour >1.0cm but ≤2.0cm in greatest dimension
T2	Tumour >2.0cm but ≤5.0cm in greatest dimension
T3	Tumour >5.0cm in greatest dimension
T4	Tumour of any size with direct extension to (a) chest wall or (b) skin, only as described below: ♦ T4a: extension to chest wall, not including pectoralis muscle ♦ T4b: oedema (including peau d'orange) or ulceration of the skin of the breast, or satellite skin nodules confined to the same breast ♦ T4c: both T4a and T4b ♦ T4d: inflammatory carcinoma
Regional lymph nodes (N)	
NX	Regional lymph nodes cannot be assessed (e.g. previously removed)
N0	No regional lymph node metastasis
N1	Metastasis to movable ipsilateral axillary lymph node(s)
N2	Metastasis to ipsilateral axillary lymph node(s) fixed or matted, or in clinically apparent* ipsilateral internal mammary nodes in the *absence* of clinically evident lymph node metastasis: ♦ N2a: metastasis in ipsilateral axillary lymph nodes fixed to one another (matted) or to other structures ♦ N2b: metastasis only in clinically apparent* ipsilateral internal mammary nodes and in the *absence* of clinically evident axillary lymph node metastasis
N3	Metastasis in ipsilateral infraclavicular lymph node(s) with or without axillary lymph node involvement, or in clinically apparent* ipsilateral internal mammary lymph node(s) and in the *presence* of clinically evident axillary lymph node metastasis; or, metastasis in ipsilateral supraclavicular lymph node(s) with or without axillary or internal mammary lymph node involvement: ♦ N3a: metastasis in ipsilateral infraclavicular lymph node(s) ♦ N3b: metastasis in ipsilateral internal mammary lymph node(s) and axillary lymph node(s) ♦ N3c: metastasis in ipsilateral supraclavicular lymph node(s)

*Note: clinically apparent is defined as detected by imaging studies (excluding lymphoscintigraphy) or by clinical examination or grossly visible pathologically.

Table 3.2 American Joint Committee on Cancer (AJCC) stage groupings

Stage 0	Tis	N0	M0
Stage I	T1	N	M0
Stage IIA	T0	N1	M0
	T1	N1	M0
	T2	N0	M0
Stage IIB	T2	N1	M0
	T3	N0	M0
Stage IIIA	T0	N2	M0
	T1	N2	M0
	T2	N2	M0
	T3	N1	M0
	T3	N2	M0
Stage IIIB	T4	N0	M0
	T4	N1	M0
	T4	N2	M0
Stage IIIC	Any T	N3	M0
Stage IV	Any T	Any N	M1

also have this appearance, eventually a node being replaced by cancer may lose its normal lobulated shape, become enlarged, rounded, and entirely hypoechoic. However, ultrasound has its limitations, particularly in the apex of the axilla. In addition, a major site of nodal spread is the internal mammary lymph node chain, which lies parasternally, and hence is not accessible to ultrasound. Usually these are involved by spread from superior and medial tumours, although axillary disease is still more common in patients with tumours at those sites. These nodes are best demonstrated by CT or PET/CT, but these investigations are not routinely performed prior to treatment, and this site is not treated surgically or by radiotherapy as standard. Thus, it remains a potential site for relapse.

Sentinel lymph node biopsy (SLNB) technology has developed in order to determine the first node draining the tumour, and hence predict if nodal metastatic disease has occurred. It has been embraced as a standard of care in many centres around the world and has revolutionized management of the axilla during the past decade[28]. Nonetheless, data for long-term outcomes remain scarce, and there are persistent variations in practice and inconsistencies in methodology[29]. SLNB is indicated for women with small invasive breast cancers and clinically negative nodes. SLNB indications are being expanded to larger breast tumors, some cases of ductal carcinoma *in situ* and selected clinically suspicious nodes. Because SLNB has fewer and less severe complications than axillary lymph node dissection, physicians are exploring more ways it can be used to improve breast cancer treatment[30]. The sentinel node is identified following an injection of blue dye and/or isotope, pre- or intraoperatively using a gamma probe or camera[31]. Three nodes are usually then excised and examined histopathologically to determine if the patient requires further axillary surgery.

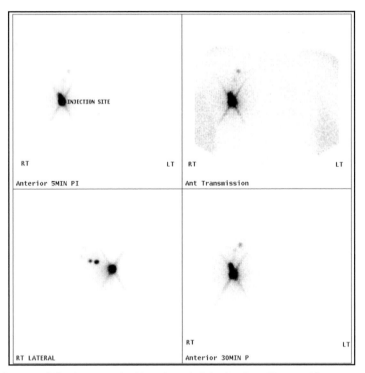

Fig. 3.3 Image following a sentinel lymph node injection in a 55-year-old woman with right-sided breast cancer. The injection site is marked with additional densities in right axilla representing the sentinel nodes.

A number of injection sites have been used, most commonly peritumoural, but dermal and periareolar sites have also had a high reported accuracy rate (Fig. 3.3)[32].

Breast cancer may present with associated secondary metastatic disease when staging investigations are not usually required at the time of diagnosis. The exception to this is where there are a number of poor prognostic factors, such as an inflammatory cancer or multiple involved axillary lymph nodes. A chest radiograph is usually performed at diagnosis in most cases, although it is not sensitive in detecting lung metastases[33]. The contralateral breast is usually evaluated with mammography as contralateral disease is present in up to 2.4%, though this figure may be much higher in patients with significant genetic risk[34,35]. In patients at moderate risk of metastatic disease, a liver ultrasound and an isotope bone scan are usually performed. Bone scans can be correlated with plain radiographs if indicated, in order to assist the differentiation of degenerative change from metastases. If this is unhelpful, then MRI or even PET/CT may be required[36,37]. CT remains the gold standard investigation for general assessment of metastatic disease, though PET/CT is being increasingly employed[38]. However, indications for such secondary staging investigations are limited to assessment of higher risk patients, e.g. patients with large, high-grade tumours, multiple involved axillary lymph nodes, or inflammatory carcinoma.

Metastatic disease of the breast can involve virtually any organ, and typically presents 2–5 years after diagnosis. While investigation of the asymptomatic patient is inappropriate, radiological tests may be used in the context of progressive symptomatology to definitively diagnose treatable metastatic disease. Chest radiography as well as a baseline test, is still the first-line investigation of chest symptoms, though in the absence of an alternative diagnosis to explain the symptom, a CT scan should be performed. This can demonstrate lung metastases, mediastinal nodes as well as a pleural effusion. Occasionally breast cancer can involve the mediastinal fat diffusely causing an ill-defined alteration in the usual fat density rather than forming a focal mass. A high-resolution CT (HRCT) may specifically demonstrate lymphangitis.

Liver disease is less common, and may present with hepatomegaly or deranged liver function tests. An ultrasound will demonstrate hypoechoic lesions, sometimes appearing as 'target' lesions. CT scanning will show low attenuation lesions, enhancing in the portal venous phase of scanning. Occasionally a more diffuse pattern of infiltrative disease is observed, which makes the liver appear cirrhotic-like or 'pseudocirrhotic'. MRI may be used if there is equivocation, but this is not usually needed. Other abdominal disease is rare and is thought to arise transcoelomically. It typically manifests as peritoneal disease, appearing very similar on CT to ovarian carcinoma.

Metastases affecting the central nervous system are unusual, but are increasing in prominence as this serves as a 'sanctuary site' since increasingly disease is becoming treated by newer chemotherapeutic agents that do not cross the blood–brain barrier[39]. Headache or convulsion is the commonest symptom, and although a CT scan is a good initial diagnostic investigation for excluding other acute pathologies, an MRI scan may provide a more definitive diagnosis. In particular, it may demonstrate more lesions, and can be employed to image the spinal cord; metastases show characteristic enhancement on gadolinium contrast-enhanced T1-weighted studies.

Increasing experience with PET/CT in breast cancer patients indicates there may be a role for this modality in: 1) evaluation of patients who are suspected of tumour recurrence; 2) identification of patients with multifocal or distant sites of malignancy who otherwise appear to have isolated, potentially curable, locoregional recurrence[40],[41]. PET/CT appears to be superior to bone scintigraphy in the detection of osteolytic lesions, but inferior (although still efficacious) in the detection of osteoblastic lesions[42]. It may show bony disease response, not usually observed on standard CT or MRI studies, which tend to show residual marrow abnormality even if the disease is treated (Fig. 3.4). PET/CT has limitations in characterizing subcentimetre lung and liver lesions, as they may not have sufficient glucose metabolism to be sufficiently FDG avid. Developments in this field include fusion of FDG PET with MRI to improve specificity of the breast MRI, but this is still in the realms of research[58]. In addition, novel PET tracers are being developed that may more specifically identify breast cancer, rather than just sites of active metabolism as FDG does. Ultimately this will help tailor therapy to the individual patient by improving our ability to quantify the therapeutic target, identify drug resistance factors, and measure and predict early response[44]. An example of this includes carbon-11 labelled sulfonanilide analogues which target aromatase, though again this remains a research area currently[45].

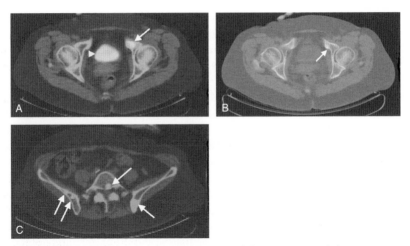

Fig. 3.4 PET/CT images of a 43-year-old woman with known metastatic breast cancer. (A) Fusion image shows abnormal uptake in the left superior pubic ramus (white arrow) and incidental physiological bladder FDG uptake (arrowhead). (B) Plain CT image does not show abnormality at this site, as a destructive lesion or sclerotic reaction has not yet formed. This was subsequently confirmed to be a new occult site of bone disease. (C) Other sites of known disease are not FDG avid on this fusion image (arrows), as they are inactive 'healed' metastases. Such bony response is not otherwise visible on any other cross-sectional imaging modality. See colour section.

3.3 **Radiotherapy planning**

All patients with primary or recurrent breast cancer should be considered for postoperative radiotherapy as it reduces local recurrence following surgery for both invasive and *in situ* disease. Higher risk patients may require chest wall and supraclavicular radiotherapy, however, axillary treatment has to be considered in the context of node positivity and surgical procedure performed. Breast-conserving surgery followed by whole-breast radiotherapy (WBRT) is currently the gold standard for the majority of patients with early breast cancer. Targeting is critical for effective radiotherapy. The aim is to better target the tumour while decreasing the dose administered to surrounding normal tissues. In the treatment of early operable breast cancer, methods of localization of the primary tumour site have previously failed to demonstrate the tumour site accurately in three dimensions.

Conventional single-plane two-dimensional radiotherapy breast plans can lead to substantial off-axis dose inhomogeneities, particularly in women with larger breasts. The gold standard imaging modality remains CT, with placement of surgical clips located in three dimensions by CT the favoured option. However, this is less than perfect in large part due to the intrinsic lack of contrast between soft tissues[36]. This can lead to high variability in target definition. The risks include a geographical miss with tumour underirradiation on the one hand, and tumour overestimation with undue normal tissue irradiation on the other hand. A more complex form of radiotherapy, intensity modulated radiotherapy (IMRT), can produce superior dosimetry compared with conventional techniques, but the planning, treatment time, and quality assurance measures are time-consuming, and the equipment is not yet universally available in the UK[47].

Parasternal radiation with standard fields does not allow for individual anatomical variability of the internal mammary lymph nodes. One possibility for individual treatment planning, taking into account the depth and lateral extension of the internal mammary lymph nodes, is to visualize this node chain by internal mammary lymphoscintigraphy (IMLS) prior to radiation[38]. Their exact localization on the simulation film allows for individual shaping of the parasternal field, thus ensuring adequate enclosure of the internal mammary lymph nodes and matching of the field margins. IMLS is easy to perform with standard equipment.

MRI allows set up in the conventional treatment position. It gives exquisite detail of the primary cavity, nodes, and surrounding tissues, and the neighbouring organs at risk, without the use of contrast. The primary site, neighbouring organs at risk, and other adjacent critical structures can be identified in three planes, and be optimally treated or avoided[64]. However, MRI has potential limitations. Patient claustrophobia and contraindications to scanning (e.g. cardiac pacemaker) can be a problem, as well as image distortion secondary to either the machine or the patient. Distortion correction algorithms can be applied in order to obtain more accurate imaging data. As MRI lacks the electron density information generated by CT, MR images are assigned bulk attenuation factors for the regions of interest, or fused with CT data for treatment planning. There may also be a future role for PET/CT in radiotherapy planning, particularly at sites of metastatic disease[50].

3.4 **Therapeutic assessment and follow-up**

Therapeutic response assessment can be made by mammography, though this is not sensitive or specific. Complete resolution of cancer can occur with residual mammographic abnormality; conversely resolution of mammographic findings but with residual active disease[53,54]. Ultrasound is an alternative but treatment often changes the tumour from a well-defined mass to an area of ill-defined distortion making it increasingly difficult to assess. MRI has the advantage that tumour-specific enhancement increases conspicuity on a pre-treatment study. However, MRI has not been validated to be efficacious for therapeutic assessment by any large prospective study. Indeed tumour vascularity often changes following treatment but morphological appearances do not. This may make the MRI more difficult to interpret as the tumour may be delineated less confidently without these vascular characteristics.

For primary breast cancer that has been treated curatively, annual mammography for 5 years although not standard, is a suitable protocol for imaging follow-up[54]. Scar tissue can be difficult to assess mammographically. As it is heterogeneous, it can take a varying time to involute and may appear quite different between mammograms due to subtle differences in the way the breast is compressed. If there is clinical or mammographic suspicion of local scar recurrence at any time, then a focused ultrasound is invaluable. Indeed this is perhaps the most useful application of breast Doppler ultrasound, in distinguishing scar tissue from recurrent disease, with the latter often showing significant vascularity. With the advent of MRI breast screening, those high-risk patients that develop a cancer should, post-treatment, continue with their annual MRI as well as annual mammography as per the NICE guidelines. The exception is the patient who has undergone bilateral mastectomy where no imaging surveillance is necessary. MRI has the advantage of being highly sensitive in detecting recurrent disease; abnormal contrast enhancement is pathognomic. In the presence of a prosthetic reconstruction, mammographic interpretation is limited—full field digital imaging to a much lesser extent than conventional film screen radiographs. Ultrasound and MRI are less affected by prostheses and can be used where appropriate.

Following radiotherapy, arm lymphoedema is common, and distinction has to be made between recurrent disease in the upper axilla and post-treatment fibrosis. Similarly, brachial plexopathy can be referable to recurrent disease or radiation fibrosis (Figs. 3.5 and 3.6). Both CT and MRI can demonstrate recurrent masses in the axilla, chest wall, infra- and supraclavicular regions. Multiplanar imaging is essential for delineating the detail of the brachial plexus. Imaging may show recurrent lymphadenopathy or be used to distinguish infiltrative tumour from non-specific thickening of the nerves following treatment (Fig. 3.7). PET/CT may also be an excellent technique in this regard and certainly has a role where there is equivocation on other imaging modalities.

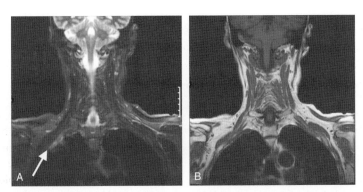

Fig. 3.5 Coronal MR images in a 70-year-old woman treated 2 years ago for right-sided breast cancer presenting with a new pain in the right arm. Axillary and chest wall radiotherapy were part of the treatment regimen. (A) STIR image shows high signal within the right lung apex and the soft tissues of the overlying chest wall (arrow). This appearance is non specific. (B) Corresponding T1-weighted image shows no abnormality, and following intravenous gadolinium (image not shown), there was no enhancement in this area. These features are entirely in keeping with post radiotherapy treatment changes only.

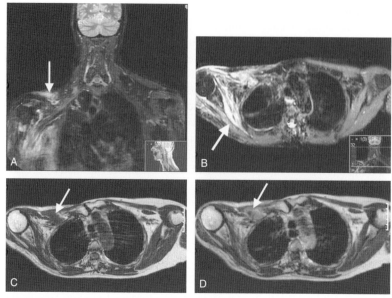

Fig. 3.6 MR images in a 61-year-old woman with new neurology in the right arm and previously treated for right breast cancer 3 years prior. Axillary and chest wall radiotherapy were part of the treatment regimen. (A) and (B) Coronal and axial STIR images show marked high signal within the soft tissues overlying the shoulder girdle that are non-specific. These appearances could be due to either treatment change or recurrent disease. (C) and (D) Axial T1-weighted images pre- and postintravenous injection of gadolinium showing an enhancing mass in the right subpectoral area that is in keeping with disease recurrence. This could not be discerned from surrounding high signal on the STIR sequences, which are highly sensitive but not specific at distinguishing recurrence from post-treatment change.

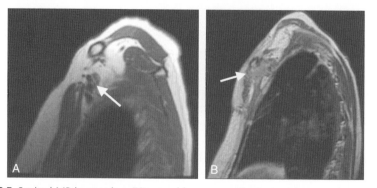

Fig. 3.7 Sagittal MR images in a 58-year-old woman with previous breast cancer and new left arm neurology. (A) Right infraclavicular area shows normal brachial plexus (arrow) just behind the subclavian vessels. (B) Left infraclavicular area shows a large mass (arrow) obliterating the normal fat planes and inseparable from the subclavian vessels and brachial plexus. This is in keeping with recurrent disease.

3.5 **Summary**

◆ Mammography and ultrasound remain the primary diagnostic tools, though MRI is being utilized increasingly.

◆ Secondary disease staging is performed typically with ultrasound or intravenous contrast enhanced CT, though MRI and PET/CT have been shown to be efficacious.

◆ Mammography and ultrasound are still performed for assessment of local recurrence, though MRI is efficacious in this area and being utilized increasingly.

◆ CT is the standard imaging modality for radiotherapy planning, but MRI may be a valuable adjunct.

References

1. Parkin DM, Bray F, Ferlay J, *et al.* Global cancer statistics, 2002. *CA Cancer J Clin* 2005; **55**: 74–108.

2. Coleman MP, Rachet B, Woods LM, *et al.* Trends and socioeconomic inequalities in cancer survival in England and Wales up to 2001. *Br J Cancer* 2004; **90**: 1367–73.

3. Programmes NCS. *NHS Breast Screening Programme Annual Review 2006.* NHS Cancer Screening Programmes, 2006.

4. Evans AJ, Pinder SE, Ellis IO, *et al.* Screen detected ductal carcinoma in situ (DCIS): overdiagnosis or an obligate precursor of invasive disease? *J Med Screen* 2001; **8**: 149–51.

5. Maxwell AJ, Hanson IM, Sutton CJ, *et al.* A study of breast cancers detected in the incident round of the UK NHS Breast Screening Programme: the importance of early detection and treatment of ductal carcinoma in situ. *Breast* 2001; **10**: 392–8.

6. Gotzsche PC, Nielsen M. Screening for breast cancer with mammography. *Cochrane Database Syst Rev* 2006; **4**: CD001877.

7. Kerlikowske K, Grady D, Rubin SM, *et al.* Efficacy of screening mammography. A metaanalysis. *JAMA* 1995; **273**: 149–54.

8. Moss SM, Cuckle H, Evans A, *et al.* Effect of mammographic screening from age 40 years on breast cancer mortality at 10 years' follow-up: a randomised controlled trial. *Lancet* 2006; **368**: 2053–60.

9. Duffy SW, Tabar L, Vitak B, *et al.* The Swedish Two-County Trial of mamthmographic screening: cluster randomisation and end point evaluation. *Ann Oncol* 2003; **14**: 1196–8.

10. Radiologists RCo. *Making the best use of clinical radiology services*, 6th edn. London: The Royal College of Radiologists, 2007.

11. Lewin JM, D'Orsi CJ, Hendrick RE, *et al.* Clinical comparison of full-field digital mammography and screen-film mammography for detection of breast cancer. *AJR Am J Roentgenol* 2002; **179**: 671–7.

12. Zuley M. How to transition to digital mammography. *J Am Coll Radiol* 2007; **4**: 178–83.

13. Feig SA. Breast masses. Mammographic and sonographic evaluation. *Radiol Clin North Am* 1992; **30**: 67–92.

14. Bassett LW. Mammographic analysis of calcifications. *Radiol Clin North Am* 1992; **30**: 93–105.

15. Raza S, Baum JK. Solid breast lesions: evaluation with power Doppler US. *Radiology* 1997; **203**: 164–8.

16. Kuhl CK. Current status of breast MR imaging. Part 2. Clinical applications. *Radiology* 2007; **244**: 672–91.

17. Kuhl CK, Schrading S, Bieling HB, *et al.* MRI for diagnosis of pure ductal carcinoma in situ: a prospective observational study. *Lancet* 2007; **370**: 485–92.

18. Kriege M, Brekelmans CT, Peterse H, *et al.* Tumor characteristics and detection method in the MRISC screening program for the early detection of hereditary breast cancer. *Breast Cancer Res Treat* 2007; **102**: 357–63.

19. Warner E, Plewes DB, Hill KA, *et al.* Surveillance of BRCA1 and BRCA2 mutation carriers with magnetic resonance imaging, ultrasound, mammography, and clinical breast examination. *JAMA* 2004; **292**: 1317–25.

20. Kuhl CK, Schrading S, Leutner CC, *et al.* Mammography, breast ultrasound, and magnetic resonance imaging for surveillance of women at high familial risk for breast cancer. *J Clin Oncol* 2005; **23**: 8469–76.

21. Griebsch I, Brown J, Boggis C, *et al.* Cost-effectiveness of screening with contrast enhanced magnetic resonance imaging vs X-ray mammography of women at a high familial risk of breast cancer. *Br J Cancer* 2006; **95**: 801–10.

22. Khoo LA, Taylor P, Given-Wilson RM. Computer-aided detection in the United Kingdom National Breast Screening Programme: prospective study. *Radiology* 2005; **237**: 444–9.

23. Niklason LT, Kopans DB, Hamberg LM. Digital breast imaging: tomosynthesis and digital subtraction mammography. *Breast Dis* 1998; **10**: 151–64.

24. Avril N, Adler LP. F-18 fluorodeoxyglucose-positron emission tomography imaging for primary breast cancer and loco-regional staging. *Radiol Clin North Am* 2007; **45**: 645–57.

25. Moinfar F. Accurate size measurement in infiltrating lobular carcinoma of the breast–gross versus microscopic evaluation. *Breast J* 2006; **12**: 509–10.

26. Sardanelli F, Giuseppetti GM, Panizza P, *et al.* Sensitivity of MRI versus mammography for detecting foci of multifocal, multicentric breast cancer in fatty and dense breasts using the whole-breast pathologic examination as a gold standard. *AJR Am J Roentgenol* 2004; **183**: 1149–57.

27. Kepple J, Layeeque R, Klimberg VS, *et al.* Correlation of magnetic resonance imaging and pathologic size of infiltrating lobular carcinoma of the breast. *Am J Surg* 2005; **190**: 623–7.

28. Krag D, Weaver D, Ashikaga T, *et al.* The sentinel node in breast cancer – a multicenter validation study. *N Engl J Med* 1998; **339**: 941–6.

29. Hazel CA, Petre KL, Armstrong RA, *et al.* Visual function and subjective quality of life compared in subjects with acquired macular disease. *Invest Ophthalmol Vis Sci* 2000; **41**: 1309–15.

30. Mabry H, Giuliano AE. Sentinel node mapping for breast cancer: progress to date and prospects for the future. *Surg Oncol Clin N Am* 2007; **16**: 55–70.

31. Motomura K, Inaji H, Komoike Y, *et al.* Combination technique is superior to dye alone in identification of the sentinel node in breast cancer patients. *J Surg Oncol* 2001; **76**: 95–9.

32. Nieweg OE. Lymphatics of the breast and the rationale for different injection techniques. *Ann Surg Oncol* 2001; **8**: S71–73.

33. Moskovic E, Parsons C, Baum M. Chest radiography in the management of breast cancer. *Br J Radiol* 1992; **65**: 30–2.

34. Chaudary MA, Millis RR, Hoskins EO, *et al.* Bilateral primary breast cancer: a prospective study of disease incidence. *Br J Surg* 1984; **71**: 711–14.

35. Shahedi K, Emanuelsson M, Wiklund F, *et al.* High risk of contralateral breast carcinoma in women with hereditary/familial non-BRCA1/BRCA2 breast carcinoma. *Cancer* 2006; **106**: 1237–42.

36. Culham LE, Ryan B, Jackson AJ, *et al*. Low vision services for vision rehabilitation in the United Kingdom. *Br J Ophthalmol* 2002; **86**: 743–7.

37. Schirrmeister H. Detection of bone metastases in breast cancer by positron emission tomography. *Radiol Clin North Am* 2007; **45**: 669–76.

38. Bartella L, Smith CS, Dershaw DD, *et al*. Imaging breast cancer. *Radiol Clin North Am* 2007; **45**: 45–67.

39. Bendell JC, Domchek SM, Burstein HJ, *et al*. Central nervous system metastases in women who receive trastuzumab-based therapy for metastatic breast carcinoma. *Cancer* 2003; **97**: 2972–7.

40. Weir L, Worsley D, Bernstein V. The value of FDG positron emission tomography in the management of patients with breast cancer. *Breast J* 2005; **11**: 204–9.

41. Isasi CR, Moadel RM, Blaufox MD. A meta-analysis of FDG-PET for the evaluation of breast cancer recurrence and metastases. *Breast Cancer Res Treat* 2005; **90**: 105–12.

42. Maruo T, Ikebukuro N, Kawanabe K, *et al*. Changes in causes of visual handicaps in Tokyo. *Jpn J Ophthalmol* 1991; **35**: 268–72.

43. Moy L, Ponzo F, Noz ME, *et al*. Improving specificity of breast MRI using prone PET and fused MRI and PET 3D volume datasets. *J Nucl Med* 2007; **48**: 528–37.

44. Eubank WB, Mankoff DA. Evolving role of positron emission tomography in breast cancer imaging. *Semin Nucl Med* 2005; **35**: 84–99.

45. Wang M, Lacy G, Gao M, *et al*. Synthesis of carbon-11 labeled sulfonanilide analogues as new potential PET agents for imaging of aromatase in breast cancer. *Bioorg Med Chem Lett* 2007; **17**: 332–6.

46. Bhatnagar AK, Brandner E, Sonnik D, *et al*. Intensity-modulated radiation therapy (IMRT) reduces the dose to the contralateral breast when compared to conventional tangential fields for primary breast irradiation: initial report. *Cancer J* 2004; **10**: 381–5.

47. Kawase K, Gayed IW, Hunt KK, *et al*. Use of lymphoscintigraphy defines lymphatic drainage patterns before sentinel lymph node biopsy for breast cancer. *J Am Coll Surg* 2006; **203**: 64–72.

48. Krauss DJ, Kestin LL, Raff G, *et al*. MRI-based volumetric assessment of cardiac anatomy and dose reduction via active breathing control during irradiation for left-sided breast cancer. *Int J Radiat Oncol Biol Phys* 2005; **61**: 1243–50.

49. Gwak HS, Youn SM, Chang U, *et al*. Usefulness of (18)F-fluorodeoxyglucose PET for radiosurgery planning and response monitoring in patients with recurrent spinal metastasis. *Minim Invasive Neurosurg* 2006; **49**: 127–34.

50. Niehoff P, Ballardini B, Polgar C, *et al*. Early European experience with the MammoSite radiation therapy system for partial breast brachytherapy following breast conservation operation in low-risk breast cancer. *Breast* 2006; **15**: 319–25.

51. Vinnicombe SJ, MacVicar AD, Guy RL, *et al*. Primary breast cancer: mammographic changes after neoadjuvant chemotherapy, with pathologic correlation. *Radiology* 1996; **198**: 333–40.

52. Therasse P, Arbuck SG, Eisenhauer EA, *et al*. New guidelines to evaluate the response to treatment in solid tumors. European Organization for Research and Treatment of Cancer, National Cancer Institute of the United States, National Cancer Institute of Canada. *J Natl Cancer Inst* 2000; **92**: 205–16.

53. Guidelines for the management of symptomatic breast disease. *Eur J Surg Oncol* 2005; **31** (Suppl. 1): 1–21.

54. Winehouse J, Douek M, Holz K, *et al*. Contrast-enhanced colour Doppler ultrasonography in suspected breast cancer recurrence. *Br J Surg* 1999; **86**: 1198–201.

Chapter 4

Lung and thorax

Noelle O'Rourke and Michael Sproule

4.1 Lung cancer

4.1.1 Clinical background

Lung cancer is the commonest cause of cancer death within the UK, with approximately 37,000 new cases per annum and 33,000 deaths. The disease is more common in men than women (3:2) and the incidence peaks at age 70–79 years[1]. It is estimated that 90% of cases are attributable to tobacco use.

The five-year survival from lung cancer worldwide varies from around 8% in the UK to 15% in the USA. Mortality is high because by the time symptoms develop approximately 75% of patients will already have locally advanced or metastatic disease. Computed tomography (CT) screening programmes for lung cancer in high-risk populations have been undertaken in both the USA and Japan, with some evidence of cost-effectiveness. However the role of screening remains controversial and clinical trials continue to address the issues of optimal imaging and scheduling and whether detecting smaller tumours will result in a meaningful reduction in disease specific mortality.

Histologically there are four main types of lung cancer: small cell lung carcinoma (SCLC, 20%); squamous carcinoma (45%); adenocarcinoma (25%); and large cell lung carcinoma (10%). For treatment purposes the latter three are taken together as non-small cell carcinoma (NSCLC). Worldwide there has been a decline in small cell carcinoma but in Japan and USA the incidence of adenocarcinoma has increased above that of squamous carcinoma.

The growth and spread of a lung tumour depends upon its pathological subtype. SCLC disseminates early beyond the thorax and for this reason the primary therapeutic approach is systemic chemotherapy. Adenocarcinoma is the slowest growing lung cancer and may be present as peripheral lung lesions sometimes for years prior to diagnosis. Squamous and large cell tumours are more rapidly growing, invading locally initially with later metastatic spread, commonly starting via the regional lymphatics. Lymphatic involvement tends to start at the ipsilateral hilum, then subcarinal area followed by paratracheal and contralateral mediastinal nodes, and then supraclavicular. The potential with all lung cancers for haematogenous dissemination means that sites of metastasis may be widespread. Most commonly involved are adrenal glands, liver, bone, contralateral lung, and brain.

The presenting symptoms of lung cancer include cough, breathlessness, chest pain, weight loss, and haemoptysis. While haemoptysis will prompt patients to seek medical attention the other symptoms can be variably pre-existent in the typical population of elderly smokers, contributing to delays in diagnosis. Failure of a chest infection to resolve in this population should warrant further investigation.

One limiting factor in survival, and indeed screening, is that the comorbidity of this population may mean that even when the cancer is diagnosed at an earlier stage, curative treatment is not an option because of the cardiac or respiratory function or general performance status of the patient. A population audit of all lung cancer patients diagnosed in Scotland in 1995 revealed that <40% of those patients presenting with early stage disease received potentially curative treatment—either surgery, chemoradiation, or radical radiotherapy[2]. The low survival in the UK has historically been attributed to the lower uptake of potentially curative therapies although there is evidence that this is now changing with the more widespread introduction of multidisciplinary team working.

4.1.2 Diagnosis and staging

Imaging plays a central role in both the diagnosis and staging of lung cancer. Types of imaging employed include plain radiographs, CT, magnetic resonance (MR) imaging, ultrasound (US), and positron emission tomography (PET) or integrated PET/CT. The chest radiograph is rarely normal in patients with lung cancer. However, the findings are very non-specific and therefore further investigations are invariably required. A CT scan of the thorax and abdomen is usually performed early in the patient's journey as this guides selection of the most appropriate investigations for confirmation of diagnosis and stage. CT has a very high sensitivity (89–100%) but relatively low specificity (56–63%). This suggests that a diagnosis of lung cancer should not be made on the basis of the CT scan alone. Histological and cytological confirmation of the diagnosis is achieved in >80% cases.

[18]F-fluorodeoxyglucose PET (FDG PET), and more recently PET/CT, has been used to investigate pulmonary nodules presenting as possible lung cancer (Fig. 4.1).

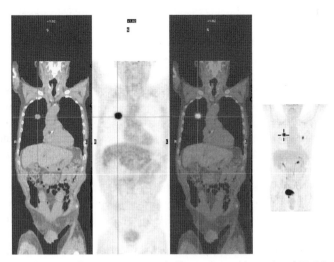

Fig. 4.1 Coronal images from a PET/CT study illustrating avid uptake of FDG in a right upper lobe nodule consistent with a bronchial carcinoma. See colour section.

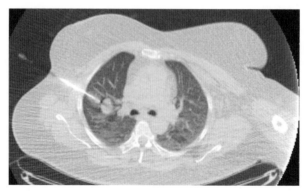

Fig. 4.2 CT-guided biopsy of right upper lobe nodule.

A meta-analysis suggests that the sensitivity of this technique is high (96%) but that the specificity is relatively low (78%)[3]. Again, this suggests that whilst FDG PET/CT may be used to investigate patients with solitary pulmonary lesions, histological/cytological confirmation of results will still be required. The specificity of FDG PET in this context varies considerably, not least due to the high incidence of granulomatous disease in parts of North America, where many of the published series arise.

The method of obtaining tissue to confirm diagnosis depends on the clinical and imaging findings. Fibreoptic bronchoscopy and biopsy is the recommended method for obtaining tissue from central lesions. CT-guided biopsy is the best method of obtaining tissue from peripheral lesions and is also indicated for central lesions if bronchoscopy has been negative (Fig. 4.2). Less commonly, mediastinoscopy, or more recently trans-bronchial fine needle aspiration can be used to obtain tissue from mediastinal nodes. This has the advantage of providing information on staging as well as diagnosis. Similarly, biopsy of extra pulmonary lesions (e.g. liver lesions, skin nodules, or neck nodes) may provide confirmation of distant metastases as well as the primary diagnosis.

4.1.2.1 Staging lung cancer

Staging is the assessment of the extent of disease and it is performed for prognostic and therapeutic purposes. Therefore, once a diagnosis of lung cancer has been made, accurate staging is the next crucial step (see Table 4.1).

The International Staging System (ISS) used to stage lung cancer was first published in 1986 by the American Joint Committee on Cancer (AJCC) and the Union Internationale Contre Cancer (UICC)[4]. It has subsequently undergone revisions, most recently in 2009[5]. The system has two major components: the anatomical extent of the disease (TNM) and confirmation of malignancy by histological/cytological examination. *T0–4* describes the primary tumour and its local complications; *N0–3* refers to regional lymph node metastases and *M0–1* refers to distant metastases. Depending on the prognosis and the therapeutic options, the TNM subsets are then categorised into one of four stages (I–IV).

Small cell lung cancer (SCLC) has traditionally been staged into limited versus extensive stage. However, based on recent survival data, the TNM classification and staging system is now recommended for SCLC[5].

Table 4.1 Staging system for lung cancer

Primary tumour (T)

T1	Tumour ≤3 cm diameter, surrounded by lung or visceral pleura, without invasion, more proximal than lobar bronchus
T1a	Tumour ≤2 cm in diameter
T1b	Tumour >2 cm in diameter
T2	Tumour >3 cm but ≤7 cm, with any of the following features: involves main bronchus ≤2 cm distal to carina; invades visceral pleura; associated with atelectasis or obstructive pneumonitis that extends to the hilar region but does not involve the entire lung
T2a	Tumour ≤5 cm
T2b	Tumour >5 cm
T3	Tumour >7 cm or any of the following: directly invades any of the following—chest wall, diaphragm, phrenic nerve, mediastinal pleura, parietal pericardium, main bronchus <2 cm from carina (without involvement of carina); atelectasis or obstructive pneumonitis of the entire lung; separate tumour nodules in the same lobe
T4	Tumour of any size that invades the mediastinum, heart, great vessels, trachea, recurrent laryngeal nerve, oesophagus, vertebral body, carina, or with separate tumour nodules in a different ipsilateral lobe

Regional lymph nodes (N)

N0	No regional lymph node metastases
N1	Metastasis in ipsilateral peribronchial and/or ipsilateral hilar lymph nodes and intrapulmonary nodes, including involvement by direct extension
N2	Metastasis in ipsilateral mediastinal and/or subcarinal lymph node(s)
N3	Metastasis in contralateral mediastinal, contralateral hilar, ipsilateral or contralateral scalene, or supraclavicular lymph node(s).

Distant metastasis (M)

M0	No distant metastasis
M1	Distant metastasis
M1a	Separate tumour nodule(s) in a contralateral lobe; tumour with pleural nodules or malignant pleural or pericardial effusion
M1b	Distant metastasis

Stage groupings

Stage IA:	T1a–T1b	N0	M0
Stage IB:	T2a	N0	M0
Stage IIA:	T1a–T2a	N1	M0
	T2b	N0	M0
Stage IIB:	T2b	N1	M0
	T3	N0	M0
Stage IIIA:	T1a–T3	N2	M0
	T3	N1	M0
	T4	N0–N1	M0
Stage IIIB:	T4	N2	M0
	T1a–T4	N3	M0
Stage IV:	Any T	Any N	M1a or M1b

Adapted from: Goldstraw P, Crowley J, Chansky K, *et al.* The IASLC Lung Cancer Staging Project: proposals for the revision of the TNM stage groups in the forthcoming (seventh) edition of the TNM classification of malignant tumours. *J Thorac Oncol* 2007; 2:706.

Clinical staging is defined as the best estimation of the extent of disease using *all* staging information that is available *prior to the initiation of any therapy*. It includes information obtained from imaging studies (*radiographic* staging) and information from biopsies (*surgical* staging). *Pathological* staging is determined after surgical *therapy*— that is, resection—has taken place. The single most important objective in staging is to identify those patients with clinical stage I–III (CI–III) as these are the patients who are potentially curable.

The imaging tools most commonly used to stage lung cancer in the Western world are CT, MR, US, PET, or integrated PET/CT. Mediastinoscopy is the most commonly performed invasive procedure. For a patient with lung cancer, overstaging the disease may wrongly exclude the patient from receiving potentially curative therapy. It is therefore acceptable to have a false negative rate (FN) although what is acceptable remains open to debate. Most clinicians would accept a rate of ~10%. False positive (FP) diagnosis leading to overstaging needs to be avoided.

4.1.2.2 T stage

Radiographic differentiation between T1 and T2 disease has little clinical importance because it does not significantly alter the choice of therapy. It is more important to be able to predict T3 and especially T4 involvement if surgical resection is being considered[6]. In Western countries, evaluation of lung cancer patients with a staging CT of the thorax and upper abdomen is standard practice. However, the reliability of CT in predicting T3 or T4 disease is suboptimal, with a FP rate of 32% and a FN rate of 18%. Therefore, patients with cT3 or cT4 disease who are fit for surgery, should not be denied surgical exploration on the basis of CT alone.

Looking specifically at chest wall invasion, the reliability of CT is very poor with a FP rate of 44% and a FN rate of 9%. However, with the exception of superior sulcus tumours, it is likely that a complete resection can be achieved in most cases. Thus accurate prediction of the extent of lateral chest wall invasion is less important preoperatively.

Mediastinal involvement by the primary tumour may be either T3 or T4 disease and it is not as likely to be resectable as chest wall involvement. As above, the reliability of CT in predicting mediastinal involvement is poor with a FP rate of 33% and FN rate of 14%.

To date, MR imaging has proven to be disappointing as a tool for staging lung cancer. Excluding superior sulcus tumours, it is not superior to CT in assessing the T stage. Approximately 50% of patients with superior sulcus tumours cannot be resected and MR has been shown to be significantly more reliable than CT in determining chest wall invasion in these cases. However, these studies pre-date multidetector CT which is probably as reliable as MR.

4.1.2.3 N stage

The most important aspect of intrathoracic staging is accurate determination of nodal involvement. CT (and MR) scans rely solely on lymph node size to predict malignant involvement. A meta-analysis found that when using a size criterion of 1cm the average sensitivity and specificity was 75% and 76% respectively. This 1cm short-axis diameter criterion has been adopted by most centres.

Overall, the reliability of CT assessment of mediastinal nodes is relatively poor. The average FP rate is high, 45%, regardless of the nodal station, histology, T stage, or tumour location. This suggests that with a CT scan positive for mediastinal lymphad-enopathy, there is no size, site, or situation in which surgical biopsy of the enlarged nodes is unnecessary, with the possible exception of extensive infiltrating disease where there is a confident diagnosis on the basis of the imaging alone.

When the CT scan is negative for mediastinal lymphadenopathy we know that it is falsely negative in 13% of cases. It is therefore reasonable to further investigate the mediastinum with mediastinoscopy or PET/CT prior to performing a thoracotomy.

Several studies have shown that conventional MR is not superior to CT in the assessment of mediastinal nodes. This may change with modern MR, particularly with the new lymph node-specific contrast agents—ultrasmall iron oxide particles (USPIO). In the meantime, there is no role for conventional MR in staging mediastinal lymphadenopathy.

The gold standard method of staging the mediastinum is mediastinoscopy. Paratracheal (stations 2R, 2L, 4R, 4L), pretracheal (stations 1 and 3), and anterior subcarinal (station 7) nodes are accessible (Fig. 4.3). The average FN rate is 9%. Although invasive, it can be done as an out patient procedure with minimal morbidity, 2.3%, and mortality, 0.05%.

To improve the accuracy of N staging it is necessary to sample the lymph node stations that cannot be reached by mediastinoscopy (aortopulmonary window, pre-aortic, paraoesophageal, inferior pulmonary ligament, and posterior subcarinal—stations 5, 6, 8, 9, and 7). This can be done by a number of techniques including transbronchial fine needle aspiration/ biopsy, thoracoscopy, percutaneous CT-guided biopsy, and, much less commonly, parasternal mediastinotomy and extended cervical mediastinoscopy.

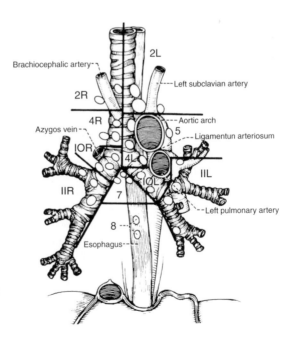

Fig. 4.3 American Thoracic Society lymph node mapping scheme.

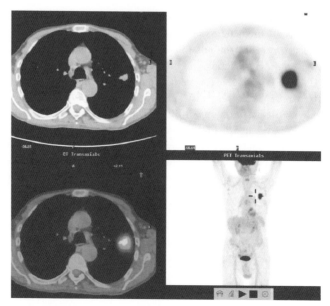

Fig. 4.4 Axial images from a PET/CT study showing avid uptake of FDG in a left upper lobe non-small cell bronchial carcinoma but no uptake in the enlarged left paratracheal lymph node; indicating that it is reactive rather than metastatic. See colour section.

It has been shown in several studies that PET scanning is more accurate than CT or MR in detecting mediastinal lymphadenopathy. In the published studies there is great variability in the FP rate (0–52%), partly due to the high prevalence of granulomatous disease in some parts of the world. The average FP figure is 16%. Therefore, if the PET scan is positive for mediastinal lymphadenopathy the patient should be considered for a biopsy via the appropriate method.

The FN rate with PET scanning is 7%, similar to mediastinoscopy at 9%. It would seem reasonable therefore to proceed directly to thoracotomy in those patients with a negative PET for mediastinal nodes (Fig. 4.4).

4.1.2.4 M stage

The most common sites of distant metastases are the brain, liver, bones, adrenal glands, and the lungs. Approximately 40% of patients with NSCLC will present with distant metastases and of these about 90% have clinical symptoms. Thorough clinical evaluation, with history (especially weight loss), physical examination, and blood tests, is crucial. If this raises suspicion of metastasis then further studies are performed. In addition, most patients with potentially curable disease based on the CT of the thorax and abdomen and the clinical examination will now have a PET/CT study.

PET/CT identifies unsuspected metastases in approximately 10–15% of patients with NSCLC. The FN rate is low, around 5%, but the FP rate is relatively high at >10%. Therefore, as with 'hot spots' in the mediastinum, a positive scan needs to be biopsied or followed up.

The use of PET leads to more accurate classification of the stage of disease. It is unproven whether this increased accuracy improves survival but it does reduce the number of futile thoracotomies and the number of patients who receive radical radiotherapy inappropriately[7].

4.1.3 Imaging for radiotherapy planning

4.1.3.1 Use of high-dose radiation treatment

The use of high-dose radiation treatment in the UK has historically been low for a number of reasons from access to care and equipment to the comorbidity of the lung cancer population. Even with the use of high-dose radiation in lung cancer, the cure rate is low and in one series routine follow-up bronchoscopy at 1 year demonstrated local control in <20% patients[8]. Some patients will relapse with distant metastases, but for most, local failure is the major obstacle to survival.

Recent decades have brought significant changes in lung radiation with the evolution of three-dimensional (3D) and now four-dimensional (4D) conformal radiotherapy and the development of altered fractionation schedules with or without concurrent chemotherapy. It is hoped that these emerging radiotherapy techniques will offer better local control for two reasons. Firstly, improved target volume definition and increased accuracy in set-up with attention to respiratory motion should reduce the likelihood of geographical misses. Secondly, better definition of tumour volume may allow the radiation dose to be escalated without being limited to the same extent by normal tissue toxicity.

High-dose radiation therapy is used as the primary management for medically inoperable stages I and II NSCLC. In these patients particularly, the respiratory and cardiac function can prove challenging in achieving an adequate dose to tumour. Radical radiotherapy is also employed, generally as part of combined modality treatment, in suitable stage III NSCLC and in limited stage SCLC. In this situation the volume of tumour can be large and will involve the mediastinum and there is the added toxicity of chemotherapy within the treatment schedule. Finally there may be a case for postoperative radiotherapy in patients with positive resection margins or concerns regarding residual disease at mediastinum or chest wall. The challenge in these patients is to reliably identify the area at risk, using pre- and postoperative images.

4.1.3.2 Treatment planning process

Radical radiotherapy to the lung is usually administered as daily fractions of treatment five times a week over 4–7 weeks. The treatment position needs to be comfortable for the patient and reproducible. The patient lies supine on a couch with their arms supported above their heads, to enable acquisition of planning images and direction of treatment beams through the chest. Techniques for immobilizing the patient vary, including polystyrene bead-filled bags shaped by vacuum suction or boards with fixed arm rests attached to support the patient. A CT scan of the whole lung from apex to diaphragm is taken with the patient in the treatment position and this is used to mark on the target volumes, in conjunction with the diagnostic imaging already performed.

Currently in development are techniques to fuse diagnostic images taken as PET or MR scans with radiotherapy planning scans. This could potentially improve the accuracy of tumour outlining, especially for circumstances such as collapse or consolidation where the PET image will much better define the gross tumour volume. However, fusion of images is complicated by differences in position of the patient between the scans and by respiratory movement which may be significant in a PET image series which has taken 20min to obtain and is done with tidal breathing compared with a helical CT series done rapidly in a single breath-hold.

ICRU (International Commission on Radiation Units and Measurements) Report 62 provides international recommendations on volume definition and nomenclature to ensure consistent reporting of radiotherapy treatment[9]. The first step in the process is to define the gross tumour volume (GTV), which then requires a margin of expansion to cover subclinical spread of disease creating a clinical tumour volume (CTV). In order to ensure that all parts of the CTV receive the prescribed dose, additional margins are required to allow for variations internally in the shape or size of the CTV. Within the lung this is of particular significance with respiratory and cardiac movement. As well as this internal margin (IM), a final margin is also required to take account of uncertainties in patient and beam positioning on set-up—the set-up margin (SM). CTV + IM + SM will define the final planning target volume (PTV) from which the selection of beam size and arrangement is made to construct a radiotherapy plan (Fig. 4.5).

Shielding conforming to the PTV is achieved using divergent customized blocks or, more commonly, by multileaf collimation (MLC). To ensure optimal positioning of the beams the planning system uses a beam's eye view (BEV) which allows the reconstructed image of the patient to be rotated on the computer screen. In this way the

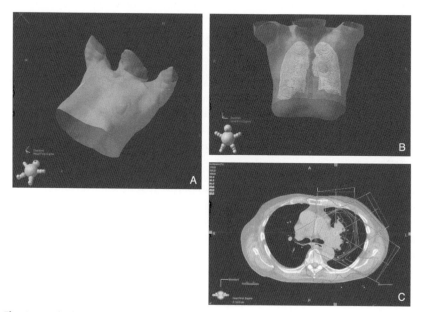

Fig. 4.5 Radiotherapy plan. (A) GTV marked in pink, surrounded by PTV in red on oblique view of body. (B) Anterior view of body with lungs marked on. (C) Transverse mid slice with field arrangement and isodose distribution marked. See colour section.

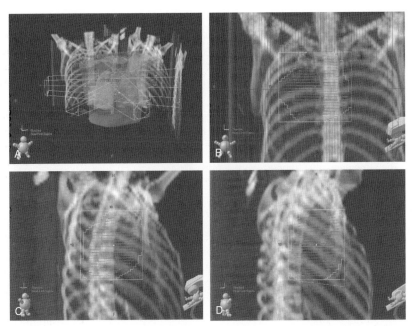

Fig. 4.6 Radiotherapy plan. (A) Three beam's eye view (BEV) images projected onto body showing orientation of fields. (B) Digitally reconstructed radiograph (DRR) of anterior field. PTV on each slice is marked in red. Blue lines show how multileaf collimator (MLC) conforms to target volume. (C) DRR for right anterior oblique field without MLC markings. (D) DRR for right posterior oblique filed without MLC markings. See colour section.

MLC can be set up to conform closely to the PTV for each individual beam, while viewing proximity to spinal cord (Fig. 4.6).

Contouring of the target volume and organs at risk is performed on each of the CT slices taken at multiple levels through the patient's chest. The GTV and CTV will be delineated by the planning physician but growth of the volume to produce PTV is usually achieved by an algorithm in the planning system to permit 3D growth in accordance with pre-set margins. The clinician can then review the volume slice by slice and modify as required. Individual radiotherapy departments may have some variation in the planning margins used and indeed there may need to be variation between patients depending upon the location of the tumour and the type of planning scan undertaken. As an approximate guide, a 5-mm margin is added to GTV to obtain CTV with a further 10-mm margin in the transverse plane to define PTV but up to 15mm craniocaudally to define PTV.

Even the contouring of GTV alone is not straightforward as evidenced by a number of studies demonstrating poor consistency achieved by groups of oncologists and radiologists all asked to volume a single tumour. One step towards achieving consistent practice is to use standardized window settings on the planning imaging with a fixed mediastinal setting and a fixed lung window setting which can be employed separately to check the tumour volume (Fig. 4.7).

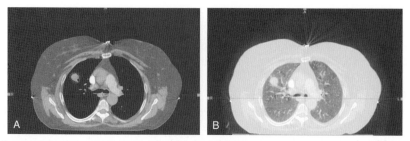

Fig. 4.7 (A) Peripheral tumour with GTV outline marked on mediastinal window setting. (B) The same peripheral tumour: this will often appear larger on lung window settings.

4.1.3.3 Dose-limiting factors in lung radiotherapy

If improved outcomes from radiation depend upon dose escalation then limiting normal tissue toxicity is essential. Moreover, tissue complication probability is increased in treatment schedules with altered fractionation or the addition of concurrent chemotherapy. For lung radiation the dose-limiting factors are pneumonitis, oesophagitis, and spinal cord tolerance. In the process of radiotherapy planning, contours are delineated for each of these organs at risk (OAR). This enables dose volume histograms (DVHs) to be generated that can be used to compare alternative radiotherapy plans with regard to not only the radiation dose to PTV, but also the relative volumes of OAR receiving radiation doses approaching defined tolerance levels (Fig. 4.8).

Symptomatic radiation pneumonitis occurs in 5–15% of patients treated with radical radiotherapy doses and depends upon total dose, volume of lung irradiated, fraction size, and use of chemotherapy. The development of DVH tools showing volumetric dose distribution to normal tissue organs opened the way for correlation of grade 3 pneumonitis with radiation dose to a given percentage of normal lung. Early work by Graham *et al.*[10] demonstrated that when 50% of total lung volume received a dose in

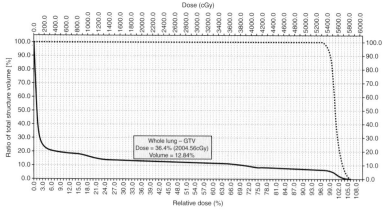

Fig. 4.8 Dose volume histogram for a patient receiving prescribed dose of 55Gy. The volume of remaining lung (whole lung subtract GTV) receiving 20Gy (V20) is <13%.

excess of 20Gy, the incidence of grade 3 pneumonitis was significantly increased. Refinement of data on normal tissue complication probabilities over the past decade has led to the use of specific parameters to assess the risk of pneumonitis and guide decisions about radiotherapy. These include the percentage of lung volume receiving >20Gy (V20), percentage of lung volume receiving >30Gy (V30) and mean lung dose (MLD). V20 in excess of 35% is associated with high risk of pneumonitis although different authors advocate the use of V30 or MLD as the most significant predictors.

Acute oesophagitis is another commonly recognized complication of radical radiation doses to the chest although with lower risk of fatal toxicity or long-term sequelae than lung damage. In practice it is increasing length of oesophagus within the treatment field which increases the risk of symptomatic oesophagitis, with caution advised for lengths >12cm.

For spinal cord, DVHs are less important as it is essential not to exceed tolerance dose at any single level within the cord. The aim is to stay below 44Gy in 2-Gy fractions although tolerance may be lowered with altered fractionation.

4.1.3.4 Respiratory motion

Tumour motion from breathing during treatment is a major challenge in planning lung radiotherapy (Fig. 4.9). Imaging the tumour on slower scanning mode gives a blurred image reflecting respiratory motion artefact. With multidetector CT imaging there is a quick 'snapshot' with the result that the extent of respiratory motion is not captured so that the target volume derived from this single point in time may geographically miss the tumour as it moves with respiration.

Shimizu et al.[11] describe mobility of lung tumours on respiration of up to 15mm in longitudinal direction and although movement of mediastinal structures is less, peripheral lower lobe tumours and tumours adjacent to the heart and diaphragm may be subject to large ranges of movement. Both physical and electronic methods have been used in attempts to overcome this. Voluntary breath-holding techniques, deep inspiration breath-hold, and active breath control are physical techniques which have

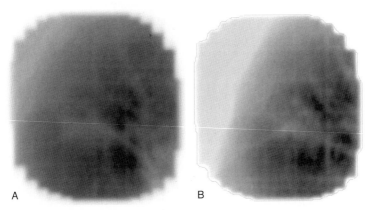

A   B

Fig. 4.9 (A) Megavoltage portal image of peripheral tumour. (B) Repeat portal image on same patient showing altered position of ribcage with respiration.

been variably successful but all rely on patient compliance and require levels of breath control which may be difficult for the majority of lung cancer patients.

The electronic methods of adjusting the radiation plan for respiration depend upon 4D imaging, with time as the fourth dimension. CT images are acquired over the whole respiratory cycle and sorted into 'bins' for each phase of respiration, so that the position of the tumour can be pinpointed for each phase. With a 'gating' radiotherapy technique the linear accelerator is set to function in an on–off mode coordinated with the phase of respiration for which the radiotherapy plan has been produced. With 'tracking' techniques there is continuous delivery throughout the breathing cycle of a 4D treatment plan which takes account of the varying position of the tumour over time.

4.1.3.5 Treatment verification

With complex radiation plans there is a need to confirm set-up and beam positions prior to the start of treatment and also to continue to monitor during the full course of treatment. Pre-treatment verification is usually achieved by fluoroscopic imaging in the treatment simulator which also allows for screening during respiratory motion. The kV radiograph produced for each beam can be compared to digitally reconstructed radiographs (DRR) derived from the treatment planning system (Fig. 4.10).

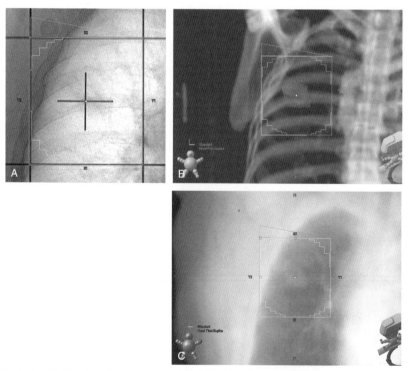

Fig. 4.10 (A) Simulator image of anterior field. (B) Reference DRR against which the simulator image can be compared. GTV is the central shaded area. This DRR image is set on bone windows. (C) DRR on soft tissue window setting.

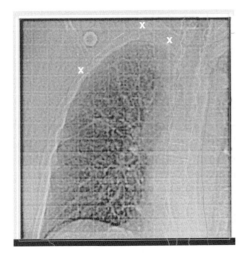

Fig. 4.11 Anterior portal image taken on treatment. Lungs outlined in green and orange. Spinal cord blue; pink GTV; red PTV. The image taken is larger than the field alone would be to allow use of reference marks (X) for comparison against simulator and DRR images. See colour section.

Traditionally, on-treatment verification was achieved by megavoltage (MV) portal imaging although this gives poor anatomical resolution of images. By this method radiographs would be produced and compared against the reference images of both the planning DRRs and the simulator radiographs. The current generation of linear accelerators have electronic portal imaging devices (EPIDs). These acquire real-time electronic images which can be stored digitally and are equipped with quantitative analysis tools for comparing the EPID image to planning DRRs. This allows on-line correction protocols with the potential for daily targeting adjustments (Fig. 4.11).

Enhanced quality of on-treatment imaging is now offered by treatment machines equipped with both kV and MV imaging with separate radiation sources and imaging panels for each energy range. Of particular importance is the cone-beam CT scanning facility which can be mounted on the treatment gantry. In this way real-time reconstructed 4D CT images can be mapped during treatment and matched to planning DRRs. This level of sophisticated imaging is required for the 4D tracking or image guided radiotherapy.

4.1.3.6 Intensity modulated radiation therapy

This radiotherapy technique works backward from a target prescribed dose with specified dose constraints for sensitive structures. Inverse planning algorithms then create a radiation plan in which there is varying intensity within each single radiation beam to conform optimally to the desired isodose distributions. This means that, in theory, with tightly conforming fields the PTV can be reduced allowing dose escalation to the tumour volume, without increasing normal tissue toxicity.

The further possible advantage of IMRT in lung treatment is that the inhomogeneous radiation dose distribution might be matched to specifically spare those parts of lung which are most useful. Functional imaging with PET, 4D CT, and perfusion MR scans can provide information on the distribution of functional lung tissue as many lung cancer patients will have emphysematous destruction or poorly perfused areas of lung which are therefore less important to spare. This opens the way for more sensitive analysis of lung DVHs than is currently available where all lung is assumed to be equal.

The drawbacks of lung IMRT, however, are that: 1) a larger total volume of lung may receive radiation, although at lower doses; and 2) there are often sharp dose gradients. This is a particular problem with tightly conforming fields such that respiratory motion may cause geographical misses. At present, IMRT has established success in head and neck, and prostate treatment but the role in lung cancer remains under investigation.

4.1.4 Therapeutic assessment and follow-up

The objectives of follow-up imaging after radiotherapy for lung cancer are threefold: to assess response to treatment; to monitor toxicity (both acute and late in onset); and to detect progression or relapse when it occurs.

Under RECIST criteria, response assessment should take place with two CT images a month apart with the first a minimum of 6 weeks following completion of radiotherapy, although outside of clinical trials usually a single investigation is undertaken. Reduction in tumour or nodal mass can be measured but it is often difficult in the presence of pneumonitic changes, or associated collapse or consolidation, to categorize response definitively. There continues to be debate about the need for and frequency of further follow-up scans. Thus this should be determined on an individual patient basis, influenced by whether second-line therapy would be feasible in case of progressive disease or relapse.

The radiological changes of acute pneumonitis commonly peak at about 3 months and as well as monitoring clinical symptoms and pulmonary function it may be worth repeating imaging several months later in these patients, to assess resolution of this toxicity (Fig. 4.12).

Tumour response after treatment assessed by PET scan is much more powerfully correlated with survival than response measured by CT[12]. This has raised the potential role of PET in early monitoring of patients to allow response adapted therapy, similar to approaches being developed in lymphoma.

4.2 Other intrathoracic malignancies

This chapter has focused on radical radiation treatment planning to the chest. Although this most often relates to NSCLC, the same principles apply in planning treatment for SCLC and other intrathoracic malignancy.

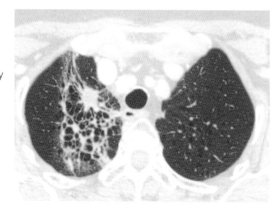

Fig. 4.12 Image from CT study of a patient previously treated with radical radiotherapy for a right upper lobe bronchial carcinoma. The scan demonstrated paramediastinal radiation fibrosis with a spiculated nodule indicating disease recurrence.

Thymoma, a tumour of the anterior mediastinum, is relatively uncommon and is characterized by its indolent course, even with macroscopic invasion. The optimal treatment is surgical resection when this can be achieved. Radiotherapy is indicated in unresectable cases and postoperatively for incomplete resection or those with high risk of local recurrence. Again the principles of radiotherapy planning and treatment delivery are similar to lung cancer but the anterior midline position of the tumour means that the field arrangement requires the majority of the dose (but staying within cord tolerance) to be delivered by anteroposterior fields in order to minimize lung toxicity. The remaining dose is then given by anterior oblique or laterally positioned fields.

Malignant pleural mesothelioma poses a therapeutic challenge as it continues to increase in incidence and is usually diffuse at presentation with relentless local progression. Until recently the standard of care has been supportive management. Radical radiotherapy is not an option for primary treatment given the lung toxicity which would be experienced with hemithorax treatment. There are a number of series and ongoing studies examining the role of multimodality therapy with extrapleural pneumonectomy followed by hemithorax radiation. Although this technique has been demonstrated to be safe and feasible in selected patients the evidence for its longer term benefit remains unclear. High dose radiation to the hemithorax in these patients is therefore not regarded as standard therapy.

4.3 **Summary**

- Lung cancer is the commonest cause of cancer death.
- Radical radiotherapy can potentially cure lung cancer.
- Local control rates following radical radiotherapy have been ≤20%.
- Functional imaging with PET and 4D imaging with CT should contribute to improved target volume definition with reduced risk of geographical miss.
- Better defined target volumes will facilitate development of IMRT for lung.
- Reducing planning margins safely and with confidence will enable dose escalation protocols aimed at better local control.
- Continued monitoring of normal tissue complication rates will better inform the use of DVH parameters to guide decisions about radiotherapy plans.
- Treatment verification techniques are evolving rapidly with real-time electronic portal imaging, kV imaging on linacs, and cone-beam CT.
- Improved on-treatment imaging will offer the potential for tracking and image-guided treatment.

References

1. Statistics from Cancer Research UK; available at http://info.cancerresearchuk.org/cancerstats/types/lung/
2. Gregor A, Thomson CS, Brewster DH, *et al*. Management and survival of patients with lung cancer in Scotland diagnosed in 1995: results of a national population based study. *Thorax* 2001; **56**: 212–17.

3. Detterbeck FC, Falen S, Rivera MP. Seeking a home for a PET, Part 1. *Chest* 2004; **125**: 2294–9.

4. Mountain CF. A new international staging system for lung cancer. *Chest* 1986; **89**: 225–33.

5. Rami-Porta R, Crowley J, Goldstraw P. The revised TNM staging system for lung cancer. *Ann Thoracic Cardiovasc Surg* 2009; **15**: 4–9.

6. Detterbeck FC, Rivera MP, Socinski MA, *et al.* (eds). *Diagnosis and treatment of lung cancer: an evidence based guide for the practicing clinician.* Chapters 5 and 6. Philadelphia, PA: WB Saunders, 2001.

7. Detterbeck FC, Falen S, Rivera MP. Seeking a home for a PET, part 2. Defining the appropriate place for positron emission tomography imaging in the staging of patients with suspected lung cancer. *Chest* 2004; **125**: 2300–8.

8. Arriagada R, Le Chevalier T, Quoix E, *et al.* ASTRO plenary: effect of chemotherapy on locally advanced non-small cell lung carcinoma: a randomized study of 353 patients. *Int J Radiat Oncol Biol Phys* 1991; **20**: 1183–90.

9. International Commission on Radiation Units and Measurements. *ICRU Report 62. Prescribing, recording and reporting photon beam therapy (supplement to ICRU report 50).* Bethseda, MD: International commission on Radiation Units and Measurements, 1999.

10. Graham MV, Purdy JA, Emami B, *et al.* Clinical dose volume histogram analysis for pneumonitis after 3D treatment for NSCLC *Int J Radiat Oncol Biol Phys* 1999; **45**: 323–9.

11. Shimizu S, Shirato H, Ogura S, *et al.* Detection of lung tumour movement in real-time tumor-tracking radiotherapy. *Int J Radiat Oncol Biol Phys* 2001; **5**: 304–10.

12. MacManus M. Role of PET in assessing response to radical chemoradiation. *Lung Cancer* 2003; **41**: S3–S65.

Chapter 5

Lymphoma

Peter Hoskin and Charlotte Fowler

Introduction

Lymphoma covers a broad spectrum of disease entities which is reflected in a wide range of imaging involved in its diagnosis and management. Whilst the pathological subtypes are of considerable importance in disease management, they do not greatly influence the staging processes in which imaging is used, although the two main groups, Hodgkin's lymphoma (HL) and non-Hodgkin's lymphoma (NHL) have very different patterns of disease distribution which can influence imaging strategies.

Computed tomography (CT) has a central role in the diagnosis, staging and follow-up of lymphoma, but it is important to recognize that extra nodal lymphoma is common, seen in approximately 40% of NHL, and these sites may have specific imaging requirements. Lymphoma is an area of particular interest for functional imaging and one of the first conditions where positron emission tomography (PET) using ^{18}F-fluorodeoxyglucose (FDG) has a defined role incorporated in international criteria for response.

The unifying feature of lymphoma is the enlargement of lymph nodes. The central role of diagnostic imaging is therefore to identify the pathological lymph node and distinguish this from the normal node which can be enlarged due to physiological reactive change. The anatomical cross sectional imaging modalities of CT, ultrasound (US), and magnetic resonance imaging (MRI) examine nodal architecture, whereas functional imaging with isotopes such as FDG PET or gallium-67 (^{67}Ga) demonstrate alteration in the physiology of the node following invasion by neoplastic disease. Both anatomical and functional imaging techniques require a substantial degree of nodal involvement before convincing abnormality can be identified and in early disease imaging may be falsely negative.

Normal nodes are ovoid in morphology with a long to short axis ratio of around 1.5–2:1, with a fatty hilum, smooth cortex, and well-defined margins (Fig. 5.1). When a node becomes involved in a neoplastic process such as lymphoma, the node enlarges particularly in the short axis, resulting in a more rounded contour, and a reduction in the long- to short-axis ratio. The cortex may become irregular and there can be loss of the fatty hilum as neoplastic tissue displaces normal nodal tissue. The margin of the cortex may be breached which results in poor definition of the nodal margins on imaging.

The minimum short-axis diameter is the standard measurement criteria. This is the minimum diameter of the node when measured at its widest point along the short

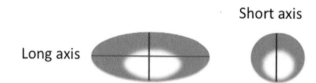

Fig. 5.1 Illustration of a normal lymph node: The lymph node has ovoid morphology with smooth cortex shown in grey and central hilar fat in white. The minimum short axis diameter is measured at the widest point of the node, at 90° to the long axis.

axis, taken at 90° to the long axis (Fig. 5.1). Nodes which measure >1cm in minimum short-axis diameter are generally considered likely to be involved in a neoplastic process, with a sensitivity and specificity of around 70%. The long-axis measurement is generally not a good indicator for presence of disease as normal nodes may be long and slender. The interporto-caval node is a good example of this, with long but slender nodes measuring up to 3cm commonly being seen draped between the portal vein and the inferior vena cava in normal patients.

5.1 **Diagnosis and staging**

5.1.1 **Diagnosis**

The two common forms of lymphoma, HL and NHL, have different patterns of disease spread and distribution and these determine the imaging modalities which are most frequently involved in making the first step towards the diagnosis. Lymphoma is the great clinical and radiological pretender and frequently mimics other aggressive conditions, such as solid neoplasms, infection, and sarcoid, and it is only after biopsy and pathological assessment that a confident diagnosis can be established. Imaging is frequently used to guide core biopsy to obtain tissue for pathological diagnosis in non-palpable cases.

HL spreads via the lymphatics resulting in a disease distribution which is contiguous along lymphatic pathways. It is more common above the diaphragm and generally involves lymph nodes within the mediastinal (70%), cervical (70%) and paraaortic (30%) groups, and the spleen (30%). Patients may present with respiratory symptoms or B symptoms which prompts a chest X-ray as part of baseline investigations, which may demonstrate mediastinal lymphadenopathy (Fig. 5.2). Alternatively, cervical lymphadenopathy will result in referral to a head and neck surgeon who may request US and/or MRI examination to establish the origin of a palpable mass. US and MRI are particularly useful imaging modalities for the definition of neck anatomy; they have higher tissue contrast than CT and do not suffer from beam-hardening artefact due to dental amalgam which frequently degrades images of the upper neck. Typical images of patients with HL are shown in Fig. 5.3.

NHL undergoes haematological spread, resulting in a more diverse and discontinguous pattern of disease distribution than HL. It is found both sides of the diaphragm with para-aortic (50%), mesenteric (50%), and mediastinal (30%) lymphadenopathy. There is also a high propensity for extra-nodal disease compared to HL including bone marrow (30%), bowel (10%), renal tract (7%), central nervous system (2%), and lung

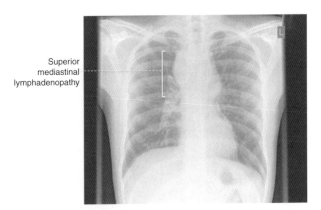

Superior
mediastinal
lymphadenopathy

Fig. 5.2 Hodgkin's lymphoma: chest radiograph showing superior mediastinal lymphadenopathy.

parenchyma (3%). This is reflected in the wider range of imaging techniques used for diagnosis including MRI for marrow and neurological lymphoma, barium contrast studies for gastrointestinal involvement, and US for testicular lymphoma. Gastrointestinal mucosa associated lymphoma (MALT) most commonly involving the stomach or large bowel can be indistinguishable on imaging from adenocarcinoma with irregular thickening of the wall and shouldering at the interface with normal anatomy. Lymphomatous involvement of the bowel can be suggested by longer segment involvement and better preserved lumen than is generally seen with carcinomas, and involvement of the terminal ileum is more frequent with lymphoma. Typical images of NHL are shown in Fig. 5.4.

5.1.2 Staging

Lymphoma staging is shown in Table 5.1; it is based on the anatomical distribution of disease. Essential investigations will include the following:

- Tissue diagnosis including full immunohistochemical profile.
- Imaging of the entire lymph node chains from base of skull to femoral regions and including the liver, spleen, and lungs.
- Peripheral blood count, erythrocyte sedimentation rate, serum lactate dehydrogenase (LDH), and markers of renal and hepatic function.
- Immunoglobulin profile and protein electrophoresis.
- Bone marrow examination in all cases of NHL and HL with stage IV disease or B symptoms.
- Cerebrospinal fluid in NHL with high-risk features in particular lymphoma affecting the paranasal sinuses and testes.

Staging aims to demonstrate the full extent of disease prior to treatment, so that the response to treatment can be accurately assessed.

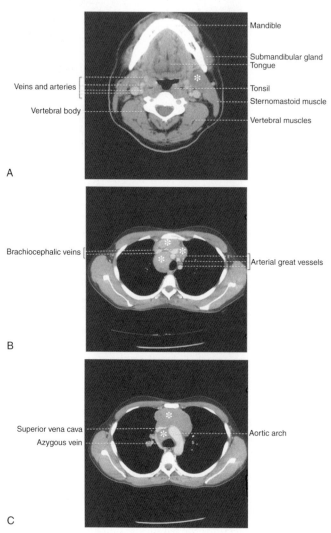

Fig. 5.3 Hodgkin's lymphoma: (A) Contrast-enhanced CT of the neck at the level of the mandible showing left cervical lymphadenopathy (shown with asterisk). (B) Contrast-enhanced CT at the level of the superior mediastinum showing gross prevascular and paratracheal mediastinal lymphadenopthy (shown with asterisks) causing displacement and compression of the branchiocephalic veins. (C) Contrast-enhanced CT at the level of the aortic arch showing gross prevascular and pretracheal mediastinal lymphadenopathy (shown with asterisks) causing compression of the superior vena cava.

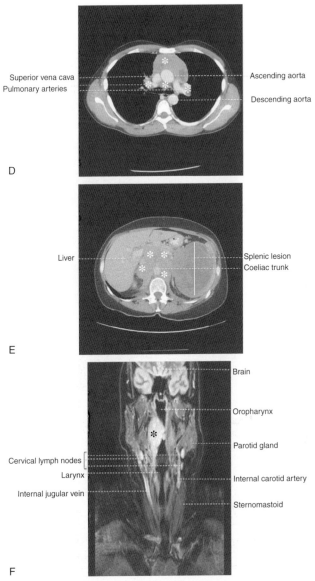

Fig. 5.3 (cont'd) (D) Contrast-enhanced CT at the level of the pulmonary artery showing gross mediastinal lymphadenopathy in prevascular, precarinal, and hilar stations (shown with asterisks). Prevascular lymphadenopathy has undergone necrotic change on the left. (E) Hodgkin's lymphoma: contrast-enhanced CT at the level of the coeliac trunk showing gross para-aortic lymphadenopathy (shown with asterisks) and very large splenic lesion. (F) Hodgkin's lymphoma: coronal STIR-weighted MRI sequence showing right tonsillar mass (shown with asterisk). It is not possible by imaging to differentiate lymphoma from adenocarcinoma; only biopsy will make the definitive diagnosis. Normal cervical lymph nodes noted.

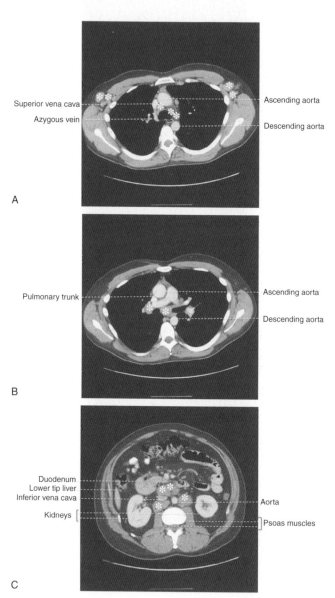

Fig. 5.4 Non-Hodgkin's lymphoma: (A) Contrast-enhanced CT at the level of azygous vein showing precarinal and axillary lymphadenopathy (shown with asterisks). (B) Contrast-enhanced CT at the level of pulmonary trunk showing right hilar and subcarinal lymphadenopathy (shown with asterisks). (C) Contrast-enhanced CT at the level of the right renal hilum showing para-aortic lymphadenopathy (shown with asterisks).

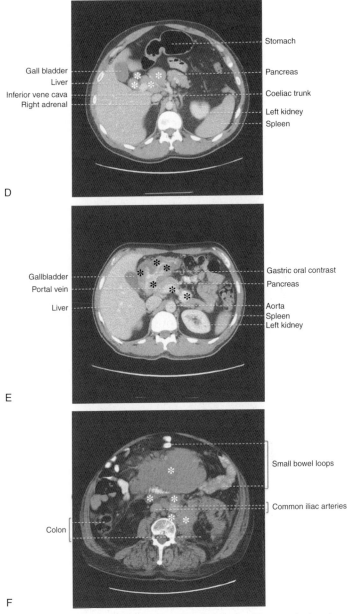

Fig. 5.4 (cont'd) (D) Contrast-enhanced CT at the level of coeliac trunk showing para-aortic and portal lymphadenopathy (shown with asterisks). (E) Contrast-enhanced CT at the level of the portal vein showing irregular mucosal thickening of the gastric body and antrum (shown with asterisks). It is not possible to differentiate lymphoma from adenocarcinoma on imaging criteria; only biopsy will make the definitive diagnosis. (F) Contrast-enhanced CT at the level of the proximal common illac arteries, showing gross mesentric and less marked para-aortic lymphadenopathy (shown by asterisks). When a loop of bowel is sandwiched between metenteric and para-aortic nodes it can resemble the filling within a bread bun, hence the term 'hamburger sign'.

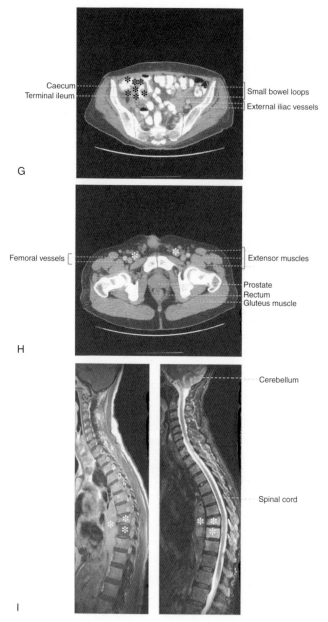

Fig. 5.4 (cont'd) (G) Contrast-enhanced CT at the level of caecum, showing irregular mucosal thickening of the caeccum and terminal ileum (shown by asterisks), over a considerable length with preservation of the lumen, features which are more suggestive of lympoma than adenocarcinoma. (H) Contrast-enhanced CT at the level of the symphysis pubis showing small volume inguinal lymphadenopathy (shown with asterisks). (I) T1- and T2-weighted sagittal acquisitions of the spinal showing bone marrow lesions and a paraspinal mass (shown by asterisks). Marrow lesions are low signal intensity on T1- and high signal intensity on T2-weighted images as fat within the marrow is replaced by neoplastic tissue. The upper vertebral body has undergone pathological fracture. The involvement of two adjacent vertebral bodies with paravertebral mass may be due to lymphoma but may also represent infection such as TB.

Table 5.1 Staging of lymphoma based on Ann Arbor system

Stage	Involved area(s)
I	One node region or extranodal site
II	Two or more node regions all on one side of the diaphragm
III	Lymph node regions both sides of diaphragm
IIIs	Spleen
III$_{(1)}$	Spleen, splenic hilar, celiac axis, and portal nodes
III$_{(2)}$	Para-aortic, mesenteric, or iliac nodes
IV	Extranodal sites (other than those designated 'E')
Qualifiers	A: no symptoms
	B: fever, sweats, or weight loss >10% body weight
	E: localized extranodal disease
	X: bulky mass: >10cm maximum dimension; >one-third thoracic diameter at T5

5.1.2.1 Anatomical imaging

5.1.2.1.1 **CT** CT is the mainstay of imaging for the staging of lymphoma. Modern helical multislice scanner protocols now allow sub-millimetre contiguous scans through the neck, chest, abdomen, and pelvis to be obtained, allowing coronal and sagittal reconstructions to be made to produce high quality images in all three dimensions. The introduction of modern equipment has increased image interpretation accuracy which is helped by the use of intravenous contrast medium which allows confident differentiation between lymph nodes and blood vessels and by the use of oral contrast medium which allows distinction between loops of bowel and neighbouring lymph nodes. CT can accurately identify not only enlarged lymph nodes and categorize these by virtue of their size, shape, and numeracy, but can also demonstrate disease in extra nodal sites, for example the brain, lungs, gastrointestinal tract, kidneys, liver, and spleen. The other cross sectional imaging modalities are used to complement CT findings in particular regions and to clarify lesions which are indeterminate on CT assessment.

5.1.2.1.2 **US** US is useful in assessing indeterminate liver and renal lesions and has a particular role in imaging splenic lymphoma. The spleen has a particularly high propensity for lymphomatous involvement, particularly in HL which has a specific staging category of IIIs for isolated splenic lymphoma. Splenic enlargement alone is common in lymphoma and based on historical series where laparotomy and splenectomy was a routine component of treatment, up to one-third of normal size spleens contain microscopic HL whereas only approximately one-third of enlarged spleens will be involved. Size criteria of the entire organ alone is therefore not helpful. US can detect splenic lesions down to 3mm in diameter with higher sensitivity than CT for the detection of splenic lymphoma (63% vs. 37%). The disadvantage of the use of US in lymphoma staging lies in the fact that it is operator dependent, making assessment of disease response less reproducible than CT or MRI.

5.1.2.1.3 **MRI** MRI has no advantage over CT in assessing lymph node chains. This is likely to change if the availability and use of intravenously administered ferromagnetic contrast agents, which are able to give information on the internal architecture of lymph nodes, becomes widespread. Where MRI currently has the advantage over CT in the staging of lymphoma is in sites where CT images are degraded by beam hardening artefacts from bone/dental amalgam or where there is poor tissue contrast, such as within the spinal canal. Assessment of the neural axis, bone marrow, head and neck, and pelvic regions particularly benefit from MRI assessment. In bone marrow assessment, MRI demonstrates the global picture of the bone marrow disease distribution more accurately than single or even paired bone marrow aspirate and trephine samples from the iliac crests, identifying bone marrow infiltration in up to 33% of patients who have negative iliac crest biopsies. False negatives may occur where there is only scanty infiltration and particularly in the case of indolent lymphomas. Bone scintigraphy tends to be unhelpful as lymphoma does not elicit a strong osteoblastic response which is necessary for the uptake of phosphate related radiotracers.

5.1.2.2 Functional Imaging

5.1.2.2.1 **^{67}Ga** ^{67}Ga was first identified in 1969 as a gamma-emitting isotope which localized in lymphoma. It gained widespread acceptance as a useful imaging modality in the staging and follow-up of lymphoma although its use has been more widespread in the USA than the UK. Gallium acts as an iron analogue physiologically. The presence of transferrin receptors which are CD 71 positive on the surface of lymphoma cells has been shown to correlate with the intensity of gallium uptake but transferrin independent mechanisms are also thought to play a role. In experienced hands gallium scanning will achieve >90% sensitivity and specificity levels in aggressive NHL and HL. It is less satisfactory for the more indolent types of lymphoma. Gallium is not specific for lymphoma, and is also taken up in granulomatous conditions such as sarcoid and tuberculosis (TB) which can result in false positive results. The use of gallium has largely being superseded by the use of FDG positron emission tomography (PET).

5.1.2.2.2 **FDG PET** FDG PET has established itself as an invaluable tool in the management of lymphoma, especially with the development of combined PET/CT where FDG PET and CT images are obtained sequentially during the same examination with image fusion to allow anatomical definition of sources of FDG uptake. The principles of FDG PET are described in Chapter 2.

In the evaluation of lymphoma, the sensitivity of PET at around 85–90% is about 15% higher than with CT. This is principally because FDG PET can identify abnormal glucose metabolism in normally sized lymph nodes as shown in Fig. 5.5. FDG PET can detect focal or multi-focal bone marrow involvement where an iliac crest sample is negative shown in Fig. 5.6. Specificity for CT and FDG PET are equivalent at about 70% for lymphomatous involvement. False positive results can result from FDG being taken up by granulomatous disorders such as sarcoid and infection (particularly TB).

There seems to be some variation between indolent lymphomas and the more aggressive lymphomas including HL, with higher levels and more reliable FDG uptake in the more aggressive type of lymphoma. Recent analyses have identified a clear cut-off in the specific uptake value (SUV) between these different types of lymphoma with values of 1–2 for indolent lymphomas and 4–5 for aggressive lymphomas reflecting the lower levels of metabolism and glucose uptake in the more indolent lymphoma.

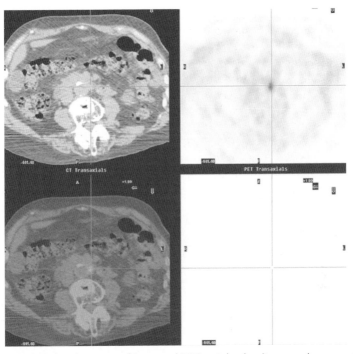

Fig. 5.5 FDG PET showing areas of increased FDG uptake despite normal para-aortic nodes on size criteria. See colour section.

This may explain the studies which have suggested that FDG PET is less useful in defining involvement with indolent lymphoma compared to the more aggressive types. Despite the observation that PET will identify more sites of lymphoma involvement in 15–20% of patients, it has yet to become the routine staging investigation in lymphoma, although the use of combined PET/CT may well bring this to the fore. One reason for this however is the analysis within these studies relating the changes to both alteration of clinical stage and management. The conventional Ann Arbor staging system for NHL and HL is shown in Table 5.1. In general, management of both types of lymphoma will depend upon stage, with patients classified into early or advanced disease. Those with early disease, that is stage Ia or IIa, will be treated with short-course chemotherapy and involved field radiotherapy whilst those with more aggressive disease, that is patients with stage Ib, IIb, III,or IV, will receive more prolonged combination chemotherapy. A change in stage therefore will only be relevant if a patient without B symptoms is moved from stage I or II to stage III or IV. Since many patients in whom PET identifies additional sites will already have stage III or IV disease this does not alter management. Similarly, where additional sites in one anatomical region are identified the added information from PET will not alter management. An additional impetus for baseline PET/CT is now emerging with the increased evidence that early response on functional imaging, in particular FDG PET, may predict outcome and further define treatment programmes (see below).

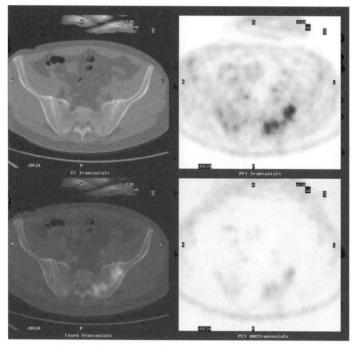

Fig. 5.6 FDG PET showing bone marrow involvement with lymphoma. See colour section.

5.2 **Radiotherapy planning**

The role of radiotherapy in the management of lymphoma has changed substantially with the advent of effective combination chemotherapy. It is, however, still the most active single modality in the management of lymphoma, and in HL involved field radiotherapy or involved lymph node radiotherapy remains an important component of treatment regimens, particularly in early disease. Similarly, in early stage NHL, involved field radiotherapy remains an important addition to short-course chemotherapy in standard management.

There have also been substantial changes in radiotherapy equipment and techniques in the last decade.

5.2.1 **Plain radiographs**

For many years lymphoma radiotherapy relied on orthogonal planning with plain X-ray identification using bone landmarks of lymph node areas. There is no doubt that such techniques resulted in high rates of tumour control and cure. However, with the advent of cross sectional imaging and increasing concerns with regard to normal tissue doses and late morbidity there has been a significant move away from radiotherapy localization using simple orthogonal fields on a treatment simulator towards CT-defined volumes. Orthogonal films remain an important component in treatment

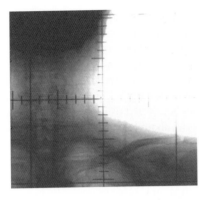

Fig. 5.7 Plain X-ray imaging of treatment field to treat left neck from conventional X-ray simulator.

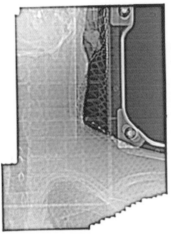

Fig. 5.8 Megavoltage image from linear accelerator beam treating left neck obtained using electronic portal imaging device (EPID). Note shaping of field using multileaf collimators and reduced contrast between bone and soft tissue seen when megavoltage beam used for imaging.

verification however, both on the treatment simulator and using megavoltage beams to produce electronic portal imaging. Examples are shown in Figs. 5.7 and 5.8.

5.2.2 CT

The use of cross sectional imaging with CT for radiotherapy planning has a number of advantages, including:

- More accurate definition of lymph node areas.
- More accurate definition of extra nodal sites.
- More accurate definition of organs at risk.
- Incorporation of tissue inhomogeneities within the planning algorithm to produce more accurate dose distributions.
- Dose volume histogram analyses for coverage of planning target volume (PTV) and organs at risk.

The widespread availability of CT simulators enables multislice 3-mm scans to be obtained in patients requiring potentially curative involved field or involved lymph node radiotherapy for lymphoma. Identification of the lymph node chains is aided by the use of contrast-enhanced scans, and numerous studies have confirmed that the use of intravenous contrast has no substantial effect upon the dosimetry algorithms for radiotherapy planning. Definition of the clinical target volume is then based on the known lymph node area to be covered using standard lymph node atlases which are now published. Organs at risk should also be outlined in this process, as shown in Fig. 5.9.

Whilst increasing the accuracy of lymph node coverage there is some evidence to suggest that, in fact, this results in an increased volume in some cases where lymph nodes are more readily identified on CT, for example the lung hilae, mediastinum, and groins. This can, however, be reconciled by more accurate planning to reduce adjacent doses to organs at risk whilst maintaining the accuracy and efficacy of treatment.

5.2.3 Functional imaging

With the availability of FDG PET and the potential to more accurately identify actual sites of involvement with lymphoma distinct from lymph node regions, there has been increasing interest in harnessing the information from PET in the radiotherapy planning process. This has resulted in the concept of involved lymph node radiotherapy rather than involved field radiotherapy which will substantially reduce the volume to be treated and, it is hoped, the sequelae of radiotherapy in later years. In general, the PET positive volume will be lower than a similarly defined CT volume. A number of controversies remain, however. It is not clear whether the radiotherapy volume should be based on a pre-chemotherapy PET scan, on the basis that even when it converts to negative there may be microscopic disease remaining, or a post-chemotherapy scan, which may contain a smaller volume but miss potential residual sites of disease.

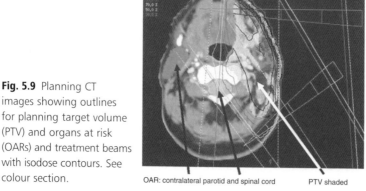

Fig. 5.9 Planning CT images showing outlines for planning target volume (PTV) and organs at risk (OARs) and treatment beams with isodose contours. See colour section.

OAR: contralateral parotid and spinal cord   PTV shaded

The incorporation of PET and PET/CT into radiotherapy planning is currently still under evaluation but is likely to have an increasing role in the future.

5.3 Therapeutic response and follow-up

Lymphomas typically respond rapidly to the introduction of appropriate treatment with resolution of enlarged lymph nodes and extra nodal deposits of lymphoma. Treatment will be tailored to response. In many protocols the convention for aggressive lymphoma and HL demands the achievement of radiological response (usually based on CT) and the addition of two further cycles of chemotherapy or radiotherapy beyond complete remission. In lymphomas showing unsatisfactory response, a change in treatment to more intensive management is often advocated. Until recently, response relied purely on morphological changes with enlarged lymph nodes returning to normal size and extranodal disease becoming no longer visible. The scene has changed further with the recent inclusion of functional imaging parameters in response criteria for lymphoma.

There remain a number of anomalies specific to certain types of lymphoma, in particular nodular sclerosing HL and sclerosing mediastinal B cell lymphoma where residual masses may contain no active lymphoma cells but simply the residual fibrotic component of the original tumour mass. These are difficult to distinguish on size criteria alone and prior to the advent of functional imaging would require repeated monitoring to ensure that progression did not occur. The management of the 'residual mass' continues to be an area of concern.

The most recent standard response criteria for lymphoma defined by the National Cancer Institute International Working Group[1] are shown in Table 5.2.

5.3.1 Timing of imaging

Conventionally imaging will be timed to identify response during treatment, define the final response, and to monitor disease in follow-up. This will usually mean investigations at the following points:

- During chemotherapy, typically midway after three or four cycles of treatment.
- At completion of chemotherapy.
- 3–6 months after completion of chemotherapy.

In addition, further imaging may be required where an ongoing response is being monitored during treatment, e.g. after three or four cycles of chemotherapy, and again after six cycles, and again after eight cycles or prior to radiotherapy. There is also interest in the prognostic value of an earlier scan after two cycles of chemotherapy to identify those patients who may require more intensive treatment.

The imaging modality of choice for assessing therapy response will be tailored depending on the distribution of disease at staging. Most lymphomas are staged by CT, so this is the most common modality of choice for post therapy follow-up. However, if initial staging revealed disease in a region which required another modality for full assessment (e.g. US for testicular, MRI for Waldeyer ring disease), then these modalities will also be required for follow-up imaging.

Table 5.2 Standard response criteria for lymphoma defined by the National Cancer Institute International Working Group[1]

Response	Physical examination	Radiological (CT)	Bone marrow examination	Lymph node masses
CR*	Normal	Normal	Normal	Normal+
Cru	Normal	Normal	Normal	Indeterminate
	Normal	Normal	>75% decrease	Normal or indeterminate
PR	Normal	Normal	Normal	Positive
	Normal	>50% decrease	>50% decrease	Irrelevant
	Palpable but decrease liver or spleen	>50% decrease	>50% decrease	Irrelevant
Relapse or progression	Enlarging or new sites	New or increased	New or increased	Reappearance

CR, complete response; Cru, CR unconfirmed; PR, partial response.

*CR: in addition any biochemical abnormality due to lymphoma, e.g. LDH, must have returned to normal.

+ Normal size for lymph nodes defined as follows:

    Any node >1.5cm before therapy must be ≤1.5cm

    Nodes 1.1–1.5cm must be <1.0cm in greatest transverse diameter or have reduced by >75% in sum of the products of the greatest diameters.

Timing: must be within 2 months of completion of all treatment.

The contribution of FDG PET to this process is under evaluation at present. At the current time, when the availability of FDG PET is limited, it has a particular role in establishing whether there is active disease in a residual mass identified on post therapy CT as shown in Fig. 5.10. This most commonly occurs in the mediastinum and may be a feature of up to 85% of patients with HL and 40% of those with NHL presenting with initial bulky mediastinal lymphadenopathy. Similar changes are seen in the abdomen particularly where there has been a large para-aortic mass and other sites of initial bulky disease. Functional imaging can help to differentiate residual mass due to post treatment fibrosis from those which contain active disease. However, FDG can be falsely positive in this clinical context, for example FDG can be taken up in thymic rebound following chemotherapy, in infection, in extra-medullary haematopoiesis and in tissues underdoing inflammatory response to radiation reaction, and these foci of uptake can be misinterpreted as representing active lymphoma. This would be less likely if there was a staging FDG PET image for comparison as foci of uptake which were not present on the staging scan could be correctly interpreted as new and therefore likely to be a consequence of treatment. Without the benefit of a staging FDG PET scan, serial imaging may be required to ensure that there is no subsequent progression within these residual masses. An International Harmonisation Project (IHP)[2] has reported consensus recommendations for the inclusion of PET criteria in defining response in lymphoma. These are shown in Table 5.3.

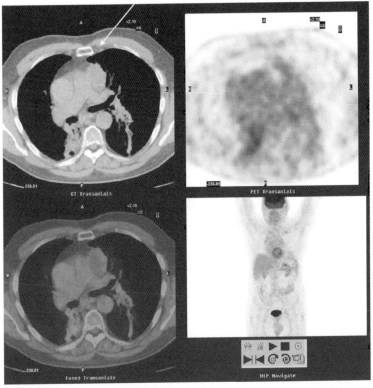

Fig. 5.10 Residual mediastinal mass on CT (arrowed) which is negative for uptake on the FDG PET image. See colour section.

5.3.2 Specific roles for PET

There are a number of specific roles for PET which are emerging which may become part of routine imaging follow-up once this modality is more widely available:

5.3.2.1 Early response assessment

There is emerging data to suggest that an early response on FDG PET in both HL and aggressive NHL after two cycles of chemotherapy is a strong predictor of subsequent outcome; those patients with negative scans at this point achieving conventional complete remissions and long-term relapse-free survival times, whereas patients with a positive scan at this point are unlikely to achieve complete remission and will subsequently progress. Whilst this data is currently limited and further studies are underway, the role of FDG PET to identify poor response patients at an early stage, prevent further futile chemotherapy, and prompt a change in management to more intensive treatment may become increasingly common and a routine part of defining management programmes in the future.

Table 5.3 International Harmonisation Project (IHP) consensus recommendations with inclusion of PET criteria in defining response in lymphoma[2]

The following changes on FDG PET should be regarded as positive for lymphoma:	
Lymph nodes:	
≥2cm diameter	Diffuse or focal uptake > mediastinal blood pool structures
<2cm diameter	Any increase in uptake over background
Lung nodules:	
>1.5cm diameter	Increase in uptake > mediastinal blood pool structures
<1.5cm diameter	Cannot be reliably assessed
Hepatic and splenic lesions:	
>1.5cm	Uptake > or = to normal liver or spleen
<1.5cm	Uptake > normal liver or spleen
Diffuse splenic disease	Diffuse uptake > normal liver (unless recent cytokine administration)
Bone marrow	Multifocal uptake

Timing of scans after therapy: 6–8 weeks after chemotherapy or chemoimmunotherapy; 8–12 weeks after radiotherapy or chemoradiotherapy.

5.3.2.2 Response at completion of treatment

FDG PET results at completion of treatment have been shown to be an important prognostic indicator for subsequent outcome. There is a very high negative predictive value for FDG PET with short-term progression-free survivals of >90% in patients with PET-negative scans at completion of treatment. The positive predictive value of a PET scan at this point however is less certain with a wide range of published figures reflecting the difficulties in interpretation of PET at an early stage after treatment. To avoid these false positive findings it is recommended that at least 6 weeks are allowed after completion of all treatment before a definitive completion FDG PET scan is taken. A positive scan in these circumstances has been associated with only a 40% 1-year progression-free survival compared to 95% for a concomitant PET negative group. Interpretation of the PET positive scan can be enhanced by reference to a staging FDG PET scan.

5.3.3 Imaging in follow-up

The role of routine imaging in the follow-up of lymphoma patients is controversial. On the one hand there is increasing concern with regard to the radiation exposure of patients who have a long prognosis, many living their natural lifespan from a relatively young age at treatment, being exposed to unnecessary irradiation, which must be balanced against the ability to detect early relapse enabling further potentially curative treatment. The predictive value of functional imaging using FDG PET therefore has considerable importance and interest in this area and the role of additional imaging in patients who are FDG PET negative at completion of treatment is questionable.

There is no role for routine imaging beyond the initial post-treatment scan at 3–6 months after completion of therapy. Patients who have residual disease, whether defined by CT criteria or positive disease on FDG PET scanning, clearly require further monitoring. Where functional imaging is not available then stable disease on two further CT scans at 6-monthly intervals is adequate to justify discontinuation of further routine imaging, and where functional imaging is available residual disease on a diagnostic CT scan followed by FDG PET which is negative, should also lead to the cessation of further routine imaging. A positive FDG PET scan should, in the absence of other criteria suggesting lymphoma relapse or progression, be followed by a biopsy of the PET-positive area.

Finally the traditional annual chest X-ray no longer has a role in the management of lymphoma patients. The only role for routine radiology following treatment and confirmation of complete remission in lymphoma is in later screening programmes. Currently UK recommendations for female patients having mediastinal radiotherapy for HL are to begin breast screening 8 years after completion of treatment. In smokers an increased risk of lung cancer is recognized and studies are underway to identify the optimal means of monitoring such patients to identify early disease for those who persist in their smoking habits.

References

1. Juweld ME, Stroobants S, Hoekstra OS, *et al.* Use of positron emission tomography for response assessment of lymphoma: consensus of the Imaging Subcommittee of International Harmonization Project in Lymphoma. *J Clin Oncol* 2007; **25**: 571–8.
2. Specht L. FDG-PET scan and treatment planning for early stage Hodgkin lymphoma. *Radiother Oncol* 2007; **85**: 176–7.

Further reading

Cheson BD, Horning SJ, Sutcliffe SB, *et al.* Report of an International workshop to standardize criteria for non Hodgkins lymphoma. *J Clin Oncol* 1999; **17**: 1244–53.

Gregoire V, Eisbruch A, Hamoir M, *et al.* Proposal for the delineation of the nodal CTV in the node-positive and the post-operative neck. *Radiother Oncol* 2006; **79**: 15–20.

Isasi CR, Lu P, Blaufox MD. A metaanalysis of 18F-2-deoxy-2-fluoro-D-glucose positron tomography in the staging and restaging of patients with lymphoma. *Cancer* 2005; **104**: 1066–74.

O'Doherty MJ, Hoskin PJ (eds). Lymphoma: diagnosis and management. *Eur J Nucl Med Mol Imaging* 2003; **30**(Suppl. 1): S1–130.

Taylor A, Rockall AG, Powell MEB. An atlas of the pelvic lymph node regions to aid radiotherapy target volume definition. *Clin Oncol* 2007; **19**: 542–50.

Chapter 6

Oesophageal tumours

R. Jane Chambers and Ian Geh

6.1 Clinical background

Oesophageal cancer is the ninth commonest cancer in the UK with >7600 new cases diagnosed per year. The incidence varies widely around the world, ranging from 5–10 per 100,000 in developed countries to 100 per 100,000 in endemic areas such as northern Iran, northern China, Kazakhstan, South Africa, and Eastern Kenya[1].

6.2 Diagnosis and staging

6.2.1 Diagnosis

The gold standard for diagnosing oesophageal cancer is with fibreoptic video endoscopy, enabling direct visualization of the tumour and biopsy for histological diagnosis. The length and location of the visible tumour (in relation to the distance from the incisors or from the oesophagogastric junction (OGJ)) can be measured and the degree of obstruction can be assessed. For OGJ tumours, the extent of gastric involvement seen on endoscopy will determine the subtyping. However, contrast studies remain useful as an initial investigation in patients with swallowing symptoms to differentiate benign from malignant lesions (Fig. 6.1). Benign lesions include strictures related to previous surgery, gastro-oesophageal reflux, long-term use of a nasogastric tube, chemical injury, and treatment of oesophageal varices. In the event of an abnormal mucosal lesion found on contrast swallow, endoscopy would still be required. The additional advantage of contrast swallow over endoscopy is the detection of motility disorders such as achalasia.

6.2.2 Staging

The purpose of staging is to assess the primary tumour for potential resectability (locoregional stage) and to identify distant metastases (commonly liver, lungs, peritoneum, and distant lymph nodes). The accepted standard for staging of oesophageal and OGJ cancers is based on the TNM staging system[2] (Table 6.1). Accurate staging of newly diagnosed patients is required to determine prognosis and management options, such as curative versus palliative intent and single versus multimodality treatment.

Commonly used imaging modalities include computed tomography (CT), endoscopic ultrasound (EUS), and magnetic resonance imaging (MRI). The use of functional imaging such as ^{18}F-fluorodeoxyglucose (FDG) positron emission tomography (PET)

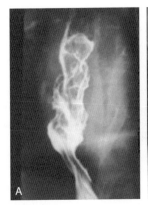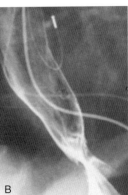

Fig. 6.1 Contrast swallow showing (A) an adenocarcinoma of lower third of oesophagus; and (B) a small adenocarcinoma at the oesophago-gastric junction.

Table 6.1 TNM staging of oesophageal cancer[6]

Primary tumour (T)

Tx	Primary tumour cannot be assessed
T0	No evidence of primary tumour
Tis	Carcinoma in situ
T1	Tumour invades lamina propria or submucosa
T2	Tumour invades muscularis propria
T3	Tumour invades adventitia
T4	Tumour invades adjacent structures

Regional lymph nodes (N)

Nx	Lymph node status cannot be assessed
N0	No regional lymph node metastases
N1	Regional lymph node metastases

Distant metastases (M)

Mx	Presence of distant metastases cannot be assessed
M0	No distant metastases
M1	Presence of distant metastases:

- ◆ Tumours of *lower* thoracic oesophagus
  - M1a: coeliac nodes
  - M1b: other distant metastases
- ◆ Tumours of *mid thoracic* oesophagus
  - M1b: distant metastases including non regional nodes
- ◆ Tumours of *upper* thoracic oesophagus
  - M1a: cervical nodes
  - M1b: other distant metastases

and FDG PET/CT can provide additional useful information. Invasive EUS-guided fine needle aspiration (EUS-FNA) is also an important diagnostic modality and can be used in conjunction with double contrast oesophagograms to differentiate superficial mucosal and submucosal tumours[3].

6.2.2.1 T stage

There is a strong correlation between the depth of tumour invasion and risk of lymph node metastases in oesophageal cancer. For intramucosal tumours the risk is 3–6%, submucosal tumours 20–30%, intramuscular tumours 45–75%, and transmural tumours 80–85%[4]. This in turn correlates with risk of distant metastases and a worsening 5-year survival[5].

Initial staging for oesophageal tumours is with CT scanning of the chest, abdomen, and pelvis. The use of CT will provide the clinician with relatively accurate information on the likely T, N, and M stage of the tumour as well as the likelihood of curative surgical resection. Although CT does not distinguish the anatomical layers of the oesophageal wall to predict T stage, it will readily identify invasion of adjacent structures such as aorta, vertebral body, pericardium, lungs, and bronchus in patients with locally advanced disease. On CT scan, fat planes can usually be seen separating the oesophagus from adjacent organs. The presence of a visible fat plane can accurately predict that there has been no invasion into the organ at that point. However, loss of the fat plane does not necessarily mean that invasion has occurred. The likelihood of irresectability is also assessed by measuring the extent of tumour surrounding the contrast-enhanced aorta. If the degree of encasement is >180°, vascular invasion is likely and if >270°, invasion is almost inevitable, both features negating the possibility of surgical resection[6]. However, loss of fat plane between tumour and pericardium is less predictive of invasion, and fat planes can be obscured following radiotherapy.

Transoesophageal EUS combines upper gastrointestinal (GI) endoscopy with ultrasonography (US) using a dedicated US probe. The five layers of the oesophageal wall can be clearly seen, each with their different echogenic appearances. The first layer corresponds to the superficial mucosa, the second layer to the muscularis mucosa, the third layer to the submusosa, the fourth layer to the muscularis propria, and the fifth layer to the adventia. Therefore EUS can be used to predict the depth of tumour invasion into the oesophageal wall prior to surgery. Multiple trials using EUS have consistently reported an overall accuracy for T stage of >80% compared to surgical pathology[7], and this accuracy improves with increasing T stage of the tumour to >90% with T3/T4 tumours [8,9] (Fig. 6.2). Meta-analysis of 27 studies demonstrated an accuracy of 89% for T staging using EUS[10]. The additional use of EUS staging information will influence the patient's management in approximately 25% of cases[11]. However, the limitations of EUS must be appreciated. Firstly, distinguishing mucosal (Tis or T1a) from submucosal lesions (T1b) in early tumours is difficult and the primary tumour will be understaged in 5% and overstaged in 6–11% with EUS[12]. Secondly, EUS will be impossible in about 30% of cases because of tumour-related stenosis preventing the probe from being passed through. However, most of these patients will have locally advanced disease (T3 or T4), which can be adequately assessed on CT. Thirdly, EUS is operator dependent with a long learning curve of experience

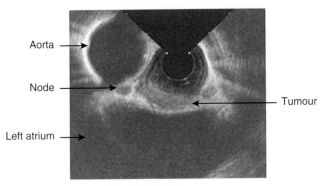

Aorta

Node

Tumour

Left atrium

Fig. 6.2 Endoscopic ultrasound image of a T3N1 tumour.

and careful audit, as accurate assessment is based on size, shape, margins, and echo pattern.

The use of FDG PET to detect oesophageal tumours is reported to be more sensitive than CT, for both squamous cell carcinoma and adenocarcinoma[13,14]. Combined analysis of seven studies (with a total of 281 patients) using FDG PET as part of initial staging, showed that in 94% the site of primary tumours could be correctly identified. In the 5% of tumours not identified, small size (most were <5mm in diameter) was the main reason for the false negative result. It is also recognized that a small subset of adenocarcinomas do not take up FDG, irrespective of size. These are usually adeno-carcinomas, either mucin-producing or poorly differentiated, or signet-ring subtype. Occasionally, the incidental finding of a small tumour arising within a hiatus hernia or Barrett's oesophagus may be seen on an FDG PET scan performed for a different purpose. In a patient who is already known to have oesophageal cancer, FDG PET does not add any further information on the T stage as determined by the CT. False positive FDG PET uptake in the oesophagus can occur with inflammatory disease, gastro-oesophageal reflux, or radiation-induced oesophagitis, often appearing as dif-fuse rather than focal uptake and confirming the need for histological diagnosis.

6.2.2.2 N stage

The oesophagus has a rich lymphatic network within the submucosa and even early T-stage tumours are at significant risk of lymph node involvement. This risk ranges from 3–6% for mucosal (T1a) to 21–24% for submucosal (T1b) tumours[15]. Using the Union Internationale Contre le Cancer (UICC) TNM staging system, the N stage refers to involvement of the lymph nodes in close proximity to the primary tumour (N1 disease) and this provides important prognostic information. This classification does not take into account involvement of lymph nodes beyond the N1 stations and if more distant lymph nodes are involved, they are classified as distant metastases (M stage).

The number, size, and location of the lymph nodes relative to the tumour site can be seen on CT, with nodes >10mm in short-axis diameter considered likely to be involved by cancer. However, enlarged nodes may also be due to non-malignant pro-cesses such as reactive hyperplasia or inflammation. Conversely, involved nodes may not appear enlarged on CT. Therefore the sensitivity and specificity of CT for detecting involved lymph nodes is poor (31–44%).

EUS provides assessment of local nodes, and several studies have compared EUS with CT and FDG PET. In a study of patients undergoing oesophagectomy and two- or three-field lymphadenectomy, Flamen and colleagues reported that EUS was more sensitive than FDG PET (81% vs. 33%) but less specific (67% vs. 89%) and combining the results of CT with EUS did not alter the cumulative specificity over FDG PET, indicating that nodal detection alone fails to differentiate benign from malignant disease[16]. The use of EUS-guided fine needle aspiration (EUS-FNA) enables histological confirmation of lymph node involvement within the diagnostic work-up and improves the sensitivity from 85% to >95%[8]. EUS-FNA of gastric and coeliac axis nodes can also be performed to stage distant lymph nodes and this procedure has been incorporated into the standard protocol for investigating potential surgical candidates in some centres.

A meta-analysis of 12 studies (including a total of 490 patients) using FDG PET to stage locoregional lymph nodes reported an overall sensitivity of 51% and specificity of 84%[17]. There are two reasons for the poor sensitivity of PET in detecting involved local lymph nodes. Firstly, FDG uptake by small volume metastases within involved nodes may be insufficient to be detected. Secondly, despite FDG uptake in involved lymph nodes being detectable, the scatter effects of FDG from the nodes and immediately adjacent primary tumour may impair the ability of the scanner to distinguish these as separate foci.

For staging of OGJ tumours, locoregional lymph nodes (N stage) would include lower para-oesophageal and pulmonary ligament nodes, diaphragmatic nodes on the dome or in retro-crural location, pericardial nodes adjacent to the oesophagus, and left gastric and coeliac axis nodes. Correct identification of lymph node metastases as coeliac axis rather than left gastric (M1a instead of N1) is critical as it can change the entire management of the patient from curative resection to palliation.

6.2.2.3 M stage

The risk of metastases increases with the T stage of the primary tumour. At presentation, 20–30% of patients have distant metastases. The UICC classification subdivides metastatic disease into M1a (non-regional lymph nodes) and M1b (distant organs). CT performed for the detection of metastatic disease has a low sensitivity of 41–83%[16], partly due to the lack of correlation between nodal size and metastatic involvement, but also due to difficulty in detecting lymph node metastases in unusual sites such as the cervical region and retroperitoneum. Small occult metastases in the liver and bone may be undetected on CT, and lesions in unexpected locations are overlooked as CT appearances often favour benign lesions, particularly those occurring in the thyroid gland, skeletal muscle and pancreas[17].

The major contribution of FDG PET in oesophageal cancer is the detection of distant metastases not identified by conventional imaging in 9–28% of patients. A meta-analysis of 12 studies by Van Westreenen and colleagues showed a pooled sensitivity and specificity for detection of distant metastases of 67% and 97% respectively[18]. The increased detection of distal lymph node and organ metastases compared with CT and EUS resulted in upstaging in 29% of patients, and downstaging in 5% of patients in one study, the latter due to exclusion of abnormal findings detected on CT images[19].

Integrated PET/CT imaging has further increased the detection of metastatic lesions compared with CT and PET performed separately, upstaging 17% of patients compared with 6% with independent imaging studies[20]. A new finding has been the detection of skeletal muscle metastases by PET not previously recognized by other imaging methods. In 5% of patients, lesions measuring <1cm (particularly in the liver or lung) may not be detected by CT or PET[21]. Whole body imaging with PET CT has also contributed to the detection of synchronous primary tumours, most often in the head and neck and large bowel, while false positive findings may be due to coincidental inflammatory disorders such as sarcoidosis.

6.3 Imaging for radiotherapy planning

The use of radiotherapy in oesophageal cancer can either be for curative or palliative intent. Intraluminal brachytherapy using radioactive iridium sources can be useful to provide palliation, but its role for curative treatment is limited.

In the curative setting, radiotherapy may be given preoperatively (neoadjuvant), as a definitive treatment modality, or postoperatively (adjuvant). Radiotherapy is often combined with synchronous chemotherapy as a radiosensitizer, known as chemoradiotherapy (CRT). Commonly used drugs in this setting are 5-fluorouracil (5FU) and cisplatin.

For the purpose of radiotherapy planning, all diagnostic information available should be taken into account in order to define the gross tumour volume (GTV). This should routinely include endoscopy, EUS, and contrast-enhanced multislice CT. Additional information from barium studies and FDG PET/CT scanning can be useful when available. For CT planning, axial slices at 3–5-mm intervals are taken with the patient immobilized appropriately. The scan should extend from the top of the apex of the lung to the iliac crest. The GTV is defined on each slice and a margin of 1–1.5cm circumferentially and 2–3cm longitudinally expanded to define the clinical target volume (CTV) to treat microscopic spread of disease and involved local lymph nodes. A further margin of 0.5–1.5cm is added to the CTV to allow for daily set up variation and internal organ motion (respiration and swallowing) to define the planning target volume (PTV).

It is recognized that there is significant inconsistency between radiation oncologists in defining target volumes[22]. Submucosal tumour extension and involved submucosal lymph nodes can be found at significant distances beyond the visible tumour. This is unlikely to be obvious on CT or endoscopy and more likely to be detected on EUS[23]. However, EUS assessment on the superior and inferior limits of the tumour has to be related to a reproducible anatomical landmark in the thorax for the purpose of radiotherapy planning. The traditional method of measuring the distance from the incisors is of little use. A suitable reference point is the top of the arch of the aorta[23] or the carina[24].

6.4 Therapeutic assessment and follow-up

Following completion of treatment for oesophageal cancer, risk of recurrence remains high and usually occurs within the first 2 years. Recurrent disease is associated with a poor prognosis and few patients can be successfully salvaged. The primary modality to detect recurrent disease and to assess response to therapy is with CT. The role of FDG PET/CT in detecting increased metabolic activity in recurrent tumours is emerging, as CT cannot reliably differentiate post-treatment changes from recurrent or residual active disease. In patients receiving neoadjuvant treatment, an early response detectable on PET/CT may predict for long-term outcome[25].

6.4.1 Assessing response to therapy

The treatment options for oesophageal cancer include surgical and non-surgical approaches. The addition of preoperative chemotherapy or CRT followed by resection improves survival when compared with surgery alone[26]. Patients who respond well to neoadjuvant CRT do not appear to benefit from surgical resection compared with continuing CRT (definitive CRT) in terms of overall survival[27,28].

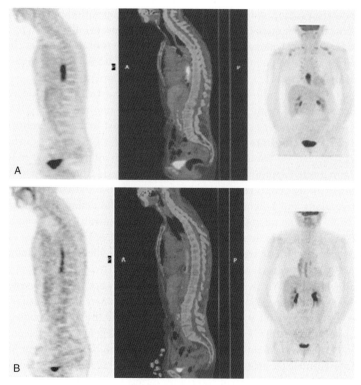

Fig. 6.3 70-year-old woman with a T3,N0,M0 squamous cell carcinoma of the lower oesophagus. Pre-treatment PET, fused PET/CT and MIP images (A) show a tumour with an SUV_{max} of 14.9. FDG uptake in brown fat in the supraclavicular fossae is a normal variant. Images 4 months later (B) following neoadjuvant chemo-radiation show a 50% reduction in tumour SUV_{max}. Note uptake in the right adjacent lung margin due to radiotherapy.

Reported pathological complete response (pCR) rates range from 8–56% (mean 24%) following preoperative CRT and resection[29]. As these patients are unlikely to benefit from surgical resection, the ability to predict pCR can contribute significantly to the patient's management.

CT is not accurate for determining tumour and lymph node response as studies have shown little correlation between reduction in tumour size and pathological response. Although EUS is a tool for preoperative staging, its use is also limited for assessing response, as it cannot differentiate residual tumour from post-treatment fibrosis[7].

Metabolic imaging using FDG PET can be used to assess response to therapy (Fig. 6.3). A baseline scan is required to compare with subsequent scans and the degree of FDG uptake within the tumour can be objectively measured using standard uptake value at 1 hour ($SUV_{max}1$ hour). Numerous studies have shown that a reduction in $SUV_{max}1$ hour at 14 days after commencement of preoperative chemotherapy or CRT correlates with good histological tumour regression and improved survival[25,30–33]. However, one study assessing FDG uptake after 7 days failed to demonstrate this correlation but this may be due to the short interval not allowing sufficient metabolic response to occur[33].

6.4.2 Follow-up

The role of regular CT imaging in the follow-up of asymptomatic patients who have completed curative treatment is unproven as recurrent disease is rarely salvaged successfully. FDG PET/CT may detect recurrent locoregional as well as distant metastatic disease (Fig. 6.4). However, like CT, this is not used routinely in the follow-up of asymptomatic patients. False positive findings can occur at the anastomotic site or in adjacent mediastinal lymph nodes due to inflammation[34].

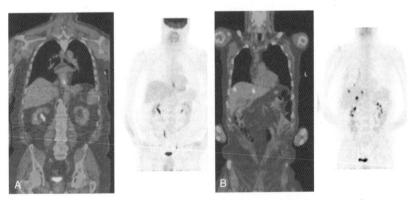

Fig. 6.4 63-year-old man with T3,N0,M0 adenocarcinoma of the lower oesophagus on baseline fused PET/CT and PET images (A). Following a complete response to neoadjuvant chemo-radiotherapy and subsequent surgery, disease has relapsed: 4 liver metastases now present (B). See colour section.

6.5 **Summary**

◆ To accurately stage oesophageal cancer a combination of imaging modalities is required.

● The most cost-effective method for overall staging is a combination of EUS-FNA plus PET/CT. However, many centres perform CT as a screening modality to identify patients with unresectable primary tumours or distant metastases before proceeding to EUS-FNA and PET/CT.

References

1. Parkin DM, Pisani P, Ferlay J. Estimates of the worldwide incidence of eighteen major cancers in 1985. *Int J Cancer* 1993; **54**: 594–606.
2. Sobin LH, Wittekind CH. Oesophagus (ICD-O C15). In: *TNM classification of malignant tumours*, 6th edn. New York: Wiley-Liss, 2002.
3. Lee SS, Ha HK, Byun JH, *et al.* Superficial esophageal cancer: esophageal findings correlated with histopathologic findings. *Radiology* 2005; **236**: 535–44.
4. Holscher AH, Bollschweiler E, Bumm R, *et al.* Prognostic factors of resected adenocarcinoma of the esophagus. *Surgery* 1995; **118**: 845–55.
5. de Meester SR. Adenocarcinoma of the esophagus and cardia: a review of the disease and its treatment. *Ann Surg Oncol* 2006; **13**: 12–30.
6. Herman SJ, Winton TL, Weisbrod GL, *et al.* Mediastinal invasion by bronchogenic carcinoma: CT signs. *Radiology* 1994; **190**: 841–6.
7. Lightdale CJ, Kulkarni KG. Role of endoscopic ultrasonography in the staging and follow-up of esophageal cancer. *J Clin Oncol* 2005; **23**: 4483–9.
8. Puli SR, Reddy JB, Bechtold ML, *et al.* Staging accuracy of esophageal cancer by endoscopic ultrasound: a meta-analysis and systematic review. *World J Gastroenterol* 2008; **14**: 1479–90.
9. Rice TW, Blackstone EH, Adelstein DJ, *et al.* Role of clinically determined depth of tumor invasion in the treatment of esophageal carcinoma. *J Thorac Cardiovasc Surg* 2003; **125**: 1091–102.
10. Rosch T. Endoscopic staging of oesophageal cancer: a review of literature results. *Gastrointest Endosc Clin N Am* 1995; **5**: 537–47.
11. Dyer SM, Levison DB, Chen RY, *et al.* Systematic review of the impact of endoscopic ultrasound on the management of patients with esophageal cancer. *Int J Technol Assess Health Care* 2008; **24**: 25–35.
12. Siewert JR, Holscher AH, Dittler HJ. Preoperative staging and risk analysis in esophageal cancer. *Hepatogastroenterology* 1990; **37**: 382–7.
13. Meltzer CC, Luketich JD, Friedman D, *et al.* Whole body FDG positron emission tomographic imaging for staging oesophageal cancer comparison with computed tomography. *Clin Nuc Med* 2000; **25**: 882–7.
14. Rasanen JV, Sihvo EI, Knuuti MJ, *et al.* Prospective analysis of accuracy of positron emission tomography, computed tomography, and endoscopic ultrasonography in staging of adenocarcinoma of the oesophagus and the oesophago-gastric junction. *Ann Surg Oncol* 2003; **10**: 954–60.
15. Sabik JF, Rice TW, Goldblum JR, *et al.* Superficial esophageal carcinoma. *Ann Thorac Surg* 1995; **6**: 896–902.
16. Flamen P, Lerut A, Van Cutsem E, *et al.* Utility of positron emission tomography for the staging of patients with potentially operable oesophageal carcinoma. *J Clin Oncol* 2000; **18**: 3202–10.

17. Flanagan FL, Dehdashti F, Siegel BA, *et al.* Staging of esophageal cancer with 18F-flourode-oxyglucose positron emission tomography. *Am J Roentgenol* 1997; **168**: 417–24.

18. van Westreenen HL, Westerterp M, Bossuyt PM, *et al.* Systematic review of the staging performance of ^{18}F-fluorodeoxyglucose positron emission tomography in oesophageal cancer. *J Clin Oncol* 2004; **22**: 3805–12.

19. Heeren PA, Jager PL, Bongaerts F, *et al.* Detection of distant metastases in oesophageal cancer with (18)F-FDG PET. *J Nucl Med* 2004; **45**: 980–7.

20. Wong WL, Chambers RJ. Role of PET/PET CT in the staging and restaging of thoracic oesophageal cancer and gastro-oesophageal cancer: a literature review. *Abdom Imag* 2008; **3**: 183–90.

21. Meyers BF, Downey RJ, Decker PA, *et al.* The utility of positron emission tomography in staging of potentially operable carcinoma of the thoracic esophagus: results of the American College of Surgeons Oncology Group Z0060 trial. *J Thorac Cardiovasc Surg* 2007; **133**: 738–45

22. Tai P, Van Dyk J, Yu E, *et al.* Variability of target volume delineation in cervical esophageal cancer. *Int J Radiat Oncol Biol Phys* 1998; **42**: 277–88.

23. Thomas E, Crellin A, Harris K, *et al.* The role of endoscopic ultrasound (EUS) in planning radiotherapy target volumes for oesophageal cancer. *Radiother Oncol* 2004; **73**: 149–51.

24. Rice PF, Crosby TLD, Roberts SA. Variability of the carina-incisor distance as assessed by endoscopic ultrasound. *Clin Oncol* 2003; **15**: 383–5.

25. Ott K, Wolfgang A, Lordick F, *et al.* Metabolic imaging predicts response, survival, and recurrence in adenocarcinomas of the esophogastric junction. *J Clin Oncol* 2006; **24**: 4692–8.

26. Gebski V, Burmeister B, Smithers BM, *et al.* Australasian Gastro-Intestinal Trials Group. Survival benefits from neoadjuvant chemoradiotherapy or chemotherapy in oesophageal cancer: a meta-analysis. *Lancet Oncology* 2007; **8**: 226–34.

27. Stahl M, Stuschke M, Lehmann N, *et al.* Chemoradiation with and without surgery in patients with locally advanced squamous cell carcinoma of the esophagus. *J Clin Oncol* 2005; **23**: 2310–17

28. Bedenne L, Michel P, Bouché O, *et al.* Chemoradiation followed by surgery compared with chemoradiation alone in squamous cancer of the esophagus: FFCD 9102. *J Clin Oncol* 2007; **25**: 1160–8.

29. Geh JI, Crellin AM, Glynne-Jones R. Preoperative (neoadjuvant) chemoradiotherapy in oesophageal cancer. *Br J Surg* 2001; **88**: 338–56.

30. Weber WA, Ott K, Becker K, *et al.* Predication of response to preoperative chemotherapy in adenocarcinomas of oesophagogastric junction by metabolic imaging. *J Clin Oncol* 2001; **19**: 3058–65.

31. Westerterp M, van Westreenen HL, Reitsma JB, *et al.* Esophageal cancer: CT, endoscopic US, and FDG PET for assessment of response to neoadjuvant therapy – systematic review. *Radiology* 2005; **236**: 841–51.

32. Weider HA, Brucher BLDM, Zimmerman F, *et al.* Time course of tumor metabolic activity during chemoradiotherapy of esophageal squamous cell carcinoma and response to treatment. *J Clin Oncol* 2004; **22**: 900–8.

33. Gillham CM, Lucey JA, Keogan M, *et al.* [18]FDG uptake during induction chemoradiation for oesophageal cancer fails to predict histomorphological tumour response. *Br J Cancer* 2006; **95**: 1174–9.

34. Kato H, Miyazaki T, Nakajima M, *et al.* Value of positron emission tomography in the diagnosis of recurrent oesophageal carcinoma. *Br J Surg* 2004; **91**: 1004–9.

Chapter 7

Gastric tumours

Ben Miller, Ian Geh, and
Shuvro Roy-Choudhury

7.1 Clinical background

The majority of malignant stomach tumours are adenocarcinomas. It is the world's second most common cancer and is the most common cancer in the Far East and South America. The incidence of adenocarcinomas of the gastric cardia has rapidly increased over the past 20 years whilst other sites have remained unchanged[1]. Adenocarcinomas of the lower oesophagus have also increased at the same rate. It is often difficult to distinguish the origin of tumours at the oesophagogastric junction (OGJ). Thus a new classification of OGJ tumours has been proposed[2] dividing the OGJ into distal oesophageal (Siewert type I), cardia (Siewert type II), and subcardial gastric cancer (Siewert type III). This classification has important management implications regarding staging wherein Siewert type III are staged as stomach cancers.

7.2 Diagnosis and staging

7.2.1 Diagnosis

Endoscopy is the modality of choice for diagnosing stomach tumours as it allows for exact localization and biopsy for histology. Double-contrast barium studies have a continued but limited role when endoscopy is not feasible or in the diagnosis of scirrhous carcinoma, which diffusely infiltrates the stomach wall (linitis plastica). In this situation, the endoscopic appearance may be normal as the infiltration is submucosal and the lack of stomach distension on barium studies may be the only radiological indication of disease[1]. More specific tailored CT protocols (see section 7.2.2) allow for higher detection rates.

7.2.2 Staging

In addition to the initial CT, endoscopic ultrasound (EUS), diagnostic laparoscopy, and occasionally ^{18}F-fluorodeoxyglucose positron emission tomography/computed tomography (FDG PET/CT) are useful modalities as problem solving tools. Staging of stomach cancers is based on the TNM (tumour, node, metastasis) staging system[3] (Table 7.1).

7.2.2.1 T stage

Initial staging is with CT of the chest, abdomen, and pelvis using oral water load to distend the stomach. Appearances of stomach cancers on CT can range from focal wall

Table 7.1 TNM classification of stomach cancer. Staging is defined according to the American Joint Committee on Cancer (AJCC) and the Union Internationale Contre le Cancer (UICC)[6]

Primary tumour (T)	
Tx	Primary tumour cannot be assessed
T0	No evidence of primary tumour
Tis	Carcinoma in situ without invasion of the lamina propria
T1	Tumour invades lamina propria or submucosa
T2	Tumour invades muscularis propria or subserosa
T2a	Tumour invades muscularis propria
T2b	Tumour invades subserosa
T3	Tumour penetrates serosa (visceral peritoneum)
T4	Tumour invades adjacent structures
Regional lymph nodes (N)	
Nx	Regional lymph nodes cannot be assessed
N0	No involvement of regional lymph nodes
N1	Metastasis in 1–6 regional lymph nodes
N2	Metastasis in 7–15 regional lymph nodes
N3	Metastasis in >15 regional lymph nodes
Distant metastases (M)	
Mx	Distant metastases cannot be assessed
M0	No distant metastases
M1	Distant metastases

thickening with or without ulceration (Fig. 7.1), a soft tissue mass, to diffuse wall thickening in linitis plastica. Tumours can show abnormally strong contrast enhancement[4]. Lower attenuation lesions correspond with fibrosis or aggressive mucinous tumours[5]. Attention to technique is important. Presence of air in the stomach causes overshooting artefacts and this can be avoided by using negative oral contrast such as water to distend the stomach. It is important to study the stomach using multiplanar reconstructions (MPRs)[5]. Curved MPRs are useful to distinguish tumours abutting adjacent organs from invading adjacent organs (Fig. 7.2). The overall accuracy of CT in staging stomach cancer ranges from 77–89%[6]. Recent studies using these specific tailored scanning and reconstruction techniques with multidetector CT and 'virtual gastroscopy', show increasing accuracy in T staging, and sensitivity for detecting the early gastric cancers (EGCs)[7]. Using these state of the art techniques, CT can detect stomach cancer (in mixed series of advanced gastric cancers (AGCs) and EGCs) with 94–98% accuracy and correctly T stage in 84–89%[8,9].

Computed tomography remains more accurate than EUS in determining advanced T3 and T4 disease, and has an accuracy of detecting serosal invasion in up to 90%[10].

Fig. 7.1 Axial contrast-enhanced CT demonstrating circumferential mid body soft tissue thickening caused by a lesser curve adenocarcinoma. The gastric wall is intact (small arrows).
A vessel in the gastrohepatic ligament simulates infiltrative disease (large arrow), which can be a pitfall.

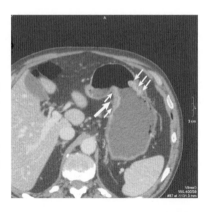

Fig. 7.2 Axial contrast-enhanced CT demonstrating an annular antral tumour (large arrows) extending into the pancreatic head. A T4 poorly differentiated adenocarcinoma was confirmed at palliative surgery.

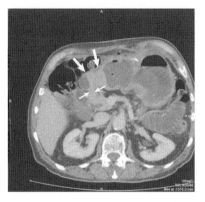

MRI has similar accuracy to CT but is limited in routine practice by artefacts and the complexity and time taken to perform the examination.

Endoscopic ultrasound (EUS) is probably the best method of predicting the pathological T stage of EGCs with series overall accuracy rates of 65–92%[6]. As in the oesophagus, the normal layers of the stomach wall can be clearly visualized on EUS. Most tumours appear hypoechoic with irregular margins, disrupting these layers. EUS is particularly sensitive for early stage tumours confined to the mucosa and submucosa (T1 and T2). However, it is operator dependent with a learning curve, hence its availability is often confined to regional centres. Where there is coexisting inflammation, the extent of disease can be overestimated.

7.2.2.2 N stage

Although current N staging depends on the number of positive lymph nodes (see Table 7.1) rather than the previously described nodal stations, the latter is important as prognosis is also dependent on extent of lymphadenectomy[11]. Involvement of the hepatoduodenal nodes, retropancreatic, mesenteric, and paraaortic nodes are considered metastatic disease (compartments 3 and 4) as these are not routinely removed even when performing D2 lymphadenectomy.

CT is the modality of choice for lymph node staging. It can detect the more distant lymph nodes (compartments 3 and 4) that may influence the surgeon to either perform an extended lymphadenectomy or not to offer curative resection at all. The overall accuracy of lymph node staging by CT is, at best, around 80%[12]. The main limitation of using CT to assess lymph node size and shape as a means of predicting tumour involvement is that this is unreliable, often over- as well as under-staging the disease.

EUS is limited to a smaller field of view (up to 6cm) and so is restricted to assessing lymph nodes close to the stomach where it has a diagnostic accuracy of 70–90%[1]. In a comparative series of 63 patients[8] similar accuracies were reported between EUS (79%) and CT (75%). There may be a role for PET/CT in the diagnosis of normal sized compartment 3 or 4 or supraclavicular nodes (M1 disease).

7.2.2.3 Distant metastases

CT is the modality of choice. Liver metastases are present in approximately 25% of newly diagnosed patients with AGC. Other sites including lung, bone, and adrenal metastases are less common but can be also detected with CT. Small peritoneal deposits can easily be missed but the presence of ascites generally indicates peritoneal disease[13]. In a female patient, it is important to include the pelvis as ovarian drop metastases, otherwise known as 'Krukenberg tumours', are often found. If there are no metastases on imaging, staging laparoscopy is indicated and can influence the clinical management in up to 20% cases[14]. FDG PET/CT is used only rarely for problem solving or to exclude suspected occult metastatic disease[15].

7.3 Imaging for radiotherapy planning

In the curative setting, radiotherapy may be given preoperatively (neoadjuvant) or postoperatively (adjuvant). It is often combined with synchronous fluoropyrimidine-based chemotherapy (chemoradiotherapy or CRT) as a radiosensitizer. Randomized trials of preoperative radiotherapy suggest possible benefit in survival but the findings are inconsistent between trials[16]. The role of preoperative CRT has not been evaluated in randomized trials and therefore remains experimental.

Following curative resection, many patients remain at high risk of locoregional recurrence. The US Intergroup 0116 Trial[17] showed that the use of postoperative CRT (45Gy in 25 fractions with synchronous 5-fluorouracil (5FU) and folinic acid) improved overall survival (50% vs. 41% at 3 years) when compared with surgery alone in patients who had curative resection (R0). Whilst this approach is standard in the USA, its adoption has been inconsistent throughout the rest of the world[18].

Following good quality surgery the role of postoperative CRT remains uncertain. If the decision is to treat the patient with postoperative CRT, preparation should include ensuring that the patient has sufficiently recovered from surgery, has an adequate nutritional intake (with or without support), and has optimal renal function. Both glomerular filtration rate (GFR) as well as differential renal function—DMSA (dimercaptosuccinic acid) or MAG3 (mercaptoacetyl triglycine)—should be assessed as the radiation dose to one kidney will often exceed tolerance and it is important to ensure that the function of the other kidney is adequate. The planning CT scan should be in the supine position with the arms raised, starting from above liver to below kidneys to allow generation of dose volume histograms (DVH) for organs at risk. Addition of intravenous contrast and dilute gastrograffin to opacify the bowel is helpful to define the various anatomical structures. The oncologist needs to be familiar with the original site and extent of tumour using information from preoperative CT, endoscopy, surgical notes, histology report, and, importantly, multidisciplinary team discussion.

In the palliative setting, short courses of radiotherapy to the stomach using parallel opposed anterior and posterior fields simulated with barium contrast can help to control bleeding or pain. In addition, radiotherapy to painful bony metastases can be effective in controlling symptoms and improving quality of life.

7.4 Therapeutic assessment and follow-up

Disease recurrence is common within the first 2 years of surgery and is associated with a poor prognosis. The benefit of postoperative imaging to identify asymptomatic recurrent disease remains unproven. When there is clinical suspicion of recurrence, CT is the imaging modality of choice. It is also used to assess response to further therapy using standard reporting criteria (Response Evaluation in Solid Tumors—RECIST)[19]. The ability of FDG PET/CT to detect abnormal metabolic function has an emerging role, as CT cannot reliably differentiate post-treatment changes from recurrent or residual active disease[15]. In the setting of neoadjuvant treatment 18-FDG PET/CT may have a role in predicting response early in the course of therapy[20].

7.5 Summary

- ◆ CT remains the main modality for staging and determining resectability but more comprehensive information is provided by a multimodality approach (CT, EUS, laparoscopy, and PET).
- ◆ The role for routine imaging following curative treatment remains unproven.

References

1. Levine MS, Megibow AJ, Kochman ML. Carcinoma of the stomach and duodenum. In: Gore RM, Levine MS (eds). *Textbook of Gastrointestinal Radiology*, pp. 619–41. Philadelphia, PA: Saunders, 2007.
2. Siewert RJ, Feith M, Werner M, *et al*. Adenocarcinoma of the esophagogastric junction: results of surgical therapy based on anatomical/topographic classification in 1,002 consecutive patients. *Ann Surg* 2000; **232**: 353–61.
3. Sobin LH, Wittekind Ch, (eds). Stomach (ICD-O C16). In: *UICC: TNM classification of malignant tumours*, 6th edn, pp. 65–8. New York: Wiley, 2002.
4. Miller FH, Kochan ML, Talamonti MS, *et al*. Gastric cancer: Radiologic staging. *Radiol Clin North Am* 2007: **35**: 331–48.
5. Shimizu K, Ito K, Matsunaga N, *et al*. Diagnosis of gastric cancer with MDCT using the water-filling method and multiplanar reconstruction: CT-histologic correlation. *AJR Am J Roentgenol* 2005; **185**: 1152–8.
6. Kwee RM, Kwee TC. Imaging in local staging of gastric cancer: a systematic review. *J Clin Oncol* 2007; **25**: 2107–16.

7. Kim JH, Eun HW, Goo DE, *et al.* Imaging of various gastric lesions with 2D MPR and CT gastrography performed with multidetector CT. *Radiographics* 2006; **26**: 1101–16, discussion 1117–18.

8. Bhandari S, Shim CS, Kim JH, *et al.* Usefulness of three-dimensional, multidetector row CT (virtual gastroscopy and multiplanar reconstruction) in the evaluation of gastric cancer: a comparison with conventional endoscopy, EUS, and histopathology. *Gastrointest Endosc* 2004; **59**: 619–26.

9. Chen CY, Hsu JS, Wu DC, *et al.* Gastric cancer: preoperative local staging with 3D multi-detector row CT-correlation with surgical and histopathologic results. *Radiology* 2007; **242**: 472–82.

10. Kumano S, Murakami T, Kim T, *et al.* T staging of gastric cancer: role of multi-detector row CT. *Radiology* 2005; **237**: 961–6.

11. Nishi M, Ohta K, Matsubara T, *et al.* [Treatment of cancer of the esophago-gastric junction with special reference to dissection of the lymphatic system] *Gan To Kagaku Ryoho* 1988; **15**(4 Pt. 1): 580–8 [Japanese].

12. Habermann CR, Weiss F, Riecken R, *et al.* Preoperative staging of gastric adenocarcinoma: Comparison of Helical CT and endoscopic US. *Radiology* 2004; **230**: 465–71.

13. Yajima K, Kanda T, Ohashi M, et al. Clinical and diagnostic significance of preoperative computed tomography findings of ascites in patients with advanced gastric cancer. *Am J Surg* 2006; **192**: 185–90.

14. de Graaf GW, Ayantunde AA, Parsons SL, *et al.* The role of staging laparoscopy in oesophagogastric cancers. *Eur J Surg Oncol* 2007; **33**: 988–92.

15. Lim JS, Yun MJ, Kim MJ, *et al.* CT and PET in stomach cancer: preoperative staging and monitoring of response to therapy. *Radiographics* 2006; **26**: 143–56.

16. Florica F, Cartel F, Enea M, *et al.* The impact of radiotherapy on survival in resectable gastric carcinoma: A meta-analysis of literature data. *Cancer Treat Rev* 2007; **33**: 729–40.

17. Macdonald JS, Smalley SR, Benedetti J, *et al.* Chemoradiotherapy after surgery compared with surgery alone for adenocarcinoma of the stomach or gastroesophageal junction. *N Engl J Med* 2001; **345**: 725–30.

18. Estes NC, MacDonald JS, Touijer K, *et al.* Inadequate documentation and resection for gastric cancer in the United States: a preliminary report. *Am Surg* 1998; **64**: 680–5.

19. Suzuki C, Jacobsson H, Hatschek T, *et al.* Radiologic measurements of tumor response to treatment: practical approaches and limitations. *Radiographics* 2008; **28**: 329–44.

20. Ott K, Weber WA, Lordick F, *et al.* Metabolic imaging predicts response, survival, and recurrence in adenocarcinomas of the esophagogastric junction. *J Clin Oncol* 2006; **24**: 4692–8.

Chapter 8

Hepatic and biliary tumours

Ben Miller, Ian Geh, and
Shuvro Roy-Choudhury

8.1 Clinical background

The liver lies in the right upper quadrant and has a dual blood supply from the portal vein (75%) and from the hepatic artery (25% of total supply). This has important implications for imaging, particularly for the timing of intravenous contrast examinations, and for vascular intervention[1].

8.1.1 Hepatocellular carcinoma (HCC)

The tumour may be solitary, multifocal, or diffusely infiltrating. It spreads locally by invasion into bile ducts, portal vein branches, and hepatic vein branches. It can metastasize to the rest of the liver via the portal vein braches. Extra hepatic metastases occur late, most often to local lymph nodes, lungs, bone, and adrenals.

8.1.2 Cholangiocarcinoma

Tumours may arise from the intrahepatic ducts (10–20%), tending to metastasize early within the liver, or from the extrahepatic ducts (80–90%), when they usually present with jaundice. Most of these arise at the hepatic hilum (Klatskin's tumours). More distal tumours are often radiologically inseparable from pancreatic, ampullary, and duodenal cancers at presentation[2].

8.1.3 Gallbladder cancer

This is rare and often associated with pre-existing cholelithiasis. Many cases are not visible and only diagnosed postoperatively in a thick-walled gall bladder.

8.1.4 Metastases

The liver is a common site of metastases. Common primaries include pancreas, stomach, bowel, breast, and lung. Most liver metastases are widespread, with 10–20% presenting with solitary or paucimetastatic disease which may be offered curative treatment.

8.1.5 Lymphoma

Liver involvement in lymphoma is most often secondary and occurs more commonly in non-Hodgkin's lymphoma.

8.1.6 **Benign lesions**

Benign lesions are common incidental findings during routine imaging and usually of no clinical significance. However in a patient undergoing staging for a known primary cancer, benign lesions, accounting for 50% of lesions[3], can cause a diagnostic conundrum. In the absence of cirrhosis or a history of malignancy almost all incidentally detected lesions measuring <2cm will be benign.

Common benign lesions include cysts, haemangiomas, hepatic adenomas, focal nodular hyperplasia (FNH), focal fat infiltration, or sparing and regenerating or siderotic nodules in cirrhosis[4].

- Simple cysts are the commonest benign lesion. They are thin-walled, well-defined, water-containing lesions with no internal septae or evidence of any enhancement on serial phases of contrast enhancement on computed tomography (CT) or magnetic resonance imaging (MRI). On ultrasound (US), these dark lesions show posterior acoustic enhancement.

- Haemangiomas are the commonest solid lesions, occurring more frequently in females, and are often multiple. They are well-defined, heterogeneous lesions that demonstrate peripheral, nodular, discontinuous enhancement with centripetal filling-in after contrast administration. Small lesions can show flash filling and large lesions may have a scar. Enhancement follows vascular density at all phases (Fig. 8.1).

- Hepatic adenomas are well circumscribed and encapsulated.

- FNH appears hyperdense on CT and hyperintense on MRI on arterial phase imaging. There is rapid wash-out and the central scar enhances in the delayed phase (Fig. 8.2). The hepatocyte specific contrast agents can be used to diagnose these with great accuracy.

- Focal fat infiltration is easily diagnosed on 'in and out of phase' MR sequences. There is no deviation of intrahepatic vessels or bile ducts.

- Hepatic abscesses appear as ring-enhancing, low-density, well-defined lesions.

- Rarer benign lesions that may present as a mass include biliary cystadenoma, sarcoidosis, rheumatoid arthritis, and histoplasmosis.

- Transient hepatic artery attenuation/intensity difference (THAD/THID) is a wedge-shaped area of increased density (simulating a lesion) due to imbalance of local blood supply from the portal system and hepatic artery[5]. This is often due to local portal vein obstruction.

8.2 **Diagnosis and staging**

8.2.1 **Imaging modalities**

8.2.1.1 US

US remains the first-line investigation in patients presenting with right upper quadrant symptoms. It is good for imaging the gall bladder and the biliary tree for radiolucent calculi, to assess for biliary obstruction, and to confirm the cystic nature of lesions. It is good for assessing the vascular structures in the liver and vascularity within lesions.

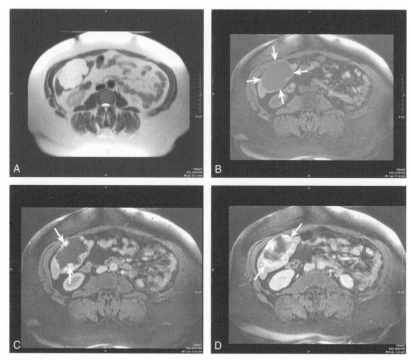

Fig. 8.1 Haemangioma picked up during a staging CT and characterized by MRI.
(A) Axial T2-weighted image shows a lobular abnormality in segment 6 markedly
hyperintense to background liver. Precontrast (B), arterial phase (C), and delayed phase
(D) T1-weighted images show nodular, discontinuous peripheral arterial enhancement
(arrows; C) with progressive centripetal filling on the delayed phase (D) typical of a
haemangioma. The enhancement follows the vascular phase and the lesion is brighter
than background liver on the delayed phase.

Contrast-enhanced US, using encapsulated microbubbles to increase the conspicuity
of vessels is excellent in helping to characterize liver lesions. This has been proven to
improve accuracy compared to unenhanced US, particularly after chemotherapy
(82% vs. 57%)[6]. It remains the modality of choice for guiding biopsy of suspicious
lesion. Intraoperative US is the most accurate modality to diagnose liver lesions. In
the setting of HCC it can detect 100% of relevant lesions and in the setting of colorectal metastasis it can detect up to 10% additional metastases than picked up by the
preoperative CT[7].

8.2.1.2 CT and MRI

These are less operator dependent, more reproducible, and have greater accuracy than
US. Newer generations of scanners have revolutionized CT imaging with their ability
to rapidly scan several phases through the liver with thin slice thickness and to perform multiplanar reformats, surface rendering, and three-dimensional (3D) vascular
reformations, for surgical planning. The additional advantage of CT over MRI is the
ability to stage the whole of the thorax, abdomen, and pelvis in one sitting.

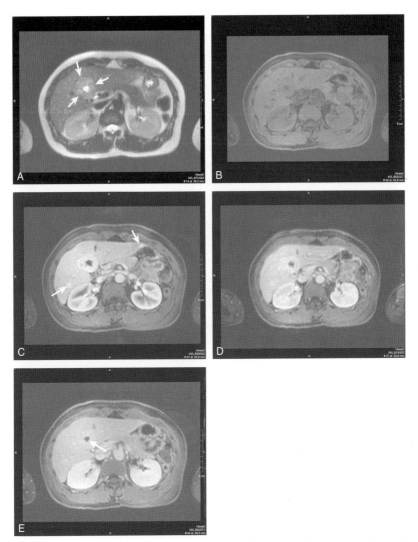

Fig. 8.2 Focal nodular hyperplasia (FNH) detected incidentally on CT and characterized by contrast-enhanced MRI. (A) Axial T2-weighted image shows a 5-cm barely hyperintense lesion in segment 4B with a bright central scar and absence of a capsule. Precontrast (B), arterial phase (C), portal venous (D), and delayed phase (E) T1-weighted images show an intensely enhancing lesion during the arterial phase (C), equilibrating with background liver rapidly on the portal phase (D), and virtually indistinguishable on the delayed phase (E). Scar enhancement in more pronounced in the delayed phase (arrow).

Contrast injection amount and protocols depend on the CT scanner, the details of which are outside the scope of this text. There are effectively five phases of enhancement possible with CT. Early arterial (15–20s), late arterial (30–35s), portal or sinusoidal (70s), equilibrium (180s), and delayed phases (5–10min). Lesions that have increased arterial flow, principally HCC and some hypervascular metastases, are best imaged in the arterial phase. Lesions without increased arterial flow, like most metastases, are usually best demonstrated on the portal phase.

MRI has the advantage of superior contrast resolution and being non-ionizing. It is limited by breathing artefacts, claustrophobia, and some contraindications. A comprehensive MRI study is deemed to be the preoperative imaging gold standard in detecting and characterizing liver lesions. Such an examination comprises of two parts: 1) non-contrast thin-section T2W sequence using the dual echo technique (where benign lesions appear very bright, malignant lesions appear moderately bright) and T1W images in and out of phase (to assess fat content of a lesion or to diagnose fatty infiltration or sparing); 2) pre- and postcontrast dynamic MRI, usually using a fat suppressed gradient echo T1W 3D volume sequence. Vascular enhancement phases on MRI are similar to CT (see above).

In practice, for routine staging of a known primary cancer, a single portal phase CT is sufficient. If there is suspicion of HCC or a hypervascular metastasis, both arterial and portal phases should be performed. To characterize a solitary liver lesion where there is no known primary, a triple or even quadruple phase approach with either CT or MRI is commonly used[8].

8.2.1.3 Positron emission tomography and staging laparoscopy

These are occasionally used as a problem solving tool in hepatobiliary tumours, particularly to exclude extrahepatic disease in patients being considered for surgical treatments.

8.2.2 Specific diseases

8.2.2.1 Hepatocellular carcinoma

US is commonly used in screening of patients with cirrhosis to look for early signs of the development of an HCC. It has fairly low sensitivity and appearances are variable. The presence of dysplastic or regenerating nodules can make interpretation difficult.

CT and MR are more accurate and are now widely available. On CT or MRI, small tumours enhance in the arterial phase (20–35s) and rapidly washout in the portal phase, becoming isoattenuating with the liver (Fig. 8.3). Larger tumours have a more heterogenous and mosaic appearance and more variable behaviour with contrast. There is often a hypoattenuating rim due to the fibrous capsule that shows delayed enhancement and often a low attenuation centre due to central necrosis.

Fibrolamellar HCC is a rare, slow growing tumour and is seen in the absence of underlying cirrhosis and can reach large sizes. The lesion enhances in the arterial phase, although less homogenously than in FNH. It commonly has a fibrous central scar that may show delayed enhancement but less well than in FNH. It is staged like HCC and mode of spread is similar to HCC.

8.2.2.2 Cholangiocarcinoma

Patients presenting with jaundice or right upper quadrant symptoms will usually have US as a first-line test. This will show duct dilatation and the extent will vary according to the level of the lesion. A mass may not be visible unless it is of a sufficient size.

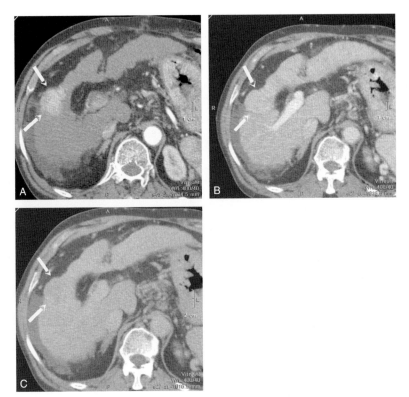

Fig. 8.3 Hepatocellular carcinoma in a 62-year-old woman with hepatitis and cirrhosis. Arterial phase CT (A) shows a 4.2-cm cortex deforming irregular, hypervascular lesion in segment 5 (arrows). The lesion becomes isodense with normal liver in the portal phase (B) and shows further 'washout' in the delayed phase (C). A hypervascular metastasis would behave similarly. Note nodular liver surface and ascites.

In the management of painless obstructive jaundice, if choledocholithiasis is excluded as the cause of the dilated ducts on US, then CT or MR is indicated.

On CT, the portal phase images will show biliary tract dilatation and there may be a mass lesion visible. When presenting as an intrahepatic mass, cholangiocarcinomas are often seen as ill-defined low or isoattenuating lesions simulating metastases and causing duct dilatation. There may be capsular retraction and/or lobar or segmental atrophy. The lesions show diagnostic delayed enhancement due to their fibrous stroma and can be the only phase on which they are identified. MR appearances are similar, most often being hypointense on T1W and mildly hyperintense on T2W images (Fig. 8.4). More commonly, cholangiocarcinomas are extrahepatic and are usually small and slow growing. Occasionally they will present as subtle focal thickening of the bile duct causing biliary duct dilatation. Longitudinal as well as lateral tumour extensions are important surgical considerations.

A pancreas protocol CT with some delayed phase images are required for staging. Dynamic MRI of the liver (with delayed phase imaging) with magnetic resonance

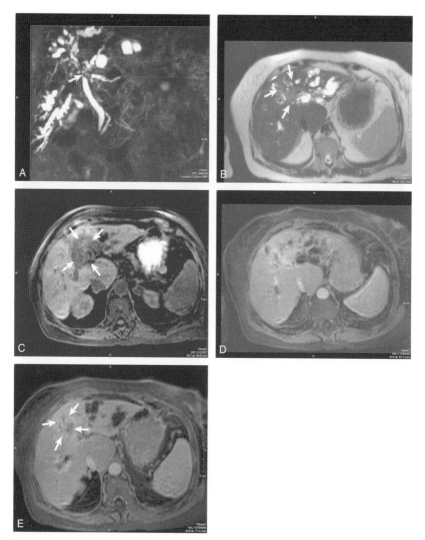

Fig. 8.4 Cholangiocarcinoma in a 72-year-old woman presenting with painless jaundice. (A) Coronal MR cholangiopancreaticography image shows bilobar intrahepatic biliary duct dilatation. The presence of a hilar mass can be inferred (arrow). (B) T2 axial image demonstrating the hilar mass. Precontrast (C) and portal venous (D) phase images show a hypointense lesion with some enhancement on the delayed phase image (E). Note the lobar atrophy. This pattern is characteristic for a cholangiocarcinoma.

cholangio-pancreatography (MRCP) is an excellent alternative and gives most relevant staging information.

Endoscopic retrograde cholangio-pancreatography (ERCP) and percutaneous transhepatic cholangiography (PTC) are invasive methods of opacifying the biliary tree to demonstrate the level and extent of any obstructing lesion. Temporary placement of plastic stents or drains at ERCP (for more distal lesions) or PTC (for more proximal lesions) can be used to decompress an obstructed biliary tree. Subsequently, a permanent metallic stent can be placed for palliation,

8.2.2.3 Metastases

On US, most appear as low echogenic, ill-defined, rounded lesions, sometimes with a low echogenic ring. On CT, most metastases appear as ill-defined, low-attenuation lesions in the portal phase. They may show ring enhancement in early phases and peripheral washout in delayed phases. Small lesions are easily confused with simple cysts or haemangiomas and US can be helpful to discriminate for superficial lesions. On MRI, metastases typically appear low to intermediate signal on T1W and moderately high signal on T2W MR images.

Hypervascular metastases, typically from neuroendocrine tumours, renal cell carcinomas, sarcomas, melanomas, and occasionally colon and breast cancers, show arterial enhancement followed by a rapid washout, leaving them isodense or hypodense to surrounding liver on the portal phase. Calcification is sometimes seen, particularly in larger metastases from mucin producing gastrointestinal tract tumours or those after chemotherapy. Cystic metastases are less common (ovary, colon, stomach) but cystic change in a larger solid lesion is quite common, as is cystic change following chemotherapy. The metastases from ovarian malignancies are commonly cystic, and are located on the peritoneal surface of the liver from trans-coelomic spread.

8.2.2.4 Gallbladder adenocarcinoma

US is often the initial imaging modality. Typical appearances are of a variably thick-walled gallbladder or of a mass either within the gallbladder or extending out into the liver. It can be used to guide biopsy.

CT will often show a soft tissue mass in the gall bladder bed. Direct spread into the liver is seen as hypodense areas. It will demonstrate any biliary tract dilatation and local lymph node spread. Accuracy of local T staging with multislice CT and multiplanar reconstructions is 84.9%[9].

8.3 Imaging for radiotherapy planning

Despite technical advances in radiotherapy delivery, including conformal planning, intensity modulated radiotherapy (IMRT), image guided radiotherapy (IGRT) and body stereotactic radiotherapy, at the present time there is no routine application of radiotherapy to primary liver tumours.

8.4 Therapeutic assessment and follow-up

CT is the main radiological modality with MRI or PET being used as problem-solving tools. Specific imaging protocols may be necessary to assess response to specialized surgical or interventional management. An example of such a protocol will include performing a pre- and postcontrast CT following radiofrequency ablation or transarterial chemoembolization of liver malignancies to assess for viable residual or recurrent disease.

Metastases show altered characteristics after treatment, for example calcification can occur in a mucus secreting adenocarcinoma metastasis or a treated metastasis from a gastrointestinal stromal tumour may masquerade as a cyst. Margins may become more ill defined and lesions may become more subtle. The background liver may become hypodense due to fatty infiltration making hypodense metastasis more difficult to define. These have implications for surgical treatment after potential downstaging of metastasis with modern multimodal chemotherapy. This is an evolving field and recent developments in molecular and perfusion imaging may well modify practice in the near future.

8.5 **Summary**

- Dynamic contrast-enhanced CT and MRI form the basis of liver lesion characterization, sometimes with specific contrast agents.
- Most lesions have typical features. Occasional large lesions and small subcentimetre lesions can be difficult to characterize. In these cases interval imaging or a biopsy may become necessary.
- Most incidentally detected lesions are benign.

References

1. Robinson, PJ. The liver. In: Husband, JE, Reznek, RH (eds). *Imaging in Oncology*, 2nd edn, pp.1059–83. London: Taylor and Francis, 2004.
2. Baron RL, Peterson MS. From the RSNA refresher courses: screening the cirrhotic liver for hepatocellular carcinoma with CT and MR imaging: opportunities and pitfalls. *Radiographics* 2001; **21**: S117–32.
3. Kreft B, Pauleit D, Bachmann R, *et al.* [Incidence and significance of small focal liver lesions in MRI.] *Rofo* 2001; **173**: 424–9.
4. The Radiology Assistant—educational web site of the Radiological Society of the Netherlands. Liver: Masses Part I: detection and characterization http://www.radiologyassistant.nl/en/446f010d8f420 Liver: Masses Part II: common liver tumors. http://www.radiologyassistant.nl/en/448eef3083354
5. Colagrande S, Centi N, Galdiero R, *et al.* Transient hepatic intensity differences: part 1, those associated with focal lesions. *AJR Am J Roentgenol* 2007; **188**: 154–9.
6. Konopke R, Bunk A, Kersting S. Contrast-enhanced ultrasonography in patients with colorectal liver metastases after chemotherapy. *Ultraschall Med* 2008; **29** (Suppl. 4): S203–9.
7. Figueras J, Planellas P, Albiol M, *et al.* [Role of intra-operative echography and computed tomography with multiple detectors in the surgery of hepatic metastases: a prospective study.] *Cir Esp* 2008; **83**: 134–8.
8. Nomura K, Kadoya M, Ueda K, *et al.* Detection of hepatic metastases from colorectal carcinoma: comparison of histopathologic features of anatomically resected liver with results of preoperative imaging. *J Clin Gastroenterol* 2007; **41**: 789–95.
9. Kim SJ, Lee JM, Lee JY, *et al.* Accuracy of preoperative T-staging of gallbladder carcinoma using MDCT. *AJR Am J Roentgenol* 2008; **190**: 74–80.

Chapter 9

Pancreatic tumours

Ben Miller, Ian Geh, and
Shuvro Roy-Choudhury

9.1 Clinical background

Ninety percent of primary pancreatic tumours are ductal adenocarcinomas, which
have a predilection for the head and neck and will be the main focus of discussion in
this chapter. Tumours of the islet cells are less common and are discussed separately
in Chapter 18.

9.2 Pancreatic adenocarcinoma

Pancreatic adenocarcinoma is a leading cause of cancer death with >7000 cases/year in
the UK. Peak incidence is between 60–80 years. The vast majority present at an advanced
stage, typical symptoms being painless jaundice, epigastric pain radiating to the back,
abdominal mass, and unexplained weight loss. Approximately 50% have evidence of
metastatic disease and a further 30% have unresectable locally advanced disease at
presentation. Of the 15–20% of patients who are suitable for curative resection (typically with a Whipple's procedure), the median survival remains poor at 15 months[1].
Radical R0 resection with negative margins offers the only realistic hope for cure. The
Whipple's procedure is associated with 1–5% mortality and 20% morbidity[2]. This
should only be performed if there is a reasonable probability of achieving R0 resection.
Therefore, accurate preoperative assessment to differentiate between surgical candidates from patients with incurable disease is of paramount importance[3].

9.2.1 Diagnosis and staging

9.2.1.1 Diagnosis

9.2.1.1.1 **Transabdominal ultrasound (TAUS)** TAUS is often the initial examination
but the retroperitoneal position of the pancreas can hinder thorough evaluation, as
part of the gland can be obscured by gas in the stomach or the transverse colon. The
role of TAUS is usually limited to confirming the presence of a mass lesion, diagnosing
a dilated biliary tree, exclusion of biliary cholelithiasis, and the detection of ascites and
hepatic metastases. This is a precursor to more sensitive and specific imaging modalities. These will usually be computed tomography (CT), magnetic resonance imaging
(MRI), and endoscopic ultrasound (EUS).

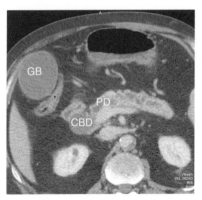

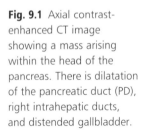

Fig. 9.1 Axial contrast-enhanced CT image showing a mass arising within the head of the pancreas. There is dilatation of the pancreatic duct (PD), right intrahepatic ducts, and distended gallbladder.

9.2.1.1.2 **CT** CT is the most commonly used diagnostic modality and new advances in its technology have widened the primary role of CT in pancreatic imaging. The advent of multidetector row CT (MDCT) has resulted in faster scanning times and improved spatial resolution. Software developments have allowed for greatly improved image manipulation, including three-dimensional (3D) surface rendering, particularly of blood vessels, maximum intensity projection (MIP), and curved multiplanar reformatting. A typical scanning protocol will use 1000mL oral water as negative intraluminal contrast with 100–150mL intravenous iodinated contrast injected at 4mL/s via a power injector. Thin (1–2mm) slices are obtained in both a pancreatic parenchymal phase (40s or using bolus tracking) and a later portal venous phase (70s) and are sent to a workstation for post processing. The main aim is to maximize the attenuation difference between the tumour and normal pancreas. Approximately 90% of tumours will be hypodense relative to surrounding the normal enhancing pancreas (Fig. 9.1). The late arterial pancreatic phase allows accurate detection of vascular involvement. An early arterial phase (20s) can be added if surgical planning of vascular anatomy is required and presented in 3D format.

A well-recognized sign of an obstructing pancreatic tumour is the classical 'double duct' sign where both the common bile and pancreatic ducts become obstructed and are dilated. In cases where the primary lesion cannot be seen, more subtle secondary signs are useful (Table 9.1). If the primary lesion cannot be identified on CT in the presence of these secondary signs, further evaluation with EUS or MRI is indicated (Fig. 9.2). Accuracy of CT in detecting pancreatic adenocarcinoma has improved from 62–91% in the helical CT era[4] to 85–100% in the MDCT era[5,6].

9.2.1.1.3 **MRI** MRI has an established role for evaluating biliary tree pathology at magnetic resonance cholangiopancreaticography (MRCP), but is less commonly used to diagnose pancreatic cancer. This is primarily due to the success of MDCT. Despite faster scanning times, advances in body coils and software developments, MR images are still susceptible to peristalsis and breathing motion artefacts. Claustrophobic patients do not tolerate MRI well and patients with certain implants, e.g. pacemakers, cannot be scanned. Nevertheless, with scrupulous technique, the intrinsic soft tissue contrast ability of MR does allow for excellent demonstration of lesions, and this is

Table 9.1 Secondary signs of a pancreatic tumour

Sign	Remark
Pancreatic duct cut-off	Subtle sign
Distal pancreatic atrophy	Subtle sign
Vascular occlusion	Look for development of collaterals
Pancreatic cortical deformity	Use gastroduodenal artery as a landmark
Double duct sign	Always abnormal but can also be seen in chronic pancreatitis

particularly useful where secondary signs are present but the primary lesion is not seen on CT. The duct penetration sign can be useful to differentiate between chronic pancreatitis and adenocarcinoma[7]. Studies have demonstrated diagnostic accuracies of 76–89%[8]. Use of T1 gradient-recalled echo (GRE) images with pancreas-specific contrast agent mangafodipir trisodium maximizes tumour–pancreas contrast and can detect 93–100% of tumours[9].

9.2.1.1.4 **EUS** EUS is sensitive for pancreatic lesions but is relatively non-specific. It is very operator dependent and its general availability in the UK is more limited. A lesion will typically appear as an irregular hypoechoic mass relative to the normal pancreatic tissue, but other causes such as pancreatitis and metastases can look similar. Nevertheless, accuracy rates for diagnosing tumours are higher than MDCT (97%), particularly for tumours <2cm in size[10]. A normal EUS can reliably exclude a tumour: in several studies negative predictive values of 100% have been reported[11]. When required, EUS-guided fine needle biopsy is the method of choice to obtain histological confirmation of malignancy. It has a lower risk of peritoneal seeding compared to other percutaneous approaches[12]. EUS-guided coeliac axis nerve block can be useful in the palliative setting[13].

9.2.1.1.5 **Endoscopic retrograde cholangiopancreatography (ERCP)** ERCP is often performed to palliate obstruction to the biliary tract by stenting. However the presence

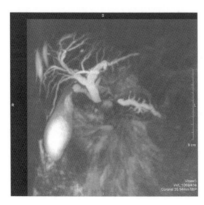

Fig. 9.2 MRCP image showing dilatation of both the common bile duct and the pancreatic duct due to a tumour.

of stents in the common bile duct and any post-procedural inflammation can hinder interpretation of subsequent staging imaging and ideally these should be performed prior to ERCP. Percutaneous biopsy should be avoided in potentially resectable cases but can be performed when palliative treatment options are being considered, including entry into clinical trials.

9.2.1.2 Staging

This is performed to assess for potential resectability of the primary tumour (locoregional stage) and to identify distant metastases (commonly peritoneum, liver, and lungs). The accepted standard for staging of pancreatic cancers is based on the TNM (tumour, node, metastasis) staging system[14] (Table 9.2).

9.2.1.2.1 **T Stage** Initial staging is with CT of the chest, abdomen, and pelvis. The accuracy of MDCT in staging and resectability ranges from 85–95% with an accuracy up to 90% to exclude unresectable disease[15]. T1 and T2 lesions are determined on the basis of size. Extension into the peripancreatic soft tissues indicates T3 disease and invasion

Table 9.2 TNM classification of pancreatic cancer. Staging defined according to the American Joint Committee on Cancer (AJCC) and the Union Internationale Contre le Cancer (UICC)

Primary tumour (T)	
Tx	Primary tumour cannot be assessed
T0	No evidence of primary tumour
Tis	Carcinoma in situ
T1	Tumour limited to the pancreas, 2 cm or less in greatest dimension
T2	Tumour limited to the pancreas, more than 2 cm in greatest dimension
T3	Tumour extends directly into any of the following: duodenum, bile duct, peripancreatic tissues
T4	Tumour extends directly into any of the following: stomach, spleen, colon, adjacent large vessels
Regional lymph nodes (N)	
Nx	Regional lymph nodes cannot be assessed
N0	No regional lymph node metastasis
N1	Regional lymph node metastasis
N1a	Metastasis in a single regional lymph node
N1b	Metastasis in multiple regional lymph nodes
Distant metastasis (M)	
Mx	Distant metastasis cannot be assessed
M0	No distant metastasis
M1	Distant metastasis

Table 9.3 Signs of irresectability in ductal pancreatic cancer[18,19]

Sign	Remark
Tumour size	Rarely is a tumour >4cm resectable
Arterial involvement	Disease apposed or surrounding SMA
Venous involvement (Tear drop sign)	Eccentric deformity of the SMV or portal vein. May not be a contraindication in some centres. Tumour often apposed rather than invading. A contact of >180° or >2cm or surface irregularity usually indicates invasion. Curved planar reformats very useful. Venous collaterals indicate invasion
Adjacent organ	Commonly stomach or liver. Duodenal involvement usually not a contraindication
Metastasis	Distant nodes, liver, or peritoneum

into the superior mesenteric artery (SMA) or coeliac axis indicates T4 disease. Because these tumours tend to spread early via the lymphatics, it is important to try to recognize subtle involvement of the peripancreatic tissue, as well as early peritoneal or perineural spread. A tumour's suitability for resection (Table 9.3) is determined by the absence of vascular invasion, spread to adjacent organs, distant metastatic disease, and ascites. In the past, catheter angiography was the only way of identifying vascular involvement but the use of new generation CT scanners with multiplanar capability has rendered this almost obsolete (Fig. 9.3).

Evidence of vascular invasion such as narrowing of vascular lumen, irregularity of wall, vessel encasement, the presence of collateral vessels and echogenic material within the lumen can also be seen on EUS[16]. The vessels most reliably assessed are the portal vein, splenic vein, and proximal superior mesenteric vein (SMV) with a reported negative predictive value of involvement of up to 90%[17]. However, most authors believe that MDCT is more reliable and accurate in excluding unresectable disease[20] with a reported accuracy for EUS around 77%[21].

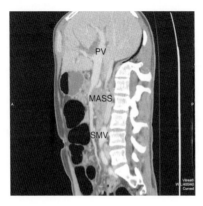

Fig. 9.3 CT curved planar reformat of the portal vein (PV) and superior mesenteric vein (SMV) in the sagittal plane. A tumour (MASS) arising from the pancreas is invading the superior mesenteric artery (not shown) and SMV.

9.2.1.2.2 **N stage** Lymph nodes are described in one of four groups according to location: 1) superior to the pancreatic head and body; 2) inferior to the head and body; 3) anterior, including anterior pancreaticoduodenal, pyloric, and proximal mesenteric nodes; and finally 4) posterior including posterior pancreaticoduodenal, common bile duct, and proximal mesenteric stations.

9.2.1.2.3 **M stage** Distant metastases in pancreatic cancer commonly occur in the liver, peritoneum, and lungs. Liver metastases generally appear as low attenuation, ill-defined lesions on CT and are solid on ultrasound. The presence of ascites is often a sign of peritoneal disease spread. Small tumour deposits on the peritoneum and liver surface will be subtle on imaging and requires a high index of suspicion, although modern thin-section CT show improved resolution for these.

The role of ^{18}F-fluorodeoxyglucose (FDG) PET/CT in routine staging of pancreatic cancer has not been defined. These imaging modalities can often provide complementary or alternative information, and to a large extent, local availability and radiologist expertise will decide which modality or combination of modalities is used[22].

9.3 Mucinous neoplasms of the pancreas

With the widespread use of CT and MRI in modern imaging, incidental cystic lesions within the pancreas are being detected with relative frequency. These are classified as mucinous cystic neoplasms (MCNs) and intraductal papillary mucinous neoplasm (IPMNs). Other benign cystic lesions include serous cystadenomas, pseudocyts, and epithelial cysts[23]. MCNs predominate in the body and tail of the pancreas and arise commonly in middle-aged females. They have an ovarian-type stroma secreting mucin and do not communicate with the pancreatic duct. The classic appearance of an MCN is of a unilocular or multilocular cystic lesion, each cyst >2cm in diameter, perhaps containing a solid or papillary nodule or exhibiting punctuate mural calcification. Serous cystadenomas, on the other hand, are usually located around the head, contains smaller cysts, and are less prone to turn malignant. IPMNs are slow growing tumours, subdivided into main duct type and side branch duct type. Side branch duct type is most commonly found in the pancreatic head, neck, and uncinate process, often appearing as a mass lesion on imaging. Main duct type IPMN has the higher risk of developing malignancy. Imaging appearances can often be very similar to those seen in chronic pancreatitis or other cystic lesions[24]. Features suggestive of IPMN include location in the head and uncinate process, communication with the main pancreatic duct, presence of solid components within the lesion[25], and bulging of the duodenal papilla with mucin secretion (Fig. 9.4). A recent study demonstrated accuracies for the diagnosis of IPMN of 76% for MDCT and 80% for MRCP[26].

Differentiation of MCN from the other cystic lesions is often not easy on CT, MRI, or US appearances alone. EUS however, is able to aid in this differentiation by enabling EUS fine needle aspiration, and obtaining fluid from these cystic lesions. This can be analysed for cytological malignancy, amylase content, and carcinoembyonic antigen (CEA) levels. Using this approach, a recent study demonstrated 100% sensitivity and 89% specificity for differentiating benign from malignant lesions[27].

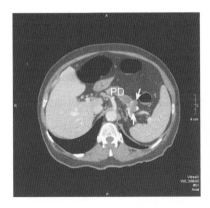

Fig. 9.4 Contrast-enhanced axial CT shows pancreatic duct dilatation along its length caused by an intraductal papillary mucinous tumour (arrows).

9.4 **Imaging for radiotherapy planning**

External beam radiotherapy can be used in pancreatic cancer as curative or as palliative intent. In the curative setting it is often combined with synchronous fluoropyrimidine-based chemotherapy (chemoradiotherapy or CRT) as a radiosensitizer and can be given as neoadjuvant (prior to surgery), definitive, or adjuvant (postoperative) treatment. Numerous randomized trials of radiotherapy in the above settings have either shown conflicting results or have been criticised for their design flaws[1,28–30]. Therefore, the role of radiotherapy for pancreatic cancer remains controversial and its use has not been incorporated into standard UK clinical practice. Intraoperative radiotherapy (IORT) has been used immediately following resection of the pancreas in an attempt to improve locoregional control but there have been no prospective trials (randomized or non-randomized) to establish its efficacy[31].

Treating pancreatic cancers with radiotherapy is technically challenging. Firstly, there are uncertainties in defining the extent of tumour and lymph node involvement and secondly, the radiation dose and volume are limited by the potential toxicity (acute and permanent) to the surrounding critical structures. The treatment delivered must take into account all these factors. For the purpose of radiotherapy planning, CT localization at 3–5-mm slice intervals with the patient immobilized (supine position, arms raised) is required. Intravenous contrast with or without opacification of the bowel will help to delineate the anatomy, particularly to distinguish bowel loops and vasculature from tumour and lymph nodes. Critical structures including liver, spinal cord, and both kidneys are outlined. The tumour and visible lymph nodes (gross tumour volume—GTV) are then identified and outlined, often with the help of a cross-sectional radiologist. A margin of 1.5–2.0cm is grown around the GTV and labelled as the planning target volume or PTV. This is to allow for microscopic spread of the tumour beyond CT resolution, organ movement, and daily variation of patient positioning. Taking into account the predefined dose constraints to the critical structures, a three- or four-field coplanar conformal plan is made and used to deliver radiotherapy.

In patients with incurable disease (unresectable locally advanced or distant metastases), radiotherapy may be given to the pancreas for palliation of pain or bleeding into the duodenum. Localization of the tumour should be performed using CT and treated with a 2–3-cm margin either using parallel opposed anterior and posterior fields or a three- to four-field plan. Painful bone and soft tissue metastatic disease can respond well to short courses of palliative radiotherapy.

9.5 **Therapeutic assessment and follow-up**

Follow-up of patients after surgical resection usually involves clinical assessment with or without tumour marker (CA19-9 and CEA) measurements. Further evaluation (usually with CT) is indicated if there is clinical suspicion of recurrent disease. Common sites of relapse include local and lymph node recurrence, peritoneal, liver, and lung metastases. The use of FDG-PET/CT scanning may be useful to distinguish recurrent disease from postoperative changes.

For selected patients who have completed definitive CRT for locally advanced unresectable pancreatic cancer, a reassessment CT may be performed at 4–8 weeks to document treatment response and to exclude metastatic disease. Curative resection may be considered in a small proportion of these patients as salvage for treatment failure.

9.6 **Summary**

♦ Ductal adenocarcinoma is the most common malignant pancreatic tumour and >80% are unresectable at diagnosis.

♦ MDCT is performed for staging and to determine resectability.

♦ EUS is useful for detecting small cancers not visible on CT and for obtaining histological confirmation of malignancy.

♦ There is no role for routine surveillance following curative treatment.

References

1. Neoptolemos JP, Dunn JA, Moffitt DD, *et al.* ESPAC-1 a European randomised controlled study of adjuvant chemoradiation and chemotherapy in resectable pancreatic cancer. *Lancet* 2001; **358**: 1576–85.

2. Alexakis N, Halloran C, Raraty M, *et al.* Current standards of surgery for pancreatic cancer. *Br J Surg* 2004; **91**: 1410–27.

3. Schima W, Ba-Ssalamah A, Kölblinger C, *et al.* Pancreatic adenocarcinoma. *Eur Radiol* 2007; **17**: 638–49.

4. Irie H, Honda H, Kaneko K, *et al.* Comparison of helical CT and MR imaging in detecting and staging small pancreatic adenocarcinoma. *Abdom Imaging* 1997; **22**: 429–33.

5. Grenacher L, Klauss M, Dukic L, *et al.* (2004). [Diagnosis and staging of pancreatic carcinoma: MRI versus multislice-CT – a prospective study.] *Rofo* 2004; **176**: 1624–33.

6. Klauss M, Mohr A, von Tengg-Kobligk H, *et al.* A new invasion score for determining the resectability of pancreatic carcinomas with contrast-enhanced multidetector computed tomography. *Pancreatology* 2008; **8**: 204–10.

7. Ichikawa T, Sou H, Araki T, *et al.* Duct-penetrating sign at MRCP: usefulness for differentiating inflammatory pancreatic mass from pancreatic carcinomas. *Radiology* 2001; **221**: 107–16.

8. Miller FH, Rini NJ, Keppke AL. MRI of adenocarcinoma of the pancreas. *AJR Am J Roentgenol* 2006; **187**: 365–74.

9. Schima W, Függer R, Schober E, *et al.* Diagnosis and staging of pancreatic cancer: comparison of mangafodipir trisodium-enhanced MR imaging and contrast-enhanced helical hydro-CT. *AJR Am J Roentgenol* 2002; **179**: 717–24.

10. DeWitt J, Devereaux B, Chriswell M, *et al.* Comparison of endoscopic ultrasonography and multidetector computed tomography for detecting and staging pancreatic cancer. *Ann Intern Med* 2004; **141**: 753–63.

11. Klapman JB, Chang KJ, Lee JG, *et al.* Negative predictive value of endoscopic ultrasound in a large series of patients with a clinical suspicion of pancreatic cancer. *Am J Gastroenterol* 2005; **100**: 2658–61.

12. Micames C, Jowell PS, White R, *et al.* Lower frequency of peritoneal carcinomatosis in patients with pancreatic cancer diagnosed by EUS-guided FNA vs. percutaneous FNA. *Gastrointest Endosc* 2003; **58**: 690–5.

13. Varadajulu S, Wallace MB. Applications of endoscopic ultrasonography in pancreatic cancer. *Cancer Control* 2004; **11**: 15–22.

15. Tamm EP, Loyer EM, Faria S, *et al.* Staging of pancreatic cancer with multidetector CT in the setting of preoperative chemoradiation therapy. *Abdom Imaging* 2006; **31**: 568–74.

16. Ahmad NA, Lewis JD, Ginsberg GG, *et al.* EUS in preoperative staging of pancreatic cancer. *Gastrointest Endosc* 2000; **52**: 463–8.

17. Rosch T, Dittler HJ, Strobel K, *et al.* Endoscopic ultrasound criteria for vascular invasion in the staging of cancer of the head of the pancreas: a blind reevaluation of videotapes. *Gastrointest Endosc* 2000; **52**: 469–77.

18. Lu DS, Reber HA, Krasny RM, *et al.* Local staging of pancreatic cancer: criteria for unresectability of major vessels as revealed by pancreatic phase thin section helical CT. *AJR Am J Roentgenol* 1997; **168**: 1439–43.

19. O'Malley ME, Boland GW, Wood BJ, *et al.* Adenocarcinoma of the head of the pancreas: determination of surgical unresectability with thin section pancreatic phase helical CT. *AJR Am J Roentgenol* 1999; **173**: 1513–18.

20. Bao PQ, Johnson JC, Lindsey EH, *et al.* Endoscopic ultrasound and computed tomography predictors of pancreatic cancer resectability. *J Gastrointest Surg* 2007; **12**: 10–16.

21. Long EE, Van Dam J, Weinstein S, *et al.* Computed tomography, endoscopic, laparoscopic, and intra-operative sonography for assessing resectability of pancreatic cancer. *Surg Oncol* 2005; **14**: 105–13.

22. Jeffrey RB. Pancreatic malignancy. In: Husband JE and Reznek RH (eds). *Imaging in oncology*, 2nd edn, pp.325–41. London: Taylor and Francis, 2004.

23. Planner AC, Anderson EM, Slater A, *et al.* An evidence based review for the management of cystic pancreatic lesions. *Clin Radiol* 2007; **62**: 930–7.

24. Megibow AJ. Pancreatic neoplasms. In: Gore and Levine (eds). *Textbook of Gastrointestinal Radiology*, pp.1915–31. Philadelphia, PA: Saunders, 2008.

25. Fukukura Y, Fujiyoshi F, Sasaki M, *et al.* Intraductal papillary mucinous tumours of the pancreas: thin section helical CT findings. *AJR Am J Roentgenol* 2000; **174**: 441–7.

26. Sahani DV, Kadavigere R, Blake M, *et al.* Intraductal papillary mucinous neoplasm of pancreas: multi-detector row CT with 2D reformations – correlation with MRCP. *Radiology* 2007; **238**: 560–9.

27. Rafique A, Freeman S, Carroll N. A clinical algorithm for the assessment of pancreatic lesions: utilization of 16- and 64-section multidetector CT and endoscopic ultrasound. *Clin Radiol* 2007; **62**: 1142–53.

28. Kalser MH, Ellenberg SS. Pancreatic cancer. Adjuvant combined radiation and chemotherapy following curative resection. *Arch Surg* 1986; **120**: 899–903. Erratum in: *Arch Surg* 1986; **121**: 1045.

29. Moertel CG, Frytak S, Hahn RG, *et al.* Therapy of locally unresectable pancreatic carcinoma: a randomized comparison of high dose (6000 rads) radiation alone, moderate dose radiation (4000 rads + 5-fluorouracil), and high dose radiation + 5-fluorouracil; The Gastrointestinal Tumor Study Group. *Cancer* 1981; **48**: 1705–10.

30. Neoptolemos JP, Stocken DD, Freiss H *et al.* A randomized trial of chemoradiotherapy and chemotherapy after resection of pancreatic cancer. *N Engl J Med* 2004; **350**: 1200–10.

31. Ruano-Ravina A, Almazan Ortega R, Guedea F. Intraoperative radiotherapy in pancreatic cancer: a systematic review. *Radiother Oncol* 2008; **87**: 318–25.

Chapter 10

Gastrointestinal stromal tumours

Brinder Mahon, Beatrice Seddon, and Ian Geh

10.1 Clinical background

Gastrointestinal stromal tumours (GISTs) are rare tumours arising from the same common mesenchymal stem cell precursor as the interstitial cells of Cajal, which are pacemaker cells of the autonomic nervous system, located within the wall of the gut and responsible for gastrointestinal (GI) tract peristalsis[1–3]. Although GISTs can arise from anywhere within the GI tract, the stomach is the most common site (50–60%), followed by the small intestine (20–30%). GIST is a relatively new disease entity characterized by activating mutations in the *c-kit* proto-oncogene (which encodes for the transmembrane glycoprotein KIT receptor CD117) in 90% of cases[4–6]. Prior to the widespread availability of detection of CD117 (KIT receptor) on tumour cells by immunohistochemistry[7], GISTs were often misdiagnosed as leiomyomas on histology, radiology, and endoscopy.

Small tumours (<2cm) are usually asymptomatic and may be encountered as incidental findings during upper GI endoscopy or surgery[8] (Fig. 10.1). These tumours can grow extraluminally to a large size without causing any symptoms and therefore the diagnosis is often made late in the pathological process[9]. In one study, the average size of tumours at presentation was 13cm[10]. Intraluminal tumours tend to present earlier and are hence smaller at presentation. The most commonly used algorithm divides patients into very low, low, intermediate, and high risk of recurrence according to the National Institute of Health workshop consensus[11] (Table 10.1).

10.2 Diagnosis and staging

10.2.1 Diagnosis

Small lesions appear as smooth, well-defined lesions with normal overlying mucosa at upper GI endoscopy. Further assessment with endoscopic ultrasound (EUS) is recommended, to assess whether the lesion is arising from within the smooth muscle wall, or is an indenting extraluminal mass (Fig. 10.2). EUS has been shown to be 100% specific in establishing this distinction, as compared with standard trans-abdominal ultrasound, which is less accurate[12].

In general, the spatial and contrast resolution of EUS is in the order of 100 times greater than MRI and about 10 times greater than CT. This advantage, combined with the ability to sample tissue deeper than can be obtained by endoscopy alone, makes EUS an essential diagnostic tool in characterizing submucosal lesions. The main

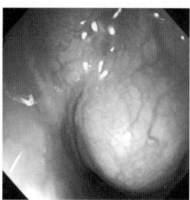

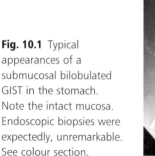

Fig. 10.1 Typical appearances of a submucosal bilobulated GIST in the stomach. Note the intact mucosa. Endoscopic biopsies were expectedly, unremarkable. See colour section.

limitation of EUS is operator variability, as it is a technique heavily dependent on training and experience.

The five layers of the gut wall can be clearly discriminated on EUS: the superficial mucosa, muscularis mucosa, submusosa, muscularis propria, and subserosa. The appreciation of a tumour arising from either of the two muscle layers (the second or the fourth layers) is the key to the diagnosis of GIST. Although GISTs are the commonest submucosal tumour, the differential diagnoses include aberrant pancreas, lipoma, neuroendocrine tumour, and intramural cyst. However, based on morphological appearance as well as the identification of gut wall layer of origin and location, the differential diagnosis can be narrowed down significantly.

When assessing the potential for aggressive behaviour of a GIST, size >4cm, anechoic spaces rather than a homogeneous appearance, and/or echogenic foci are between 80–100% sensitive[13]. However, aggressive behaviour cannot be excluded when these features are not present, and EUS-fine needle aspiration (EUS-FNA) may be performed to make a diagnosis. In two studies the accuracy of EUS-FNA has been shown to be 79% and 91%[14,15].

Table 10.1 National institute of health workshop consensus for assessing risk of malignancy of GISTs[11]

Risk	Size	Mitotic count
Very low	<2cm	<5 per 50 HPF
Low	2–5cm	<5 per 50 HPF
Intermediate	<5cm	6–10 per 50 HPF
	5–10cm	<5 per 50 HPF
High	5–10cm	>5 per 50 HPF
	>10cm	Any
	Any	>10 per 50 HPF

HPF, high-power fields.

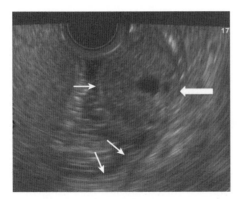

Fig. 10.2 EUS appearances of a typical GIST. Note the normal intact mucosa (small arrows). 2.5-cm GIST lesion arises from the first muscle layer (large arrow) and contains an anechoic space suggesting that this is a more aggressive lesion.

In larger primary tumours, the diagnosis may be suspected on cross-sectional imaging on the basis of site and morphological appearance. Although obtaining tissue via image-guided percutaneous biopsy is feasible in most cases, it is often not deemed necessary unless a non-surgical disease such as lymphoma is suspected, because patients will proceed directly to surgical resection on the basis of a radiological diagnosis. However, when disease is locally advanced or metastatic, tissue sampling is mandatory to confirm the diagnosis prior to commencing drug treatment with imatinib. The potential risk of tumour seeding in the abdominal wall biopsy tract is of concern, but remains unquantified. The safest technique to obtain a tissue diagnosis is via EUS-FNA as usually only a single tissue plain is crossed. However, for advanced or metastatic disease, EUS-FNA may not be feasible, and percutaneous biopsy is frequently utilized as potential tumour seeding is considered to be less relevant.

10.2.2 Staging

Complete surgical resection (R0) is considered to be the only curative treatment for GISTs. CT scanning is widely available and is used for detection, characterization, and staging of GISTs. The location, size, and extent of local invasion of adjacent structures by the primary tumour and the presence of distant disease, including liver and peritoneal metastases, can be detected.

Although MRI scanning can provide similar information to CT for locoregional assessment and detection of distant metastases, it is not commonly used for this indication. This is because separate body compartments need to be scanned independently, meaning that a significantly longer time is required for imaging. In addition, movement artefacts can occur in all but the most cooperative patients due to the long duration of image acquisition. However, there are some exceptions, which include the assessment of rectal and pelvic GISTs where MRI provides better tissue plane definition than CT, and for the characterization of liver lesions that are equivocal for metastatic disease on CT.

Functional imaging with ^{18}F-fluorodeoxyglucose (FDG) PET has become increasingly important in the assessment of GISTs[16,17]. Tumour cells preferentially take up FDG due to altered glucose metabolism. The degree of uptake appears to be related to the malignant potential of the tumours[18]. PET has been shown to be as sensitive as CT in the staging of patients with advanced and metastatic disease, prior to starting systemic therapy[19]. A small percentage of GISTs do not take up sufficient FDG and appear negative on PET, so-called FDG-negative tumours. More recently, PET has been combined with CT (PET/CT) to gain more accurate information on the exact location of the abnormal FDG uptake and also to evaluate FDG-negative tumours[20].

10.2.2.1 Locoregional stage

Small tumours measuring <2cm may not be visible on CT. Tumours <4cm usually appear as well-defined, rounded masses with regular margins. They may be polypoid or endoluminal and tend to enhance homogenously with intravenous contrast. Larger tumours appear as lobulated masses, which frequently grow exophytically from the bowel wall into the abdominal cavity, and may displace adjacent structures[21] (Fig. 10.3). With intravenous contrast they often enhance heterogeneously due to cystic degeneration, central liquefactive necrosis. Calcification, ulceration, and fistulation are usually associated with larger, more aggressive tumours[10,20,21]. Although these degenerative changes frequently occur in large tumours, they are occasionally seen in smaller lesions. Rare complications such as intussusception and intestinal obstruction can be readily diagnosed on CT. Despite the large size of many tumours at presentation, direct invasion of adjacent organs is relatively uncommon.

MRI features are similar to the CT appearances, with either homogeneous or heterogeneous enhancement following administration of gadolinium. Heterogeneous enhancement may be either patchy, intratumoural, or peripheral in appearance. On T1-weighted images, the tumour is usually of low signal intensity possibly with focal areas of slightly higher signal intensity corresponding to hemorrhagic areas. On T2-weighted images, high signal changes are seen in areas of viable tumour without haemorrhage or in areas of intratumoural necrosis. However none of these findings are specific for GISTs and can be seen in many other tumours.

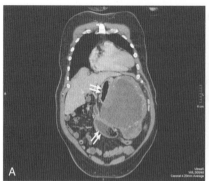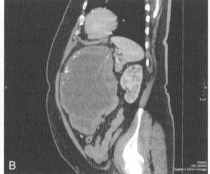

Fig. 10.3 Contrast-enhanced CT: coronal (A) and sagittal (B) images show a large well-defined GIST with small foci of calcification. The adjacent stomach (arrows; A) is displaced medially. In a large GIST, it can often be difficult to establish the site of origin on CT as many parts of the bowel can be in contact with the tumour.

10.2.2.2 Distant metastases

Approximately 50% of GISTs have metastasized by the time of diagnosis[22]. The liver is the most frequent site, followed by peritoneum. Liver metastases can have a variable appearance, although often appear as large necrotic lesions. On CT scan they usually appear hypervascular, and feeding arterial vessels may be identified on arterial phase imaging with a vascular blush or early washout seen on portal venous phase imaging, possibly with some retained peripheral enhancement. MRI can have an important role when assessing for liver metastases, as it is more sensitive than CT in this situation. With the recent advent of liver-specific contrast agents (Kupffer cell uptake agents and hepatobiliary specific agents), indeterminate liver lesions can be characterized with higher specificity. MRI is particularly used when there is uncertainty about the presence of liver metastases on CT.

Peritoneal metastases usually appear as multiple, smooth, rounded, and homogeneously-enhancing lesions of variable size. Lymph node involvement and complications such as organ obstruction are uncommon, even in advanced stages of the disease, but are all easily recognized on CT. Rare cases of lung and bone metastases have been described.

10.3 Imaging for radiotherapy planning

There is virtually no role for radiotherapy in the locoregional management of early stage GISTs, the management of which is surgical resection[24,25]. The management of widespread metastatic disease is with systemic therapy with imatinib, and usually radiotherapy will have no role. While painful soft tissue or bony metastases may be palliated with radiotherapy, these are a rare occurrence.

10.4 Post-surgical follow-up and therapeutic assessment

10.4.1 Follow-up after surgical resection

Small lesions <2cm are of very low metastatic potential and may be kept under surveillance. Annual EUS follow-up is probably advisable, although there is no clear evidence for the optimal interval and duration of reassessment. Lesions >2cm should be considered for resection, to provide a definitive histological diagnosis as well as important information on risk of future recurrence[11]. Following resection of a GIST, the optimal method of follow-up has yet to be defined by prospective studies, but should be based on risk stratification. Recurrent disease is usually asymptomatic for a long time until a significant burden of disease develops. Therefore routine imaging with CT is probably the only feasible investigation to detect early recurrent disease. The use of FDG PET/CT scanning for surveillance is limited by availability and cost issues. In addition, the patient is exposed to significantly higher radiation doses from PET/CT compared with CT alone.

The current UK guidelines[25] for the follow-up of resected GISTs are based on the Fletcher risk stratification criteria[11]. For very low-risk GISTs, no further follow up is required. Low-risk GISTs require a single CT of the abdomen and pelvis at 12 months. Intermediate-risk GISTs require a baseline CT at 3 months and follow-up CTs at 12, 24, 36, 48, and 60 months from resection. High-risk GISTs require a baseline CT at 3 months, then 6-monthly CTs for the first 3 years, and 12-monthly CTs to 5 years.

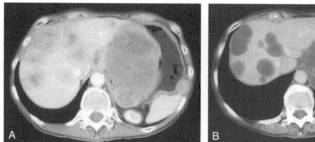
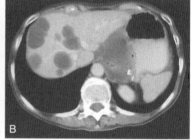

Fig. 10.4 Contrast-enhanced CT before (A) and following commencement of imatinib therapy (B). Responding liver metastases show a reduction in size and enhancement.

10.4.2 **Therapeutic assessment during treatment with tyrosine kinase inhibitors**

For patients receiving therapy with tyrosine kinase inhibitors, serial CT scans are used to monitor response to treatment. In the assessment of response, the radiologist and the oncologist need to be aware of a number of radiological pitfalls, which are unique to GISTs. The transition of tumours from heterogeneously enhancing masses to homogenous, low attenuation masses on contrasted CT is characteristic of tumour response[26] (Fig. 10.4). Reduction in both size and density is often seen in responding lesions (partial response), but equally, in many patients responding lesions do not change in size (stable disease), merely in density, and indeed paradoxical enlargement of the apparent disease due to necrosis or haemorrhage within the lesions may also be observed (pseudo-progressive disease). Therefore one must be wary of using conventional size criteria within response assessment tools such as RECIST (Response Evaluation Criteria In Solid Tumors)[27] to report treatment response in GISTs[28]. This may explain why when using RECIST, overall survival of patients with stable disease is identical to patients with partial response. Although partial and complete response rates as defined by RECIST do occur with imatinib therapy, in approximately 35% of patients, these responses can take a long time to achieve (median of 14 weeks)[29]. For this reason it is important that a patient's treatment is not terminated or altered prematurely if an initial reassessment CT at 3 months fails to show tumour shrinkage. A more recent set of treatment response criteria developed specifically for GISTs—the Choi criteria—which combine a decrease in tumour density as well as size, appear to correlate better with disease-specific survival[16]. However, response rates using the Choi criteria become more similar to those assessed by RECIST at 18 months of follow-up, as the presence of perforation, calcification, or haemorrhage makes density measurement more unreliable[30].

Another recognized pitfall in the radiological assessment of treatment response to tyrosine kinases is the development of apparently 'new' low-density liver lesions[31]. Prior to commencing treatment, small liver metastases may assume a similar density in the portal venous phase to normal surrounding liver tissue, and therefore may not be visible. These will appear as hyperdense (hypervascular) lesions on the arterial phase of

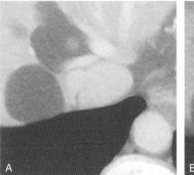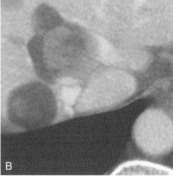

Fig. 10.5 Contrast-enhanced CT: disease progression is shown with development of a 'nodule within a mass'.

a contrast-enhanced CT. However as arterial phase imaging is not routinely acquired, hepatic metastases can be understaged. Following some weeks of imatinib therapy, these lesions undergo myxoid degeneration resulting in the appearance of apparently 'new' hypodense liver lesions. The clinician needs to be aware of this pitfall to avoid unnecessarily withdrawing or changing treatment on the basis of this pseudo-disease progression.

Following a period of response to imatinib therapy, which is on average 18–24 months, most patients will eventually develop disease resistance. This may occur as an initial area of localized progression when a small and often subtle nodule develops within a low-density metastasis which had previously responded and undergone myxoid degeneration (Fig. 10.5), the so-called 'nodule within a mass'[32]. As the diameter of the existing metastasis may not yet have increased in this situation, this situation would not be defined as disease progression using RECIST criteria.

The main utility of functional imaging (FDG PET or PET/CT) is in the follow-up of patients treated by tyrosine kinase inhibitors[16,17,33]. Because PET scanning is evaluating tumour metabolism over time, it is essential to obtain a baseline scan prior to initiating treatment. The subsequent lack of FDG uptake within the tumours is closely related to

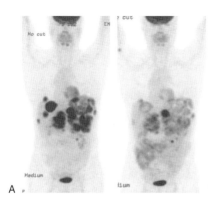

Fig. 10.6 FDG PET before (A) and after (B) commencement of imatinib therapy: liver and peritoneal metastases show a reduction in FDG uptake with treatment. Physiological bowel uptake is present (B).

the metabolic response to treatment and can be seen as early as 24 hours after treatment initiation[15,18,32] (Fig. 10.6). However, PET scanning may also allow early identification of patients with primary imatinib resistance, when a scan may show no decrease, or indeed even an early increase, in FGD uptake. When there is uncertainty concerning treatment response on CT scanning, the use of PET-CT may be useful to help differentiate active tumour from an inactive necrotic mass, and is more specific than with CT alone[19].

10.5 Summary

+ CT scanning is the mainstay for locoregional and metastatic staging, follow-up, and assessment of response to tyrosine kinase inhibitor treatment.

+ There are pitfalls in the radiological interpretation of response to imatinib therapy. Pseudo-progression with 'enlarging' lesions and 'new' liver lesions are well-recognized features of responding disease. Maximum tumour shrinkage may not be reached until, on average, 14 weeks of treatment. Absence of tumour shrinkage does not indicate treatment failure.

+ When disease response to tyrosine kinase treatment is uncertain, FDG PET or PET-CT may provide additional information in accurate determination of response.

References

1. Hirota S, Isozaki K, Moriyama Y, *et al*. Gain-of-function mutations of c-kit in human gastrointestinal stromal tumors. *Science* 1998; **279**: 577–80.

2. Kindblom LG, Remotti HE, Aldenborg F, *et al*. Gastrointestinal pacemaker cell tumor (GIPACT): gastrointestinal stromal tumors show phenotypic characteristics of the interstitial cells of Cajal. *Am J Pathol* 1998; **152**: 1259–69.

3. Sircar K, Hewlett BR, Huizinga JD, *et al*. Interstitial cells of Cajal as precursors of gastrointestinal stromal tumors. *Am J Surg Pathol* 1999; **23**: 377–89.

4. Rubin BP, Singer S, Tsao C, *et al*. KIT activation is a ubiquitous feature of gastrointestinal stromal tumors. *Cancer Res* 2001; **61**: 8118–21.

5. Heinrich MC, Corless CL, Demetri GD, *et al*. Kinase mutations and imatinib response in patients with metastatic gastrointestinal stromal tumor. *J Clin Oncol* 2003; **21**: 4342–9.

6. Debiec-Rychter M, Dumez H, Judson I, *et al*. Use of c-KIT/PDGFRA mutational analysis to predict the clinical response to imatinib in patients with advanced gastrointestinal stromal tumours entered on phase I and II studies of the EORTC Soft Tissue and Bone Sarcoma Group. *Eur J Cancer* 2004; **40**: 689–95.

7. Sarlamo-Rikala M, Kovatich AJ, Barusevicius A, *et al*. CD117: a sensitive marker for gastrointestinal stromal tumors that is more specific than CD34. *Mod Pathol* 1998; **11**: 728–34.

8. Miettinen M, Lasota J. Gastrointestinal stromal tumors: definition, clinical, histological, immunohistochemical, and molecular genetic features and differential diagnosis. *Virchows Arch* 2001; **438**: 1–12.

9. He LJ, Wang BS, Chen CC. Smooth muscle tumours of the digestive tract: report of 160 cases. *Br J Surg* 1998; **75**: 184–6.

10. Burkill GJ, Badran M, Al-Muderis O, *et al*. Malignant gastrointestinal stromal tumor: distribution, imaging features, and pattern of metastatic spread. *Radiology* 2003; **226**: 527–32.

11. Fletcher CD, Berman JJ, Corless C, *et al*. Diagnosis of gastrointestinal stromal tumors: a consensus approach (2002). *Hum Pathol* 2002; **33**: 459–65.

12. Motoo Y, Okai T, Ohta H, *et al*. Endoscopic ultrasonography in the diagnosis of extraluminal compression in gastric submucosal tumours. *Endoscopy* 1994; **26**: 239–42.

13. Chak A, Canto MI, Rosch T, *et al*. Endosonographic differentiation of benign and malignant stromal cell tumours. *Gastrointest Endosc* 1997; **45**: 468–73.

14. Okubo K, Yamao K, Nakamura T, *et al*. Endoscopic ultrasound fine-needle aspiration biopsy for the diagnosis of gastrointestinal stromal tumours in the stomach. *J Gastroenterol* 2004; **39**: 747–53.

15. Ando N, Goto H, Niwa Y *et al*. The diagnosis of GI stromal tumours in EUS-guided fine needle aspiration with immunohistochemical analysis. *Gastrointest Endosc* 2002; **52**: 37–43.

16. Choi H, Charnsangavej C, de Castro Faria S, *et al*. CT evaluation of the response of gastrointestinal stromal tumors after imatinib mesylate treatment: a quantitative analysis correlated with FDG PET findings. *AJR Am J Roentgenol* 2004; **183**: 1619–28.

17. Van den Abbeele AD, for the GIST Collaborative PET Study Group. F18-FDG- PET provides early evidence of biological response to STI571 in patients with malignant gastrointestinal stromal tumors. *Proc Am Soc Clin Oncol* 2001; **20**: 362a.

18. Yamada M, Niwa Y, Matsuura T, *et al*. Gastric GIST malignancy evaluated by 18FDG-PET as compared with EUS-FNA and endoscopic biopsy. *Scand J Gastroenterol* 2007; **42**: 633–41.

19. Gayed I, Vu T, Iyer R, *et al*. The role of 18F-FDG PET in staging and early prediction of response to therapy of recurrent gastrointestinal stromal tumors. *J Nucl Med* 2004; **45**, 17–21.

20. Goerres GW, Stupp R, Barghouth G. The value of PET, CT and in-line PET/ CT in patients with gastrointestinal stromal tumours: long term outcome of treatment with imatinib mesylate. *Eur J Nucl Med Mol Imaging* 2005; **32**: 153–62.

21. Lee CM, Chen HC, Leung TK, *et al*. Gastrointestinal stromal tumor: computed tomographic features. *World J Gastroenterol* 2004; **10**: 2417–18.

22. Levy AD, Remotti HE, Thompson WM, *et al*. Gastrointestinal stromal tumors: radiologic features with pathologic correlation. *Radiographics* 2003; **23**: 283–304.

23. Heinrich MC, Corless CL. Gastric GI stromal tumors (GISTs): the role of surgery in the era of targeted therapy. *J Surg Oncol* 2005; **90**: 195–207.

24. DeMatteo RP, Lewis JJ, Leung D, *et al*. Two hundred gastrointestinal stromal tumors: recurrence patterns and prognostic factors for survival. *Ann Surg* 2000; **231**: 51–8.

25. Reid R, Bulusu R, Buckels J, *et al*. *Guidelines for the management of gastrointesintal stromal tumours*. Novartis Pharmaceuticals UK Limited, October 2004.

26. Hong X, Choi H, Loyer EM, *et al*. Gastrointestinal stromal tumor: Role of CT in diagnosis and in response evaluation and surveillance after treatment with imatinib. *Radiographics* 2006; **26**: 481–95.

27. Benjamin RS, Choi H, Macapinlac HA, *et al*. We should desist using RECIST, at least in GIST. *J Clin Oncol* 2007; **25**: 1760–4.

28. Therasse P, Arbuck SG, Eisenhauer EA, *et al*. New guidelines to evaluate the response to treatment in solid tumors. European Organisation for Research and Treatment of Cancer, National Cancer Institute of the United States, National Cancer Institute of Canada. *J Intl Cancer Inst* 2000; **92**: 205–16.

29. Verweij J, Casali P, Zalcberg J, *et al*. Progression-free survival in gastrointestinal stromal tumours with high-dose imatinib: randomised trial. *Lancet* 2004; **364**: 1127–34.

30. Bulusu VR, Jephcott CR, Fawcett S, *et al.* RECIST and Choi criteria for response assessment (RA) in patients with inoperable and metastatic gastrointestinal stromal tumours (GISTs) on imatinib mesylate. Cambridge GIST study group experience. *J Clin Oncol* 2007; **25** (Suppl. 18): 10019.

31. Linton KM, Taylor MB, Radford JA. Response evaluation in gastrointestinal stromal tumours treated with imatinib: misdiagnosis of disease progression on CT due to cystic change in liver metastases. *Br J Radiol* 2006; **79**: 40–4.

32. Shankar S, van Sonnenberg E, Desai J, *et al.* Gastrointestinal stromal tumor: new nodule-within-a-mass pattern of recurrence after partial response to imatinib mesylate. *Radiology* 2005; **235**: 892–8.

33. Van den Abbeele A. The lessons of GIST - PET and PET/CT: a new paradigm for imaging. *Oncologist* 2008; **13** (Suppl. 2): 8–13.

Chapter 11

Rectal cancer

Vicky Goh and Rob Glynne-Jones

11.1 **Clinical background**

Rectal cancer is one of the commonest malignancies, with approximately 37500 new patients yearly in the UK[1]. Adenocarcinomas account for 98% of tumours, the remainder consist of squamous carcinomas, carcinoid, lymphoma, melanoma, and gastrointestinal stromal tumours. Peak incidence is in the fifth decade. Presentation includes rectal bleeding, change in bowel habit, frequency of defecation, tenesmus, rectal fullness, and pelvic pain. Distant spread occurs to the liver, lung, retroperitoneum, ovary, and peritoneal cavity.

Advances in surgical technique and more accurate radiotherapy planning and delivery have improved rectal cancer treatment in the past two decades. Anterior resection combined with total mesorectal excision (TME) has become the standard surgical procedure, facilitating the radial clearance of the primary tumour, mesorectal tissue, and associated vascular, lymphatic, and perineural deposits, thus improving local recurrence rates[2,3]. Abdomino-perineal resection has become reserved for the lowest rectal tumours when sphincter integrity cannot be preserved. In the UK preoperative radiotherapy (RT) or chemoradiotherapy (CRT) prior to surgery is standard care for locally advanced tumours[4].

Accurate staging is essential to ensure the correct therapeutic approach is undertaken. Imaging plays a pivotal role, defining which patients may benefit from radical surgery, selecting the most relevant surgical procedure, and identifying patients in whom a R0 resection is not possible with surgery alone, and for whom pre-operative RT or CRT may be appropriate.

11.2 **Diagnosis and staging**

11.2.1 **Diagnosis**

The diagnosis of rectal cancer is made typically by clinical examination, proctoscopy, fibreoptic endoscopy, and biopsy, although imaging has a role. Barium enema has been the commonest imaging investigation but computed tomography (CT) colonography is being applied increasingly for diagnosis. Its capability to reconstruct images into dynamic navigable three-dimensional views of the colon simulating fibreoptic colonoscopy has popularized the technique.

A systematic review has suggested that CT colonography has high average sensitivity and specificity for large and medium colorectal polyps (>10mm and 6–10mm respectively), and excellent sensitivity for cancer in the symptomatic population with >96% of cancers detected[5]. The most recent National Institute for Health and Clinical Excellence (NICE) guidance supports the use of CT colonography as an alternative to barium enema as a diagnostic test for symptomatic patients in the UK.

11.2.2 Staging

A clear understanding of the anatomy and pathway of spread is important for accurate disease assessment. The rectum extends over 12–14cm from the rectosigmoid junction down to the anorectal junction, enclosed within the mesorectum. The upper 3–4cm of the rectum is peritonealized on the anterior and lateral surface, but the vast majority of the rectum lies below the pelvic peritoneal reflection (Fig. 11.1). Once a tumour has penetrated through the muscularis propria, tumour growth can extend rapidly deep into perirectal fat. Below the supporting structures of the anus, tumour can extend into the ischiorectal fossa, a potential space around the anal canal and sphincter. Hence, there is a high risk of locoregional failure for low tumours.

Lymphatic drainage to regional nodes is dependent on site. Mid-upper rectal tumours drain to perirectal nodes and along the superior rectal vessels to the inferior mesenteric vessels. Low-mid rectal tumours drain to perirectal nodes and along mid rectal vessels to the internal iliac vessels. Most involved perirectal nodes within the mesorectum lie either at the level of, or within 5cm proximal to, the primary tumour[6]. Lateral pelvic lymph nodes (external iliac and obturator nodes) may be involved in 10–25% of patients with rectal cancer[7–10]. As lateral pelvic and internal iliac nodes are not removed with a standard TME, there is risk of local recurrence at these sites with surgery alone. Venous drainage of the upper rectum is via the superior rectal vein to the inferior mesenteric vein and portal system, while drainage of the mid and lower

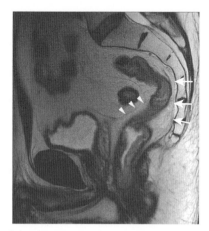

Fig. 11.1 Sagittal T2-weighted MR image demonstrating the rectum enclosed within the mesorectum extending from S3 to the level of the levator plate. Anteriorly the peritonealized surface of the upper rectum can be identified (arrowheads). Posteriorly the mesorectal fascia and presacral aponeurosis can be identified (arrow).

Table 11.1 TNM and Dukes' staging of rectal cancer

TNM classification		Dukes' classification	
T1	Tumour involves submucosa	A	Tumour confined to bowel wall
T2	Tumour involves muscularis propria		
T3	Tumour beyond the mucularis propria	B	Tumour penetrates bowel wall
T4	Tumour directly invades other organs or structures		
N0	No regional lymphadenopathy		
N1	Up to 3 regional nodes involved	C	Regional lymph nodes involved
N2	4 or more regional nodes involved		
M0	No distant metastases		
M1	Distant metastases	D	Distant metastases

rectum is to the iliac veins and inferior vena cava, thus metastases can develop either in the liver or lungs depending on tumour site.

Accurate staging is essential for defining the most appropriate treatment strategy. Commonly used classifications are the American Joint Committee on Cancer (AJCC)/ Union Internationale Contre le Cancer (UICC) TNM (tumour, node, metastasis), Dukes', or clinical stage classification (Tables 11.1 and 11.2). The distance of tumour to the CRM is also a prognostic factor for overall 5-year survival[11]. Patients with tumours that extend to within a small distance of the mesorectal fascia (e.g. 1mm), that lie outside the mesorectum, or that extend inferiorly to the anorectal junction should be offered adjuvant RT.

Magnetic resonance imaging (MRI) provides excellent depiction of the relationship of tumour and nodes to the potential surgical circumferential resection margin (CRM) (Fig. 11.2). T-staging accuracies ranging from 71–91% have been reported although differentiation between T2 and early T3 tumours may be challenging due to desmoplasia and microscopic disease. Recently MRI has been validated prospectively in a large European multicentre study (MERCURY)[12]: an accuracy of 87% and specificity of 92% in predicting a clear circumferential resection margin was reported.

Table 11.2 Clinical stage classification of rectal cancer

Stage	Description	Location from anorectal junction
I	Mobile: movable in all directions	>6cm
II	Partially fixed: movable in at least one direction (cephalocaudad or lateral)	3–6cm
III	Fixed: immovable due to fixation, perforation or deep ulceration	0–3cm
IV	Frozen pelvis: invasion of pelvic sidewall or sacrum	<0cm; into anal canal

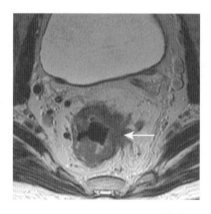

Fig. 11.2 Transaxial T2-weighted MR image showing a T3 rectal cancer extending beyond the hypointense muscularis propria layer into the mesorectal fat with evidence of macroscopic vascular invasion (arrow).

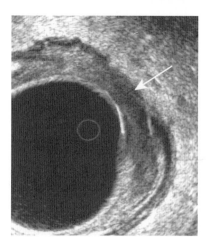

Fig. 11.3 Transrectal US image showing a T2 rectal tumour confined to the muscularis propria (arrow).

Nevertheless transrectal ultrasound (TRUS) is preferred for small early tumours (T1N0 or T2N0; <3cm; within 8cm of anal verge) to assess if local excision is appropriate. Infiltration of the rectal wall layers by tumour is well demonstrated (Fig. 11.3). However, T2 tumours may be overstaged due to peritumoural inflammation[13] and the technique is inferior to MRI for depiction of the potential surgical CRM due to its limited field of view. A recent meta-analysis examining the accuracy of TRUS, MRI, and CT for local staging has suggested that TRUS has better diagnostic accuracy for perirectal tissue invasion than CT or MRI with sensitivities of 90% vs. 79% and 82%, but comparable accuracy for invasion of adjacent organs (sensitivities of 70–74%)[14].

Reliable detection of nodal involvement remains a challenge for imaging. The majority of histologically involved lymph nodes are <5mm and will not raise suspicion on size criteria alone[15]. Furthermore, many involved nodes are <3mm and may not be seen on imaging. Accuracies varying from 62–83% have been reported for TRUS while accuracies varying from 39–95% have been reported for MRI. The use of morphological appearances in addition to size may improve specificity, e.g. mixed signal intensity and an irregular nodal border.

MR lymphangiography with ultrasmall superparamagnetic iron oxide particles (USPIO) may improve detection of nodal metastases in clinical practice in the future. However, it should be borne in mind that even USPIO administration will be useless if involved nodes are too small to be imaged in the first place. During radiotherapy planning the position of these potentially involved nodes can be estimated from their projected proximity to major vessels[16,17]. MR lymphangiography involves imaging prior to intravenous infusion of USPIO and re-imaging 24 hours later. Following infusion these particles pass into the interstitial space and drain via the lymphatics to regional lymph nodes where they are taken up by macrophages. The susceptibility effect of the iron oxide particles causes a reduction in MR signal intensity on susceptibility-weighted sequences (T2* weighting): metastatic nodes maintain a uniform or eccentric bright signal while normal nodes darken by 24 hours (Fig. 11.4). Preliminary study in rectal cancer has shown promise but findings have yet to be validated with larger studies[18].

CT is the preferred imaging modality for distant staging as metastatic disease can be readily depicted. It is superior to hepatic US for detecting hepatic metastatic disease with sensitivities of 70–90% versus 35–75% but has similar specificity (>90%)[19–21]. There may be a role for ^{18}F-fluorodeoxyglucose positron emission tomography (FDG PET)/CT as the technique is more sensitive than CT for detection of distant metastatic disease[22,23] (Fig. 11.5). However, to date FDG PET/CT has not been shown to be superior to conventional imaging for nodal staging with sensitivity of only 29%[24,25].

11.3 **Imaging for radiotherapy**

Three approaches are commonly employed: 1) short-course preoperative RT; 2) long-course preoperative CRT; and 3) postoperative CRT. A preoperative approach reduces the risk of tumour seeding, increases the likelihood of a R0 resection, and has less acute toxicity and enhanced radiosensitivity due to better oxygenated cells, and is favoured in the UK.

The radiation fields have to encompass the gross tumour in terms of primary and discontinuous spread, the lymph nodes that are suspected of being involved, and

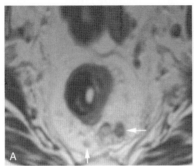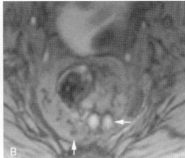

Fig. 11.4 T2-weighted axial MR image showing a normal node before (A) and T2*-weighted axial MR image 24 hours (B) after administration of USPIO. Normal nodes become homogenously darker due to the susceptibility effect of iron oxide (arrow). Nodes containing metastases remain bright (arrow).

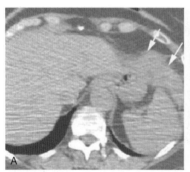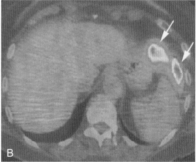

Fig. 11.5 FDG PET/CT image demonstrating uptake in a peritoneal metastasis. See colour section.

potential areas of microscopic spread. In the past, standardized radiation fields were based on patterns of locoregional relapse documented in historical series[5] predating the widespread use of TME. The conventional reference points for two standardized fields for upper and low rectum have been the bony landmarks within the pelvis (particularly the sacrum) but these fields would be considered excessively large nowadays.

The fields used currently are based on fields used in previous and current phase III trials; patterns of spread and local failure. However, different philosophies towards radiation field size remain.

11.3.1 **Treatment planning**

Different approaches to planning are employed in practice. The standard approach uses the bony pelvis to define the fields, the lateral field border lying 1cm outside the lateral bony pelvis, the posterior field border encompassing the entire sacrum, the superior border by the sacral promontory, anterior border 2–3cm anterior to the sacral promontory, and inferior border 2–3cm distal to the inferior margin of the primary tumour. These large fields do not attempt to individualize radiotherapy planning, but were useful for conformity in the context of large randomized trials. Most radiation oncologists now agree that conventional fields placed at simulation according to the bony anatomy are inferior to those derived from CT planning[26]. Individualized CT planning enhances coverage particularly on the anterior aspect which is most marked for tumours in the low rectum.

The individualized planning CT is performed from the superior aspect of L5 to 2cm beyond the anal marker to cover the entire pelvis. Images of 3mm slice thickness or less are acquired. Oral contrast (dilute gastrograffin or barium) to opacify the bowel, and intravenous contrast to highlight vessels such as the superior rectal artery, internal and external iliac arteries, and also the ureters

The CT-based volume approach (Fig. 11.6) marks areas of macroscopic tumour (gross target volume, GTV), and adds anatomical areas of potential tumour spread (nodes, mesorectum, and ischiorectal fossa) to form a *clinical target volume* (CTV). The relevant groups of lymph nodes, which should be included in the CTV depend on whether the local tumour site is in the upper middle or lower rectum, whether the tumour is circumferential, and whether the stage and grade indicate a significant risk of

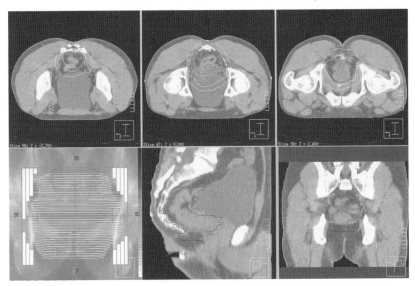

Fig. 11.6 Planning CT demonstrating definition of GTV, CTV expanded, CTV2, and PTV for a mid rectal cancer from its superior to inferior aspect. See colour section.

microscopic nodal metastases. The expanded GTV and CTV are combined with agreed margins added in all directions subsequently to convert the volume to a *planning target volume* (PTV) to account for the systematic and random set up errors.

Preliminary study using MR lymphangiography to map out lymph node pathways in patients with gynaecological malignancies has suggested that a 7-mm margin around pelvic vessels offers a good surrogate target for pelvic nodes[17]. In the future, MR lymphangiography using USPIO may have a role on an individual patient basis particularly in the context of IMRT.

11.4 **Therapeutic assessment and follow-up**

11.4.1 **Therapeutic assessment**

Imaging is performed typically 4–6 weeks following the completion of RT to assess therapeutic response. MRI is used most commonly to demonstrate tumour shrinkage and regression from the potential surgical CRM and nodal downstaging[27]. However, the presence of diffuse wall thickening and blurring of wall layers following RT may reduce T-staging accuracy. Small studies using PET have demonstrated a decrease in flurodeoxyglucose uptake following chemoradiation, which may predict for long term outcome[28–30]. Dynamic contrast-enhanced MRI[31,32] and dynamic contrast-enhanced CT (also known as perfusion CT)[33,34] which provide surrogate assessment of angiogenesis have also shown a decrease in vascularity following radiotherapy. Diffusion-weighted MRI which provides a surrogate measure of tumour cellularity has demonstrated an increase in apparent diffusion coefficient (ADC) following chemo-radiation suggesting a decrease in cellularity with treatment[35].

11.4.2 **Surveillance**

There has been debate over the best approach for surveillance. An American Society of Clinical Oncology (ASCO) expert panel convened in 1999 to develop evidence-based guidelines concluded that periodic clinical evaluation with carcinoembryonic antigen (CEA) and colonoscopy were justifiable but other testing added little benefit[36]. Randomized trials of more intensive versus less intensive strategies have been difficult to conduct. Trials mainly from the 1990s[37–40] have included colon and rectal cancers, a range of stages from early to advanced, less well-defined indications for adjuvant therapy, and differing frequency and content of screening for intensive and less intensive groups. Results from these studies have suggested that the number of recurrences is similar for either group but are detected earlier with more intensive surveillance. The impact on overall 5-year survival is less clear with only two studies showing a significant improvement in overall survival with intensive surveillance; a more recent study (clinical examination and blood tests + abdominal CT (or ultrasound), chest plain film, and colonoscopy versus clinical examination and blood tests only) again has shown no survival difference[41]. A meta-analysis has suggested that CT every 3–12 months may provide a survival benefit. In practice, yearly body CT scans are commonly performed for surveillance for at least 3 years in the United Kingdom but clearly further clarification is needed.

11.5 **Summary**

- ◆ MRI is the modality of choice for assessing primary tumour extent and potential resectability. TRUS is preferred for early (T1/T2) tumours.
- ◆ CT is advocated for staging metastatic disease; however FDG PET/CT is more sensitive and may play a greater role in the future, particularly if surgical excision of metastases is being considered.
- ◆ RT planning performed using CT has limitations that CT/MRI fusion, PET/CT, or MRI planning may overcome, but these techniques require further study and clinical validation.
- ◆ MRI is the preferred modality for therapeutic assessment typically at 4–6 weeks following completion of RT.
- ◆ Debate continues as to the optimum method for surveillance. Yearly body CT is advocated. PET/CT is a sensitive alternative but has the disadvantage of being more expensive, and imposes a higher radiation. MRI is preferred for suspected pelvic recurrence.

References

1. Statistics from Cancer Research UK available at http://info.cancerresearchuk.org/cancerstats
2. Heald RJ, Ryall RDH. Recurrence and survival after total mesorectal excision for rectal cancer. *Lancet* 1986; **1**: 1479–12.
3. Heald RJ. Total mesorectal excision is optimal surgery for rectal cancer: a Scandinavian consensus. *Br J Surg* 1995; **82**: 1297–9.
4. Swedish rectal cancer trial. Improved survival with preoperative radiotherapy in resectable rectal cancer. *N Engl J Med* 1997; **336**: 980–7.

5. Halligan S, Altman DG, Taylor SA, *et al.* CT colonography in the detection of colorectal polyps and cancer: systematic review, meta-analysis and proposed minimum dataset for study level reporting. *Radiology* 2005; **237**: 893–904.

6. Koh DM, Brown G, Temple L, *et al.* Distribution of lymph nodes in rectal cancer: in vivo MR imaging compared with histopathological examination. Initial observations. *Eur Radiol* 2005; **15**: 1650–7.

7. Takahashi T, Ueno M, Azekura K. Lateral node dissection and total mesorectal excision for rectal cancer. *Dis Colon Rectum* 2000; **43**: S59–68.

8. Ueno H, Mochizuki H, Hashifuchi Y, *et al.* Prognostic determinants of patients with lateral node involvement by rectal cancer. *Ann Surg* 2001; **234**: 190–7.

9. Hida J, Yasutomi M, Fujimoto K, *et al.* Does lateral lymph node dissection improve survival in rectal carcinoma? Examination of node metastases by the clearing method. *J Am Coll Surg* 1997; **184**: 475–80.

10. Nagawa H, Muto T, Sunouchi K, *et al.* Randomized controlled trial of lateral node dissection vs. nerve–preserving resection in patients with rectal cancer after preoperative radiotherapy. *Dis Colon Rectum* 2001; **44**: 312–18.

11. Birbeck KF, Macklin CP, Tiffin NJ. Rates of circumferential resection margin involvement vary between surgeons and predict outcomes in rectal cancer surgery. *Ann Surg* 2002; **235**: 449–57.

12. Mercury study group. Diagnostic accuracy of preoperative magnetic resonance imaging in predicting curative resection of rectal cancer: prospective observational study. *BMJ* 2006; **333**: 779–84.

13. Maier AG, Barton PP, Neuhold NR, *et al.* Peritumoral tissue reaction at transrectal ultrasound as a possible cause of overstaging: histopathological correlation. *Radiology* 1997; **203**: 785–9.

14. Bipat S, Glas AS, Slors FJM, *et al.* Rectal cancer: Local staging and assessment of lymph node involvement with endoluminal US, CT and MR imaging-a meta-analysis. *Radiology* 2004; **232**: 773–83.

15. Zheng Y-C, Zhou Z-G, Li L, *et al.*, Distribution and patterns of lymph nodes metastases and micrometastases in the mesorectum of rectal cancer. *J Surg Oncol* 2007; **96**: 213–19.

16. Chao KS, Lin M. Lymphangiogram-assisted lymph node target delineation for patients with gynecologic malignancies. *Int J Radiat Oncol Biol Phys* 2002; **54**: 1147–52.

17. Taylor A, Rockall AG, Reznek RH, *et al.* Mapping pelvic lymph nodes: guidelines for delineation in intensity-modulated radiotherapy. *Int J Radiat Oncol Biol Phys* 2005; **63**: 1604–12.

18. Koh DM, Brown G, Temple L, *et al.* Rectal cancer: mesorectal lymph nodes at MR imaging with USPIO versus histopathologic findings – initial observations. *Radiology* 2004; **231**: 91–9.

19. Charnley RM, Morris DL, Dennison AR, *et al.* Detection of colorectal liver metastases using intraoperative ultrasonography. *Br J Surg* 1991; **78**: 45–8.

20. Carter R, Hemingway D, Cooke TG, *et al.* A prospective study of six methods for detection of hepatic colorectal metastases. *Ann R Coll Surg Engl* 1996; **78**: 27–30.

21. Leen E, Angerson WJ, Wotherspoon H, *et al.* Detection of colorectal liver metastases: comparison of laparotomy, CT, US, and Doppler perfusion index and evaluation of post-operative follow-up results. *Radiology* 1995; **195**: 113–16.

22. Park IJ, Kim HC, Yu CS, *et al.* Efficacy of PET/CT in the accurate evaluation of primary colorectal carcinoma. *Eur J Surg Oncol* 2006; **32**: 941–7.

23. Gearhart SL, Frassica D, Rosen R, *et al.* Improved staging with pretreatment positron emission tomography/computed tomography in low rectal cancer. *Ann Surg Oncol* 2006; **13**: 397–404.

24. Kantarova I, Lipska L, Belohlavek O, *et al.* Routine 18F-FDG PET preoperative staging of colorectal cancer: comparison with conventional staging and its impact on treatment decision making. *J Nucl Med* 2003; **44**: 1784–8.

25. Abdel-Nabi H, Doerr RJ, Lamonica DM, *et al.* Staging of primary colorectal carcinomas with fluorine-18 fluorodeoxyglucose whole-body PET: correlation with histopathologic and CT findings. *Radiology* 1998; **206**: 755–60.

26. Gopaul D, Richer J, Powers KK, *et al.* Evaluation of CT planning versus conventional simulation for preoperative treatment of rectal cancer. *Radiother Oncol* 2007; **84** (Suppl. 2): S66 (abstract 230).

27. Allen SD, Padhani AR, Dzik-Jurasz AS, *et al.* Rectal carcinoma: MRI with histologic correlation before and after chemoradiation therapy. *AJR Am J Roentgenol* 2007; **188**: 442–51.

28. Konski A, Hoffman J, Sigurdson E, *et al.* Can molecular imaging predict response to preoperative chemoradiation in patients with rectal cancer? A Fox Chase Cancer Center prospective experience. *Semin Oncol* 2005; **32**: S63–7.

29. Guillem JG, Moore HG, Akhurst T, *et al.* Sequential preoperative fluorodeoxyglucose-positron emission tomography assessment of response to preoperative chemoradiation: a means for determining long term outcomes of rectal cancer. *J Am Coll Surg* 2004; **199**: 1–7.

30. Kalff V, Duong C, Drummond EG, *et al.* Findings on 18F-FDG PET scans after neoadjuvant chemoradiation provides prognostic stratification in patients with locally advanced rectal carcinoma subsequently treated by radical surgery. *J Nucl Med* 2006; **47**: 14–22.

31. De Vries A, Griebel J, Kremser C, *et al.* Monitoring of tumor microcirculation during fractionated radiation therapy in patients with rectal carcinoma: preliminary results and implications for therapy. *Radiology* 2000; **217**: 385–91.

32. DeVries AF, Griebel J, Kremser C, *et al.* Tumor microcirculation evaluated by dynamic contrast enhanced magnetic resonance imaging predicts therapy outcome for primary rectal carcinoma. *Cancer Res* 2001; **61**: 2513–16.

33. Sahani DV, Kalva SP, Hamberg LM, *et al.* Assessing tumor perfusion and treatment response in rectal cancer with multisection CT: initial observations. *Radiology* 2005; **234**: 785–92.

34. Bellomi M, Petralia G, Sonzogni A, *et al.* CT perfusion for the monitoring of neo-adjuvant chemoradiation therapy in rectal carcinoma. *Radiology* 2007; **244**: 486–93.

35. Dzik-Jurasz A, Domenig C, George M, *et al.* Diffusion MRI for prediction of response of rectal cancer to chemoradiation. *Lancet* 2002; **360**: 307–8.

36. Desch CE, Benson AB 3rd, Smith TJ, *et al.* Recommended colorectal cancer surveillance guidelines by the American Society of Clinical Oncology. *J Clin Oncol* 1999; **17**: 1312.

37. Pietra N, Sarli L, Costi R, *et al.* Role of follow-up in management of local recurrences of colorectal cancer: a prospective randomized trial. *Dis Colon Rectum* 1998; **41**: 1127–33.

38. Kjeldsen BJ, Kronborg O, Fenger C, *et al.* A prospective randomized study of follow-up after radical surgery for colorectal cancer. *Br J Surg* 1997; **84**: 666–9.

39. Ohlsson B, Breland U, Ekberg H, *et al.* Follow-up after curative surgery for colorectal carcinoma. Randomized comparison with no follow-up. *Dis Colon Rectum* 1995; **38**: 619–26.

40. Mäkelä JT, Latinen SO, Kairaluoma MI. Five-year follow up after radical surgery for colorectal cancer: results of a prospective randomized trial. *Arch Surg* 1995; **130**: 1062–7.

41. Rodriguez-Moranta F, Salo J, Arcusa A, *et al.* Postoperative surveillance in patients with colorectal cancer who have undergone curative resection: a prospective, multicenter, randomized, controlled trial. *J Clin Oncol* 2006; **24**: 386–93.

Chapter 12

Anal cancer

Vicky Goh and Rob Glynne-Jones

12.1 Clinical background

Anal cancer is rare, representing only 1.5% of lower gastrointestinal tract malignancies[1], but its incidence is increasing. Anal canal tumours constitute 75% of cancers. Squamous cell carcinomas are the commonest type, the remainder consist of adenocarcinomas, neuroendocrine tumours, undifferentiated carcinomas, melanomas, gastrointestinal stromal tumours, and lymphomas.

Peak incidence is in the sixth decade of life. The pathogenesis is multifactorial. Sexually transmitted viruses, cigarette smoking, chronic inflammation, immunosuppression, and genetic susceptibility have been implicated. Patients with anal cancer are more likely to have had a previous malignancy and more likely to develop a further malignancy (e.g. lung, bladder, vulva, vagina, or breast). Small early cancers may cause few symptoms, and are sometimes diagnosed serendipitously with the removal of anal tags. More advanced lesions present as non-healing ulcers, perineal pain, sensation of a mass, rectal bleeding, itching, discharge, and faecal incontinence. Tumours may be diagnosed concomitantly with a benign anal condition such as haemorrhoids, anal fissure or fistula.

Anal cancer is predominantly a locoregional disease; metastases are relatively rare. Less than 10% of patients have disease outside the pelvis at presentation; <20% of patients will have distant relapse following 'curative' treatment. The risk of distant metastases increases with T stage and number of regional nodes involved, and may be higher in basaloid histology. Definitive chemoradiation (RT with concomitant 5-fluorouracil and mitomycin C) with curative intent has replaced abdomino-perineal resection (APR) as the standard of care and offers survival rates similar to surgical approaches, but with preserved sphincter function[2-4]. Nevertheless small tumours of the anal margin (<2cm) may be treated with surgery if there is no canal involvement and a strong likelihood of a clear resection margin.

12.2 Diagnosis and staging

Diagnosis is made typically by clinical examination, proctoscopy, and biopsy. Direct proctoscopy is often difficult in more advanced lesions because of pain; patients then undergo examination under anaesthetic (EUA) and biopsy. Digital rectal examination (DRE) remains a valuable method for staging disease extent; nevertheless imaging is being used increasingly as it provides information such as tumour length, degree of circumferential extent, involvement of adjacent structures, and extension above the dentate line and below the anal margin. Magnetic resonance imaging (MRI) is the imaging modality of choice to assess locoregional disease extent although transrectal ultrasound (TRUS) and computed tomography (CT) continue to provide useful information. CT of the thorax and abdomen is preferred to a chest radiograph and liver US for assessing metastatic disease due to its higher sensitivity.

More recently 18-F fluorodeoxyglucose positron emission tomography/CT (FDG PET/CT) has been advocated for staging[5] as positive lymph nodes in the pelvis and inguinal regions may be identified more easily than with other imaging modalities. PET offers high sensitivity[6,7], and high specificity in immunocompetent patients with anal cancer[6-8]. However, HIV (human immunodeficiency virus) patients appear to have a higher incidence of PET-positive inguinal nodes (44% vs. 16%). More accurate staging of lymph nodes is important as treatment is potentially influenced in terms of the radiation fields and the need for a boost to these sites. FDG PET/CT is also recommended by some authors for target definition and delineation of the primary tumour.

Staging is based on the TNM (tumour, node, metastasis) classification (Table 12.1). Because few cancers are resected surgically this classification is based on clinical factors such as tumour size (assessed by clinical examination and imaging studies). This is applicable to all carcinomas arising from the canal apart from melanoma. Nodal status is based on distance from the primary site rather than the number of nodes involved, as this has more prognostic significance, and it should be noted that the definition is different for cancers in the anal canal and margin.

Table 12.1 TNM classification and stage grouping of anal cancer

Stage	T*	N+	M
0	T_{is}	N0	M0
I	T1	N0	M0
II	T2	N0	M0
	T3	N0	M0
IIIA	T1	N1	M0
	T2	N1	M0
	T3	N1	M0
	T4	N0	M0
IIIB	T4	N1	M0
	Any	N2	M0
	Any	N3	M0
IV	Any	Any	M1

*Tumour stages: Tis, carcinoma in situ; T1, <2cm; T2, 2–5cm; T3, >5cm; T4, invading adjacent organs but not anal sphincter.
+Nodal stages: N0, no regional nodes; N1, preirectal nodes; N2, unilateral internal iliac or inguinal nodes; N3, perirectal and inguinal, or bilateral internal iliac, or bilaieral inguinal nodes.

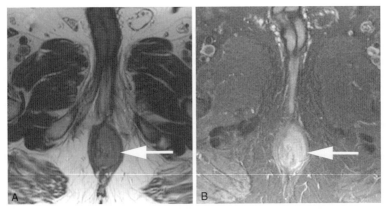

Fig. 12.1 T2W (A) and STIR (B) axial MR images demonstrating the intermediate to high signal squamous carcinoma in the mid canal.

There are few imaging data of staging accuracy as there is the lack of gold standard histopathological correlation given that definitive chemoradiation is the standard of care. MRI provides good contrast resolution and multiplanar anatomical detail. The anal canal surrounding structures and pelvic nodes are well demonstrated. The intermediate to high signal intensity tumour is well delineated on T2 and STIR-weighted sequences (Fig. 12.1) as is primary tumour extension into surrounding structures, e.g. anterior urogenital triangle[9]. TRUS provides excellent detail of the anal canal (Fig. 12.2) and may demonstrate tumour infiltration through the layers of the anal canal wall[10] but is inferior to MRI for assessing invasion of adjacent structures and nodal involvement because of its restricted field of view.

Contrast enhanced CT is inferior to MRI for depicting the primary tumour due to its inferior contrast resolution; the anal canal wall layers are not well visualized even with multidetector CT. However CT is essentially equivalent to MRI for demonstrating invasion of adjacent organs and regional nodes. As nodal involvement is predicted by size criteria, it remains limited for both MRI and CT. Approximately 30% of patients present with palpable enlarged inguinal-femoral nodes (>1cm) but only 50%

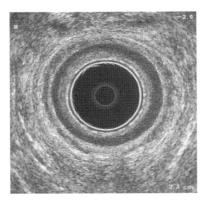

Fig. 12.2 TRUS image demonstrating appearances of a normal anal canal.

of these will be positive for disease on biopsy; the remainder are reactive secondary to infection. MR lymphangiography with ultrasmall superparamagnetic iron oxide particles (USPIO) may potentially improve nodal assessment in clinical practice in the future, but remains investigational[11]. Preliminary studies in rectal cancer[11] and gynaecological cancers[12,13] have shown promise but studies have yet to be published for anal cancer.

CT is preferred for staging metastatic disease currently as it is more sensitive than plain radiographs or US. However, usage of FDG PET/CT may increase in the future as it appears to be superior to CT, offering high sensitivity and specificity for nodal and distant disease in immunocompetent patients with anal cancer. In one study PET detected nodal metastases in 24% of patients considered node negative on CT[14]. In another PET correctly identified 91% of primary tumours compared with 59% on CT, and detected nodal metastases in 17% of patients considered node negative on CT[6]. Comparative studies of PET with MRI have yet to be published.

12.3 Imaging for radiotherapy

12.3.1 Radiation treatment

In the UK National ACT II trial external beam radiotherapy is delivered in two phases. Phase I uses large parallel opposed fields and encompasses the gross target volume (GTV) and all inguinal-femoral and pelvic lymph node groups at risk of microscopic disease. The recommended dose is 30.6Gy in 17 fractions of 1.8Gy per fraction. Phase II techniques vary depending on the presence or absence of lymphadenopathy. The recommended dose is 19.8Gy in 11 daily fractions.

Intensity modulated radiation therapy (IMRT) is a novel technology which allows the delivery of high doses of radiotherapy. It is possible to target the tumour while sparing normal surrounding structures to a greater degree than conventional two- (2D) or three-dimensional (3D) planning—specifying a desired dose distribution with an optimal intensity. Using IMRT in anal cancer to deliver the same dose as in ACT II may allow some sparing of sensitive tissues such as perineal skin, the external genitalia, the bony pelvis (sacrum and pubis), the femoral head and neck, the bladder, and small bowel. This sparing of normal tissues may lower acute toxicities particularly of skin and genitalia, and allow improved compliance to treatment (particularly to concurrent and consolidation chemotherapy after chemoradiation) and lessen late morbidity.

12.3.2 Treatment planning process

3D-conformal approaches to treatment planning using CT have overtaken 2D approaches where treatment fields were defined using orthogonal radiographs and known anatomical landmarks. For planning purposes a single visit to CT simulator will allow subsequent field placement for phase I and delineation and definition of GTV and CTV for the second planned phases of treatment. Patients are imaged with a full bladder in the prone position. Immobilization devices such as a belly board may be used. Rectal contrast is administered prior to imaging.

Intravenous contrast may be useful for localization of vessels and hence lymph node groups. The CT study is performed from the superior aspect of L5 to 3cm beyond the anal marker or perianal tumour marker to cover the entire pelvis

12.3.3 Target volume definition

The *GTV* includes all areas of macroscopic tumour visible on planning CT. Multiple GTVs may have to be defined to include clinically or radiologically apparent inguinal-femoral or pelvic lymphadenopathy. The tumour extent within the anal canal can be difficult to ascertain on planning CT due to its poor contrast resolution, even with intravenous contrast administration. To overcome this, measurements of tumour length and distance from the anal verge from clinical examination and comparison with MRI have been used to define the superior border of the GTV.

However this is less than optimal, as different patient positioning is often used in staging and planning (prone or supine), and the tumour may also potentially move with peristalsis—although this movement is lessened if a defunctioning stoma has been fashioned. There may be a role for MRI/CT co-registration to improve tumour delineation on a planning CT or MRI for planning but further study is required in anal cancer. There is little data on PET for planning. One study has published data on anorectal cancers which included three anal cancers limiting its generalizability but suggested that GTVs were smaller on PET than CT, and in one case of anal cancer, the PTV was altered to include metabolically active disease[15].

Definition of the *clinical target volume* (CTV) and *planning target volume* (PTV) is not as straightforward as for rectal cancer as there is little information on the pattern of failure which is essential for CTV definition, and the extent of organ motion and departmental set up errors for anal cancer techniques. A current approach, for example used in the phase III ACT 2 trial, is to define the GTV and treatment fields used (Fig. 12.3).

12.4 Therapeutic assessment and follow-up

Patients who do not respond to chemoradiotherapy (CRT) are usually treated with APR, hence it is important to assess patients following treatment. MRI is performed most commonly 6–8 weeks following treatment although there is little data of its accuracy or predictive value. One study has suggested MRI appearances such as tumour size reduction and signal intensity change are predictive of a good outcome (Fig. 12.4).

There is little PET data. Schwarz and colleagues have suggested that a complete or partial metabolic response in the primary anal tumour at the completion of treatment can distinguish patients with an excellent or poor progression free and cause specific survival[16]. A partial reduction in standardized uptake value at a mean of 2 months following treatment is a predictor of poor outcome, with a significantly reduced progression free and cause specific survival after CRT. CT is of little use for assessing the primary tumour following CRT but will be able to demonstrate nodal downstaging. Likewise data have suggested that TRUS is poor for therapeutic assessment due to the presence of radiotherapy change[17].

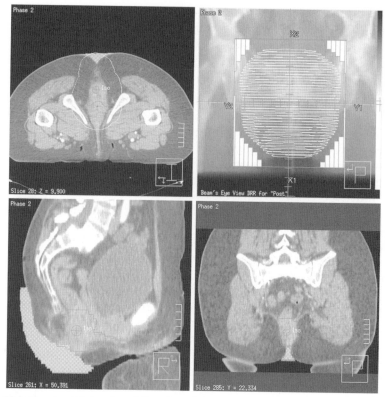

Fig. 12.3 Planning CT showing delineation of the GTV and treatment fields. See colour section.

Surveillance is typically performed by clinical examination, proctoscopy, and CT of the thorax, abdomen, and pelvis. There appears to be no benefit in performing TRUS. Given that disease relapse is uncommon, particularly metastatic relapse, the scheduling of CT for metastatic surveillance outside trials remains controversial.

12.5 **Summary**

- MRI is the preferred modality for local staging due to its superior contrast resolution. CT is the preferred modality for assessing metastatic disease due to its superior sensitivity. PET/CT will play a greater role in the future.

- CT for planning has its limitations. There may be a role for CT/MRI fusion or PET to improve tumour and nodal delineation.

- Following treatment, MRI is performed to assess therapeutic response; PET/CT may play a greater role in the future due to its perceived greater sensitivity and predictive value.

- CT of the thorax, abdomen, and pelvis is performed for metastatic surveillance currently but frequency of scheduling remains controversial.

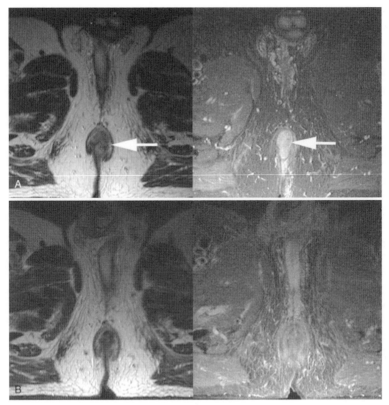

Fig. 12.4 Axial MR images pre- (A) and post-chemoradiation (B) demonstrating resolution of the anal canal tumour following treatment.

References

1. Jemal A, Siegel R, Ward E, *et al*. Cancer statistics, 2008. *CA Cancer J Clin* 2008; **58**: 71–96.

2. Nigro ND, Vaitkevicus VK, Considine B, Jr. Combined therapy for cancer of the anal canal: a preliminary report. *Dis Colon Rectum* 1974; **17**: 354–56.

3. Nigro ND, Seydel HG, Considine B, Jr., *et al*. Combined radiotherapy and chemotherapy for squamous cell carcinoma of the anal canal. *Cancer* 1983; **51**: 1826–9.

4. Cummings BJ, Keane TJ, O'Sullivan B, *et al*. Epidermoid anal cancer: treatment by radiation alone or by radiation and 5-flurouracil with and without mitomycin C. *Int J Radiat Oncol Biol Phys* 1991; **21**: 1115–25.

5. Engstrom PF, Benson AB 3rd, Chen YJ, *et al*. Anal canal cancer clinical practice guidelines in oncology. *J Natl Compr Canc Netw* 2005; **3**: 510–15 or www. NCCN.org for 2008 version.

6. De Winton E, Heriot A, Ng M, *et al*. Utility of 18-fluorodeoxyglucose positron emission tomography (FDG-PET) in the staging, radiotherapy planning and prognostication of anal cancer. *J Clin Oncol* 2007; **25**: (abstract 4559).

7. Cotter SE, Grigsby PW, Siegel BA, *et al*. FDG-PET/CT in the evaluation of anal carcinoma. *Int J Radiat Oncol Biol Phys* 2006; **65**: 720–5.

8. Brust D, Polis M, Davey R, *et al.* Fluorodeoxyglucose imaging in healthy subjects with HIV infection: impact of disease stage and therapy on pattern of nodal activation. *AIDS* 2006; **20**: 985–93.

9. Koh DM, Dzik Jurasz A, O'Neill B, *et al.* Pelvic phased array MR imaging of anal carcinoma before and after chemoradiation. *Br J Radiol* 2008; **81**: 91–8.

10. Goldman S, Norming U, Svensson C, *et al.* Transanorectal ultrasonography in the staging of anal epidermoid carcinoma. *Int J Coloretcal Dis* 1991; **6**: 152–7.

11. Koh DM, Brown G, Temple L, *et al.* Rectal cancer: mesorectal lymph nodes at MR imaging with USPIO versus histopathologic findings – initial observations. *Radiology* 2004; **231**: 91–9.

12. Taylor A, Rockall AG, Reznek RH, *et al.* Mapping pelvic lymph nodes: guidelines for delineation in intensity-modulated radiotherapy. *Int J Radiat Oncol Biol Phys* 2005; **63**: 1604–12.

13. Rockall AG, Sohaib SA, Hairisinghani MG, *et al.* Diagnostic performance of nanoparticle-enhanced magnetic resonance imaging in the diagnosis of lymph node metastases in patients with endometrial and cervical cancer. *J Clin Oncol* 2005; **23**: 2813–21.

14. Trautmann TG, Zuger JH. Positron emission tomography for pretreatment staging and posttreatment evaluation in cancer of the anal canal. *Mol Imaging Biol* 2005; **7**: 309–13.

15. Anderson C, Koshy M, Staley C, *et al.* PET-CT fusion in radiation management of patients with anorectal tumors. *Int J Radiat Oncol Biol Phys* 2007; **69**: 155–62.

16. Schwarz JK, Siegel BA, Dehdashti F, *et al.* Tumor response and survival predicted by post therapy FDG-PET/CT in anal cancer. *Int J Radiat Oncol Biol Phys* 2008; **71**: 180–6.

17. Lund JA, Sundstrom SH, Haaverstad R, *et al.* Endoanal ultrasound is of little value in follow up of anal carcinomas. *Dis Colon Rectum* 2004; **47**: 839–42.

Chapter 13

Urological cancers

Oliver Wignall, Vincent Khoo, and
S. Aslam Sohaib

13.1 Prostate cancer

13.1.1 Clinical background

Prostate cancer is the most common cancer in males and is the second leading cause of cancer deaths in the Western world[1]. In the UK there are about 23,000 new cases diagnosed annually and approximately 10,000 deaths[1,2]. The incidence of prostate cancer increased sharply in the early 1990s due to the use of prostate-specific antigen (PSA) testing in asymptomatic individuals but more recently the incidence declined and has now levelled off[3]. The most important risk factors implicated in the development of prostate cancer include age, ethnic origin, and family history[2].

For patients with organ-confined prostate cancer, management options include observation, active surveillance, radical prostatectomy, or radiotherapy (external beam or brachytherapy). For patients with locally advanced or metastatic disease treatment, options include a combination of hormone therapy, radiotherapy, or chemotherapy.

13.1.2 Diagnosis and staging

13.1.2.1 Diagnosis

The diagnosis of prostate cancer is usually made by needle biopsy performed using trans-rectal ultrasound (TRUS) guidance. TRUS involves a high-frequency endorectal transducer to produce high-resolution images of the prostate. In conjunction with local anaesthetic and antibiotic prophylaxis, sampling of the prostate is performed with a 18G trucut needle[4,5]. The diagnostic yield of TRUS-guided biopsy increases with the number of cores taken and the standard is now 12. Although prostatic cancer classically appears hypoechoic in comparison to the surrounding peripheral zone, its ultrasonic appearance is variable[6,7]. For this reason TRUS is not used to detect or direct biopsies to malignant lesions but to target the gland for systematic sampling.

13.1.2.2 Staging

Staging in prostate cancer may be clinical staging with digital rectal examination (DRE), imaging based, or pathological staging (tumour, node, metastasis, TNM) following prostatectomy (Table 13.1). Though DRE is poor at local staging and underestimates the local extent of tumour in 40–60% of cases[8] it is widely used and forms part of

Table 13.1 TNM classification for prostate cancer

Primary tumour (T)	
TX	Primary tumour cannot be assessed
T0	No evidence of primary tumour
T1	Clinically inapparent tumour not palpable or visible by imaging: ◆ T1a: tumour incidental histological finding in ≤5% of tissue resected ◆ T1b: tumour incidental histological finding in >5% of tissue resected ◆ T1c: tumour identified by needle biopsy, e.g. because of elevated PSA level
T2	Tumour confined within the prostate: ◆ T2a: tumour involves one half of one lobe or less ◆ T2b: tumour involves more than one half of one lobe, but not both lobes ◆ T2c: tumour involves both lobes
T3	Tumour extends through the prostatic capsule: ◆ T3a: extracapsular extension (unilateral or bilateral) ◆ T3b: tumour invades seminal vesicle(s)
T4	Tumour is fixed or invades adjacent structures other than the seminal vesicles: bladder neck, external sphincter, rectum, levator muscles or pelvic wall
Regional lymph nodes (N)	
NX	Regional lymph nodes cannot be assessed
N0	No regional lymph node metastasis
N1	Regional lymph node metastasis
Distant metastasis (M)	
MX	Distant metastasis cannot be assessed
M0	No distant metastasis
M1	Distant metastasis: ◆ M1a: non-regional lymph node(s) ◆ M1b: bone(s) ◆ M1c: other site(s)

Partin's nonograms. TRUS is not used for staging as its accuracy is no better than DRE and there is significant interoperator variability[9]. Computed tomography (CT) lacks soft tissue contrast resolution and does not allow reliable tumour visualization but gross disease extension or enlarged adenopathy may be seen[10].

13.1.2.2.1 **T stage** MRI is the imaging modality of choice for local staging due to its superior soft-tissue contrast resolution. A variety of coils have been used in magnetic resonance imaging (MRI) of prostate cancer, but combined endorectal and pelvic phased-array coils has been shown to be the most accurate compared to pelvic phased array or endorectal coils alone[11]. Intraprostatic visualization and zonal anatomy are best demonstrated on T2-weighted images (Fig. 13.1). The prostate has a fibrous capsule and is divided into five histologically distinct zones; peripheral zone (PZ), central

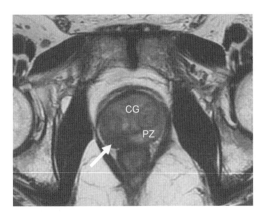

Fig. 13.1 Prostate cancer. Axial T2-weighted MR images through the prostate showing the zonal anatomy; central gland (CG) and peripheral zone (PZ). Prostate cancer is seen as the low signal area (arrow) in the right PZ.

zone (CZ), transition zone (TZ), periurethral glandular tissue, and anterior fibromuscular stroma[12]. The CZ, TZ, and periurethral glandular tissue cannot be distinguished separately at imaging and are referred to as the central gland (CG). Approximately 70% of prostate cancers arise in the PZ, 30% in the central gland.

Prostate cancer regions are typically of low signal intensity within the PZ on T2-weighted images (Fig. 13.1). However, low signal intensity lesions in the PZ can also be caused by prostatitis, scarring, and post-biopsy haemorrhage. To avoid post-biopsy changes it is recommended to delay the MRI for a minimum of 3-4 weeks after biopsy[13]. In terms of staging accuracy the reported sensitivity and specificity of MRI in detecting extracapsular spread is highly variable[14,15]. The sensitivity and specificity of MRI in detecting seminal vesicle invasion (Fig. 13.2) is also variable ranging from 85–97% and 21–63% respectively[16].

Functional MRI techniques, such dynamic contrast-enhanced MRI and MR spectroscopy, have been described in the assessment of prostate cancer[16]. Dynamic contrast-enhanced MRI provides a means of assessing tissue perfusion and permeability by

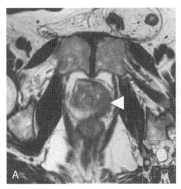
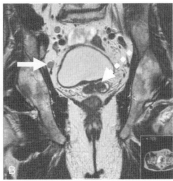

Fig. 13.2 Prostate cancer. T2-weighted MR images (A) axially through the prostate, and (B) coronally through the seminal vesicles shows prostate cancer with extraprostatic spread (arrowhead), and seminal vesicle invasion (dashed arrow) (stage T3b) and nodal disease (arrow).

imaging the passage of intravenous gadolinium through the tissues. Recently, MR spectroscopy (MRS) integrated with MRI has been reported in prostate cancer[17]. In prostate cancer, MR spectra from protons in choline and citrate are assessed. High levels of citrate and intermediate levels of choline are observed within the normal PZ. However, prostate cancer cells have a reduced capacity for citrate production and increased cell turnover results in higher choline levels. The combination of MRS and MRI may improve the localization of cancer and preliminary data suggests that it may also be able to assess tumour aggressiveness.

13.1.2.2.2 **N stage** Lymph node staging is performed in patients with a significant risk of nodal metastases in whom a potentially curative treatment is planned. CT and MRI are the principal imaging modalities used in the detection lymph node spread (Fig. 13.2). The detection of lymph node metastases by CT is based on size (Table 13.1) as CT cannot detect microinvasion in normal sized nodes. In addition hyperplastic or reactive nodes with no tumour involvement will give rise to false positive results. The sensitivity and specificity of CT in the detection of node metastases range from 25–78% and 77–98% respectively[18].

The detection of lymph node metastases by MRI is also based on size resulting in similar limitations as CT. The sensitivity and specificity of MRI in the detection of lymph node metastases range from 0–100% and 94–100% respectively[19]. Recently lymph node-specific contrast agents, ultrasmall particles of iron oxide (USPIO), have been evaluated in the detection of node involvement with malignancy. The USPIO are taken up by macrophages in the reticuloendothelial system causing loss of signal on T2- and T2*-weighted sequences in normal nodes. A portion of the nodes infiltrated with metastatic disease do not take up the USPIO and hence remain of high signal intensity. A study of 80 patients with prostate cancer showed that the use of USPIO significantly increased the sensitivity of detection of node metastases when compared to conventional MRI[20].

13.1.2.2.3 **M stage** Distant metastasis in prostate cancer is most commonly to the bone with the axial skeleton involved in 85% of patients dying from prostate cancer[21]. Bone scintigraphy with technetium 99m diphosphonate is the main imaging modality used in the detection of metastatic bone disease (Fig. 13.3) [22]. Bone metastases demonstrate increased uptake of tracer, however plain film correlation may be needed to exclude other causes of increased tracer uptake, such as degenerative disease or Paget disease. MRI may be helpful in the evaluation of lesions which are equivocal on both radionuclide scanning and plain films[23]. Other sites of distant disease include distant lymph nodes, lung, and liver, and CT is the primary imaging modality used in their evaluation. Other sites of metastatic disease are extremely rare and occur late.

13.1.3 Imaging for radiotherapy planning

Cross sectional imaging plays a central role in the definition of target volumes, organization of treatment planning, and verification of treatment. Irrespective of the radiotherapy technique, it is vital that there is optimal visualization of the planning volumes and adjacent critical structures or organs in order to avoid a geographical miss of the tumour and to minimize unnecessary irradiation of any organs at risk (OARs).

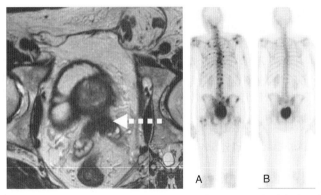

Fig. 13.3 Metastatic prostate cancer. Whole body bone scintigraphy (A) showing multiple bone metastases. (B) Following treatment with hormone therapy there has been resolution of the metastatic disease.

Modern external beam radiotherapy relies on CT for treatment planning and it is the basis for chemoradiotherapy (CRT) and intensity modulated radiation therapy (IMRT) techniques[24]. However, it is clear that MRI has replaced CT as the diagnostic imaging modality of choice and can offer advantages for radiotherapy treatment planning (RTP)[25]. In prostate planning studies of co-registered CT-MRI, investigators have reported better definition of prostate boundaries and substantially smaller treatment volumes by up to 40%[26–28]. MRI can substantially reduce the clinician's uncertainty in target volume definition compared to CT, especially at the prostatic apex[26,29]. The smaller but more appropriate treatment volumes may also enhance the therapeutic ratio when dose escalation schemes are employed. The use of USPIO imaging may aid the radiotherapeutic management of prostate cancer patients by improving detection of node involvement and thus either excluding patients from radical radiotherapy or including them into clinical trials addressing the treatment of pelvic nodes. MRI can also provide complementary information for both localization and characterization of prostate tissue through the use of the newer functional MRI techniques that may provide new therapeutic opportunities such as intraprostatic boosts[30].

In order to use MRI information for RTP, several important issues need to be addressed. These include defining and correcting for MR image distortions, overcoming the lack of electron density information in MR images which are needed for dose computation as well as other potential limitations such as patient claustrophobia, and other contraindications (e.g. *in situ* pacemakers)[31]. Sources of MR image distortion include system-related and object-induced (i.e. patient dependent) effects. These effects are important as accurate geometric imaging data is needed for RTP and they can now be assessed, quantified, and minimized through the use of correction algorithms[32,33]. After distortion correction, MR images can be either be assigned bulk attenuation factors for the relevant volumes of interest or co-registered and fused with CT images so that the superior tissue definition from MRI can be transferred to the CT data for treatment planning and subsequent treatment verification procedures.

More details on these processes can be found in standard radiotherapy physics text-books[25].

Irrespective of the imaging modality used, quality assurance of the applied processes is crucial to maintain information integrity. This is especially pertinent with the recent advances in radiotherapy such as extra-cranial stereotactic treatment and image-guided radiotherapy (IGRT) of prostate cancer whereby sequential and/or real-time imaging is used to provide four-dimensional information[34,35].

13.1.4 Therapeutic assessment and follow-up

Routine follow-up of patients following treatment of prostate cancer usually involves clinical assessment (including DRE) and serial PSA monitoring. Further evaluation including imaging then depends on these findings, previous therapy, and subsequent clinical findings. In patients who have had previous prostatectomy, MRI is used to detect local tumour recurrence. Recurrent disease is seen as asymmetrical soft tissue in the prostate bed or pelvis. TRUS in this setting may be used to obtain a biopsy and get pathological confirmation of recurrence[36].

After external beam radiotherapy (EBRT), detection of recurrent disease is made more difficult by post-radiotherapy change within the gland. Imaging is performed to look for nodal or bony disease. In general, the role of CT is in the evaluation of lymph-adenopathy as well as the detection of distant visceral metastases.

Bone scintigraphy is the gold standard for skeletal imaging after treatment (Fig. 13.3). It is indicated in patients with bone pain irrespective of PSA level as metastatic disease may occur even if PSA is undetectable[37,38]. The use of bone scintigraphy in asymptomatic patients with biochemical disease relapse depends on PSA level. It is of no added diagnostic value unless the PSA serum levels are >20ng/mL or unless the PSA velocity is >20ng/mL/year[39].

The routine use of positron-emission tomography (PET) in assessing recurrence of prostate cancer is not currently recommended; however, one study has shown that PET is able to yield true positive findings in recurrent prostate cancer even with serum PSA levels <5ng/mL[40]. In addition, PET can monitor response to chemotherapy and hormonal therapy and may be helpful in identifying hormone-refractory aggressive tumours.

13.1.5 Summary

- The most important prognostic factors in prostate cancer are PSA level, tumour stage, and Gleason score.
- TRUS is used to direct systematic sampling of the prostate.
- MRI is the imaging modality of choice for staging of the primary tumour.
- CT and MRI have a similar sensitivity and specificity for the detection of lymph node metastases. New MRI lymph node specific contrast agents (USPIO) may aid this diagnosis.
- CT is the current standard for radiotherapy treatment planning but MRI-assisted planning can add complementary information.

13.2 **Bladder cancer**

13.2.1 **Clinical background**

Bladder cancer is the commonest tumour of the urinary tract and comprises 6–8% of all male malignancies and 2–3% of all female malignancies[1].

13.2.2 **Diagnosis and staging**

13.2.2.1 Diagnosis

Diagnosis of bladder cancer is made at cystoscopy and biopsy. Imaging is used to assess upper urinary tracts and includes ultrasound (US), intravenous urography (IVU), and CT urography (CTU). US is used to identify masses in the upper renal tracts while IVU is used to image the pelvi-calyceal system and ureters. More recently with the advent of multidetector CT the combination of US and IVU is being replaced by CTU. CTU images are obtained of the bladder and renal tract when contrast media has reached the renal collecting system and bladder. CTU protocols usually incorporate pre-contrast as well as images in the nephrographic phase of enhancement, i.e. parenchymal enhancement of the kidney. These techniques therefore allows for detailed view of the renal parenchyma and the collecting systems. Mass lesions of the bladder and renal tract as well as pelvi-calyceal abnormality can all be evaluated simultaneously.

13.2.2.2 Staging

13.2.2.2.1 **T stage** Primary tumour staging with cystoscopy and transurethral resection (TUR) is accurate in the evaluation of superficial tumours (Table 13.2). For muscle-invasive tumours, however, clinical staging is inaccurate with error rates as high as 50%[41]. In these cases imaging is required to assess the extent of tumour spread[41]. US (Fig. 13.4) is not routinely used in primary tumour staging as the assessment of peri-vesical tumour spread is limited and it does not allow assessment of local lymph nodes[42,43].

CT imaging of the abdomen and pelvis is performed with a full bladder and intravenous contrast as tumours show enhancement. Delayed images with contrast in the ureters and bladder are useful in defining the extent of tumour at the bladder base and dome and spread into the ureters. CT cannot differentiate between the bladder wall layers and therefore cannot differentiate between stage T1, T2a, and T2b tumours[44]. In addition, residual bladder wall thickening following TURBT for T1 and T2a tumours is indistinguishable from muscle-invasive disease on CT. The main role of CT is to distinguish bladder tumours confined to the bladder wall from those that extend into the perivesical fat (Fig. 13.5)[45]. However, the correlation between CT findings and tumour extent in cystectomy specimens is only 65–80%[46]. Pelvic sidewall and local organ invasion is demonstrated by soft tissue extension from the main tumour.

MR is inaccurate in the evaluation of stage T1 and T2a tumours, however, there is some evidence to suggest that MR can distinguish between T2a and T2b tumours[45,47]. Invasion of the deep muscle layer by T2b tumours on T2-weighted imaging is demonstrated by disruption of the normal low signal intensity bladder wall (Fig. 13.6)[45]. Both T1- and T2-weighted sequences demonstrate T3b disease due to the contrast between tumour and perivesical fat[44,47,48]. As with CT, however, MRI cannot detect microscopic

Table 13.2 TNM classification for bladder carcinoma

Primary tumour (T)	
TX	Primary tumour cannot be assessed
T0	No evidence of primary tumour
	♦ Ta: non-invasive papillary carcinoma
	♦ Tis: carcinoma in situ: 'flat tumour'
T1	Tumour invades subepithelial connective tissue
T2	Tumour invades muscle:
	♦ T2a: tumour invades superficial muscle (inner half)
	♦ T2b: tumour invades deep muscle (outer half)
T3	Tumour invades perivesical tissue:
	♦ T3a: microscopically
	♦ T3b: macroscopically (extravesical mass)
T4	Tumour invades any of following: prostate, uterus, vagina, pelvic wall, abdominal wall
	♦ T4a: tumour invades prostate, uterus or vagina
	♦ T4b: tumour invades pelvic wall or abdominal wall
Regional lymph nodes (N)	
NX	Regional lymph nodes cannot be assessed
N0	No regional lymph node metastasis
N1	Metastasis in a single lymph node ≤2cm in greatest dimension
N2	Metastasis in a single lymph node >2cm but ≤5 cm in greatest dimension, or multiple lymph nodes, none >5cm in greatest dimension
N3	Metastasis in a lymph node >5cm in greatest dimension
Distant metastasis (M)	
MX	Distant metastasis cannot be assessed
M0	No distant metastasis
M1	Distant metastasis:

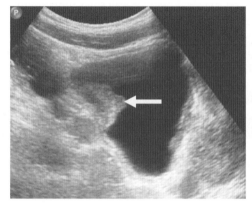

Fig. 13.4 Transitional cell carcinoma of the bladder. Longitudinal ultrasound image showing large mass (arrow) at the dome of the bladder.

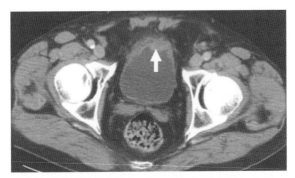

Fig. 13.5 Transitional cell carcinoma of the bladder. CT showing an enhancing soft tissue mass (arrow) arising from the anterior bladder wall with stranding in the peri-vesical fat suspicious of extra-vesical spread.

(T3a) extension into the perivesical fat. The staging error is similar for CT in the region of 30%[44,49]. MR is superior to CT in the assessment of local organ invasion due to superior contrast resolution[41,44,45] and multiplanar imaging capability. Gadolinium-enhanced dynamic scanning techniques may improve visualization of depth of bladder wall and organ invasion. MRI is therefore the imaging modality of choice for local staging of bladder cancer.

13.2.2.2.2 **N stage** Lymphatic spread of bladder cancer occurs to the perivesical, presacral, hypogastric, obturator, and external iliac nodes followed by common iliac and para-aortic nodes. In bladder cancer, CT and MR will miss microscopic nodal disease in up to 70%[19,44]. This is due to tumour infiltration without nodal enlargement. Preliminary results of MRI with USPIO in patients with bladder cancer have shown increased sensitivity in detection of nodal metastases when compared to conventional MRI[20].

13.2.2.2.3 **M stage** Distant metastases occur in advanced disease to bone, lungs, brain, and liver. Chest radiography is routinely performed in all patients to assess for lung metastases. Bone scintigraphy is not routinely indicated in asymptomatic patients[50].

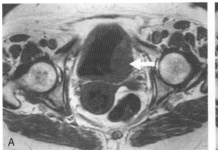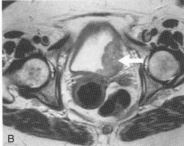

Fig. 13.6 Transitional cell carcinoma of the bladder. Axial (A) T1-weighted and (B) T2-weighted MR images showing a large intraluminal tumour (arrow) involving the left lateral bladder wall.

However, high-risk patients and those with symptoms suggestive of bone involvement should have a bone scintigram, with suspicious findings confirmed on plain radiographs or MRI[51].

13.2.3 Imaging for radiotherapy planning

Similar to prostate radiotherapy, CT is the standard imaging method used for RTP whereby three-dimensional construction permits proper identification of the whole bladder in relation to the surrounding critical organs and normal tissue such as the bowel and rectum. Extra tumour localization information is also obtained from clinical maps of the bladder during cystoscopy and MRI. The issues of utilizing MR images directly for RTP are outlined in section 13.1.3. The main issue for bladder radiotherapy is that there is substantial variation on a day-to-day basis of bladder position and size due to bladder filling and emptying[52]. This substantial organ variation often requires a larger planning margin of up to 1.5–2cm to avoid a geographical miss. A variety of IGRT methods are being evaluated to compensate for this bladder variation and can potentially reduce the size of the planning margin needed. These methods necessitates the use of multiple serial CT/MRI scans to assess for a composite bladder volume (adaptive IGRT) or cine MR with cone beam CT to predict for the daily volume bladder volumes (predictive IGRT)[34,53]. Fiducial markers have also been implanted into the bladder wall as another means of providing image guidance or to enable boosting of the bladder[54]. These IGRT strategies are currently being extensively investigated.

13.2.4 Therapeutic assessment and follow-up

After treatment of muscle-invasive bladder carcinoma with radical EBRT, follow-up serial cystoscopy and imaging is recommended to assess disease response and detect local recurrence and distant metastases. As recurrent disease may be local or metastatic, imaging of both the pelvis and abdomen is recommended[55]. Although retroperitoneal recurrence usually occurs in association with pelvic node metastases, it may be an isolated finding in 10% of patients[56].

CT performed following EBRT has been shown to be relatively inaccurate in local tumour assessment due to the difficulty in distinguishing tumour from bladder wall thickening due to radiation fibrosis[57,58]. MRI of the bladder performed following EBRT demonstrates abnormal signal intensity of the outer muscle layer on T2-weighted sequences and enhancement on contrast-enhanced T1-weighted images. Contrast enhancement cannot therefore reliably distinguish between tumour recurrence and post-radiotherapy change[59]. Using dynamic contrast-enhanced MRI, residual or recurrent tumour has an earlier onset of enhancement than fibrotic tissue which may improve accuracy in follow-up MRI post-EBRT[60].

13.2.5 Summary

- ◆ Clinical staging is accurate in early stage disease but inaccurate for evaluating invasive tumours spreading beyond the bladder.
- ◆ CT is unreliable for staging tumours confined to the bladder wall but accurate for staging advanced disease.

- MR is superior to CT for staging early tumours.
- Standard radiotherapy uses CT for treatment planning. New strategies such as IGRT are needed to deal with the substantial variation in daily bladder size and position.
- Serial cystoscopy with CT and MR are used for monitoring response and detecting recurrent disease.

13.3 Upper urinary tract urothelial tumours

13.3.1 Clinical background

Tumours of the upper urinary tract urothelium are much less common than either bladder or renal cell carcinomas. Ureteric transitional cell carcinomas (TCCs) are less common still, arising most commonly in the distal ureter. Upper urinary tract TCCs are commonly multifocal. Multifocal, ipsilateral TCCs develop in between 14–30% of patients[61].

13.3.2 Diagnosis and staging

The diagnostic evaluation of the upper tract urothelial cancer forms part of the assessment of haematuria as described for bladder tumours in section 13.2. Staging is performed with contrast enhanced CT (Table 13.3). Though MRI is comparable to CT it is not used in routine staging TCC of the renal collecting system but is useful in assessing vascular invasion by infiltrating tumours. The multi-focal nature of the disease means the whole urinary tract needs to be studied. The accuracy of CT for staging upper tract TCC has been shown to be 50% or less and it is unable to differentiate T1 and T2 tumours[62,63]. The lymphatic spread depends on the site of the primary lesion which due to the periureteric lymphatics can be to nodes in the retroperitoneum or pelvis.

13.3.3 Imaging for radiotherapy planning

Radiotherapy has only a palliative role in controlling pain and haemorrhage associated with advanced disease using simple CT-based techniques.

13.3.4 Therapeutic assessment and follow-up

Post-surgery, follow-up CT of the abdomen and pelvis is performed to assess for evidence of tumour recurrence. The contralateral collecting system is studied radiographically with retrograde pyelography or IVU and cytology.

13.3.5 Summary

- Urothelial tumours are often multi-focal and hence require imaging and evaluation of the whole renal tract.
- Staging is performed with CT but this is relatively inaccurate.

Table 13.3 TNM classification and group staging of upper tract transitional cell carcinoma

Primary tumour (T)	
TX	Primary tumour cannot be assessed
T0	No evidence of primary tumour
Ta	Non-invasive papillary carcinoma
Tis	Carcinoma *in situ*
T1	Tumour invades subepithelial connective tissue
T2	Tumour invades muscularis
T3	◆ Renal pelvis: tumour invades beyond muscularis into peripelvic fat or renal parenchyma
	◆ Ureter: tumour invades beyond muscularis into periureteric fat
T4	Tumour invades adjacent organs or through the kidney into the perinephric fat

Regional lymph nodes (N)	
NX	Regional lymph nodes cannot be assessed
N0	No regional lymph node metastasis
N1	Metastasis in a single lymph node ≤2cm in greatest dimension
N2	Metastasis in a single lymph node >2cm but ≤5 cm in greatest dimension, or multiple lymph nodes, none >5cm in greatest dimension
N3	Metastasis in a lymph node >5cm in greatest dimension

Distant metastasis (M)	
MX	Distant metastasis cannot be assessed
M0	No distant metastasis
M1	Distant metastasis

Group staging criteria			
Stage 0	Ta–Tis	N0	M0
Stage I	T1	N0	M0
Stage II	T2	N0	M0
Stage III	T3	N0	M0
Stage IV	T4	N0	M0
	Any T	N1–N3	M0
	Any T	Any N	M1

13.4 **Testicular cancer**

13.4.1 **Clinical background**

Testicular cancers comprise 1–1.5% of all male neoplasms but are the most common neoplasm in young men[64]. They are important because >95% are curable. Germ cell tumours (GCT) comprise 95% of testicular neoplasms and are subdivided into seminomas (40%) and non-seminomatous germ cell tumours (NSGCT) (60%)[65]. Patients with

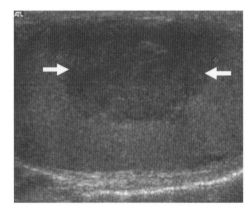

Fig. 13.7 Testicular cancer. US showing ill-defined hypoechoic intratesticular tumour (arrows).

testicular tumours typically present with a painless scrotal mass although occasionally they may present with features of metastatic disease.

13.4.2 **Diagnosis and staging**

13.4.2.1 Diagnosis

Diagnosis of testicular GCT is at biopsy or orchidectomy. Scrotal US is used to confirm diagnosis and look for other abnormalities such as microlithiasis in the contralateral testis. Scrotal US has a sensitivity of almost 100% on the detection of testicular tumours (Fig. 13.7)[66].

13.4.2.2 Staging

Staging is based on the TNM classification (Table 13.4) and patients are categorized into good, intermediate, and poor prognostic groups using the international germ cell cancer collaborative group (IGCCCG) classification (Table 13.5). Initial staging is with a contrast-enhanced CT of the thorax, abdomen, and pelvis[67].

Testicular GCT spreads via the lymphatics to the retroperitoneal nodes in a predictable pattern. Right-sided tumours initially spread to the aorto-caval nodes and nodes around the inferior vena cava. Left-sided tumours initially spread to the left para-aortic and pre-aortic nodes (Fig. 13.8)[68]. Spread to the iliac and inguinal nodes usually occurs only in association with large volume retroperitoneal disease or with a history of testicular maldescent or surgery interfering with the lymphatic drainage, e.g. pelvic surgery.

Haematogenous spread occurs most commonly to the lungs; other sites include brain, bone, and liver. CT of the brain is only indicated in those patients where there is clinical suspicion or with high-risk factors such as multiple lung metastases or HCG >10000 as brain metastases may be asymptomatic.

MRI is not used routinely in staging but has a role in the investigation of suspected brain metastases, meningeal disease, and spinal cord involvement and in problem-solving if CT images are indeterminate. PET with 18-F fluorodeoxyglucose (FDG) is not recommended for primary staging and does not improve staging in patients with clinical stage I disease[69].

Table 13.4 TNM classification and group staging of testicular cancer

Primary tumour (pT)	
pTX	Primary tumour cannot be assessed
pT0	No evidence of primary tumour
pTis	Intratubular germ cell neoplasia (carcinoma in situ)
pT1	Tumour limited to testis and epididymis without vascular/lymphatic invasion: tumour may invade tunica albuginea but not tunica vaginalis
pT2	Tumour limited to testis and epididymis with vascular/lymphatic invasion, or tumour extending through tunica albuginea with involvement of tunica vaginalis
pT3	Tumour invades spermatic cord with or without vascular/lymphatic invasion
pT4	Tumour invades scrotum or without vascular/lymphatic invasion

Regional lymph nodes (N)	
Clinical involvement	
pNX	Regional lymph nodes cannot be assessed
pN0	No regional lymph node metastasis
pN1	Metastasis with a lymph node mass ≤2cm in greatest dimension or multiple lymph nodes, none >2cm in greatest dimension
pN2	Metastasis with a single lymph node >2 cm but ≤5 cm in greatest dimension, or multiple lymph nodes, any one mass >2cm but ≤5cm in greatest dimension
pN3	Metastasis with a lymph node >5 cm in greatest dimension
Pathological involvement	
pN0	No regional lymph node metastasis
pN1	Metastasis with a lymph node mass ≤2cm in greatest dimension and ≤5 positive nodes, none >2cm in greatest dimension
pN2	Metastasis with a lymph node mass >2cm but ≤5cm in greatest dimension; or moe than 5 nodes positive, none >5cm; or evidence of extranodal extension of tumour
pN3	Metastasis with a lymph node mass >5cm in greatest dimension

Distant metastasis (M)	
MX	Distant metastasis cannot be assessed
M0	No distant metastasis
M1	Distant metastasis
	◆ M1a: non-regional lymph node or pulmonary metastasis
	◆ M1b: other sites

Group staging criteria in testicular germ cell tumours	
Stage	Definition
I	No evidence of metastases
IM	Rising serum markers with no other evidence of metastases

Table 13.4 (continued) TNM classification and group staging of testicular cancer

Stage	Definition
II	Abdominal node metastases: ♦ A: <2cm in diameter ♦ B: 2–5cm in diameter ♦ C: >5cm in diameter
III	Supradiaphragmatic node metastases: ♦ M: mediastinal ♦ N: supraclavicular cervical axillary ♦ O: no abdominal node metastases ♦ ABC: node size defined as in stage II

IV	Extralymphatic metastases:
	♦ Lung:
	  • L1: ≤3 metastases
	  • L2: >3 metastases all <2 cm in diameter
	  • L3: >3 metastases, one or more >2cm in diameter
	♦ H+: liver metastases
	♦ Br+: brain metastases
	♦ Bo+: bone metastases

Table 13.5 International Germ Cell Tumour Consensus Conference (IGCCCG) classification

NSGCT	Seminoma
Good prognosis—all of the following:	**Good prognosis:**
♦ AFP <1000ng/mL and HCG <5000IU/L (1000ng/mL) and LDH <1.5 × N *and*	♦ No NPVM
♦ Non-mediastinal primary	♦ Any primary site
♦ No NPVM	♦ Normal AFP, any HCG, any LDH
Intermediate prognosis—all of the following:	**Intermediate prognosis:**
♦ AFP 1000–10,000ng/mL, or HCG 5000–50,000IU/L, or LDH 1.5–10 × N *and*	♦ NPVM present
♦ Non-mediastinal primary site *and*	
♦ No NPVM	
Poor prognosis—any of the following:	
♦ AFP >10,000ng/mL or HCG >50,000IU/L or LDH >10 × N *or*	
♦ Mediastinal primary site *or*	
♦ NPVM	

AFP, alpha feto-protein; HCG, human gonadotrophin; LDH, lactate dehydrogenase; N, upper limit of normal; NPVM, non-pulmonary visceral metastases.

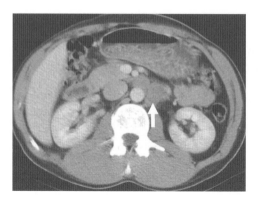

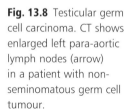

Fig. 13.8 Testicular germ cell carcinoma. CT shows enlarged left para-aortic lymph nodes (arrow) in a patient with non-seminomatous germ cell tumour.

13.4.3 **Imaging for radiotherapy planning**

Radiotherapy to a para-aortic region is an important treatment option for patients with seminoma[70] and if there has been previous inguinal or scrotal surgery or if patient follow-up is difficult, then 'dog-leg' radiotherapy fields which cover the para-aortic, ipsilateral renal hilum, and ipsilateral pelvic/inguinal nodes are recommended. Para-aortic irradiation should be tailored according to the site of primary tumour as defined on CT[70]. Surgical template fields can optimize radiotherapy.

13.4.4 **Therapeutic assessment and follow-up**

CT is the main imaging modality used in routine follow-up. Change in size or appearance of metastases and/or residual masses on CT are the main criteria used to assess response to therapy (Fig. 13.9). Cystic and fatty change which is readily assessed using CT is associated with mature differentiated teratoma and may indicate the need for surgical removal.

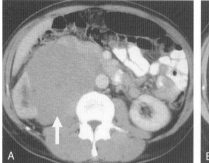 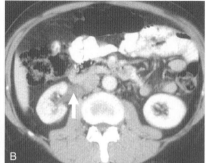

Fig. 13.9 Testicular germ cell carcinoma. (A) CT showing extensive paraortic nodal disease (arrow) in a patient with metastatic seminoma; (B) CT following chemotherapy shows a significant reduction in the volume of nodal disease (arrow).

Seminoma is extremely sensitive to chemo- and radiotherapy, such that a residual mass post-treatment usually only constitute fibrosis or necrosis. The CT findings may be allied to reduction in serum marker levels. In seminoma, FDG PET may have a role in the assessment of residual masses after chemotherapy. A negative FDG PET is 100% sensitive for absence of residual disease.

In NSGCT, FDG PET is less useful for evaluation of patients with residual masses as differentiated teratoma has variable low or no uptake and cannot be distinguished from fibrosis or necrosis.

Detection of recurrent disease relies on careful follow-up with a combination of clinical assessment, serum markers, chest radiographs, and abdominal CT. Follow-up protocols vary depending on the type of tumour, stage, treatments given, and individual institutions. They are based on the known patterns of disease relapse in testicular GCT.

13.4.5 Summary

- ◆ CT is the imaging modality of choice for staging testicular tumours.
- ◆ Regular CT monitoring is essential in the follow-up of testicular GCTs.
- ◆ FDG PET may have a role in the evaluation of a residual mass following treatment.

13.5 Penile cancer

13.5.1 Clinical background

Penile cancer is an uncommon malignancy with an incidence of 1.3 per 100,000 men in the UK in 2003.

13.5.2 Diagnosis and staging

13.5.2.1 Diagnosis

Diagnosis of the primary lesion is with a biopsy and imaging is not needed because the tumour is visible on examination.

13.5.2.2 Staging

Local staging is with US or MRI (Table 13.6). Both can assist in identifying the depth of tumour invasion, particularly with regard to corpora cavernosa infiltration[71,72]. US is often used as the initial imaging modality with MRI as an alternative if US is inconclusive. MRI is more accurate at demonstrating corporal invasion or urogenital diaphragm involvement than US, and can also help determine the extent of tumour along the surface of the penis, when the tumour is >2cm.

Lymphatic spread occurs first to inguinal nodes then pelvic nodes. US allows evaluation of the inguinal nodes and also gives an opportunity to sample them with fine needle aspiration. If inguinal lymph nodes are malignant then further imaging to look for metastases with CT of the abdomen and pelvis (Fig. 13.10)[73] and a plain chest radiograph are recommended.

Table 13.6 TNM classification of penile cancer

Primary tumour (T)	
TX	Primary tumour cannot be assessed
T0	No evidence of primary tumour
Tis	Carcinoma *in situ*
Ta	Non-invasive verrucous carcinoma
T1	Tumour invades subepithelial connective tissue
T2	Tumour invades corpus spongiosum or cavernosum
T3	Tumour invades urethra or prostate
T4	Tumour invades other adjacent organs
Regional lymph nodes (N)	
NX	Regional lymph nodes cannot be assessed
N0	No evidence of lymph node metastasis
N1	Metastasis in a single inguinal lymph node
N2	Metastasis in multiple or bilateral superficial lymph nodes
N3	Metastasis in deep inguinal or pelvic lymph nodes, unilateral or bilateral
Distant metastasis (M)	
MX	Distant metastasis cannot be assessed
M0	No evidence of distant metastasis
M1	Distant metastasis

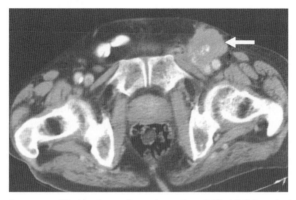

Fig. 13.10 Penile cancer. CT showing enlarged, partly-calcified left inguinal nodal mass (arrow) in a patient with carcinoma of the penis.

13.5.3 Imaging for radiotherapy planning

Once the tumour has been accurately staged then suitability for radiotherapy can be assessed. EBRT or brachytherapy are used in the treatment of infiltrating tumours T1–2 <4cm in diameter with good results. Techniques typically use orthogonal films or CT planned volumes. Irradiation of regional lymph nodes is indicated postoperatively if there is extensive nodal involvement or in patients with recurrent or inoperable metastatic nodal disease[74,75].

13.5.4 Therapeutic assessment and follow-up

Regular clinical follow-up of all patients is recommended. Local recurrence is best visualized with MRI. CT of the abdomen and pelvis are performed in the follow-up of patients with positive nodes at pelvic node dissection.

13.5.5 Summary

- US is often the first imaging modality to assess disease extent, and allows for fine needle aspiration of the inguinal nodes.
- MRI provides the greatest anatomical definition of local disease extent especially with reference to cavernosa and urogenital diaphragm infiltration.

13.6 Renal cell carcinoma

13.6.1 Clinical background

Renal cell carcinoma (RCC) is the eighth most common malignancy. Renal tumours are often detected incidentally on imaging. This has resulted in increased incidence of renal tumours which are also now smaller at presentation. For patients with renal tumour without evidence of metastases, surgery with radical nephrectomy is the treatment of choice. Imaging plays an important part in deciding surgical approach. In patients that are poor surgical candidates, various image-guided ablation techniques have been described, e.g. radiofrequency and cryoablation, but their role remains to be determined.

13.6.2 Diagnosis and staging

13.6.2.1 Characterizing renal mass lesions

In suspected RCC the first investigation performed is CT as staging information is also obtained. Traditionally it has been thought that a solid lesion most likely represents a RCC. More recently, however, there has been increasing evidence that not all solid lesions are RCC, especially smaller lesion <3cm. Some features might suggest alternative diagnoses, e.g. a central scar in oncocytomas. If a lesion remains indeterminate on CT, US or MRI may be helpful for further characterization. If despite this the lesion remains indeterminate then image-guided biopsy or surgical excision may be undertaken.

13.6.2.2 Staging

Staging in renal cancer is performed with CT (Table 13.7 and Fig. 13.11), with US and MRI reserved for problem-solving e.g. venous extension of tumour (stage T3b-c disease). Sonography is highly accurate at assessing tumour thrombus within the IVC if the examination is technically adequate. Transoesophageal echocardiography may be helpful if tumour thrombus is suspected to extend into the right atrium. MRI is

Table 13.7 TNM classification and group staging of renal cell carcinoma

Primary tumour (T)	
TX	Primary tumour cannot be assessed
T0	No evidence of primary tumour
T1	◆ T1a: tumour <4cm in greatest dimension, limited to the kidney
	◆ T1b: tumour >4cm but ≤7cm in greatest dimension, limited to the kidney
T2	Tumour >7cm in greatest dimension, limited to the kidney
T3	Tumour extends into major veins or directly invades adrenal gland or perinephric tissues but not beyond Gerota's fascia:
	◆ T3a: invades adrenal gland or perinephric tissues but not beyond Gerota's fascia
	◆ T3b: grossly extends into renal vein(s) or vena cava below diaphragm
	◆ T3c: grossly extends into vena cava above diaphragm
T4	Tumour invades beyond Gerota's fascia

Regional lymph nodes (N)	
NX	Regional lymph nodes cannot be assessed
N0	No regional lymph node metastasis
N1	Metastasis in a single regional lymph node
N2	Metastasis in more than one regional lymph node

Distant metastasis (M)	
MX	Distant metastasis cannot be assessed
M0	No distant metastasis
M1	Distant metastasis

Group staging criteria			
Stage I	T1	N0	M0
Stage II	T2	N0	M0
Stage III	T3	N0	M0
	T1–T3	N1	M0
Stage IV	T4	N0,N1	M0
	Any T	N2	M0
	Any T	Any N	M1

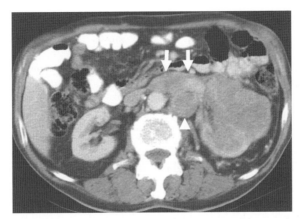

Fig. 13.11 Renal cell cancer. CT shows large left renal cancer with extension into the renal vein (arrows) and enlarged left para-aortic nodes (arrowhead).

extremely useful in delineating the extent of IVC thrombus and tumoral invasion of the IVC wall[76].

The presence of lymph node disease is a poor prognostic factor. On both CT and MRI the diagnosis of lymph node involvement is based on size criteria, which has well-known limitations. In the assessment of metastatic disease a combination of CT and MRI of the body and brain and bone scintigraphy are performed as clinically indicated. Distant metastases occur most frequently in the lungs, and other sites include bone, liver, contralateral kidney, adrenal, and brain. The role of FDG PET in assessment for metastases in advanced renal cancer is unclear as some renal tumours can have variable FDG uptake.

13.6.3 Imaging for radiotherapy planning

RCC are relatively radio-insensitive, therefore radiotherapy does not form part of the primary treatment. Radiotherapy following a radical nephrectomy has not been shown to improve survival[77]. However, radiotherapy is effective in the palliation of local symptoms due to metastatic disease[78] and has a role in the treatment of locally recurrent disease.

13.6.4 Therapeutic assessment and follow-up

Regular CT is used in the follow-up of patients post-nephrectomy. Relapse rates post-radical nephrectomy in patients with apparently localized disease range from 20–30%[82]. In the majority this involves distant disease and isolated local recurrence occurs in <5%[79].

13.6.5 Summary

- Renal mass lesions are best evaluated with CT; US, MRI, or biopsy are used where lesion remains indeterminate.
- Staging and follow-up is with CT.

13.7 **Urethral cancer**

13.7.1 **Clinical background**

Urethral cancer is very rare, occurring more commonly in women and has a peak incidence in the seventh decade.

13.7.2 **Diagnosis and staging**

Urethral cancer is diagnosed clinically with cystoscopy and transurethral biopsy. Local staging evaluation is best made using MRI, again due to its excellent soft tissue contrast resolution (Table 13.8)[80,81]. T2-weighted sequences are used to define the primary tumour and local invasion. Contrast-enhanced T1-weighted sequences may be helpful and demonstrate a moderately enhancing tumour, local invasion, and fistulae. Urethral cancer principally spreads by local invasion and lymphatic spread is to the inguinal nodes if the distal urethra is involved and to the pelvic nodes if the proximal urethra is involved. Distant metastases are rare.

13.7.3 **Imaging for radiotherapy planning**

Local staging with MRI is used to assess tumour size, location, and local extension, and to plan radiotherapy treatment (Fig. 13.12), usually based on CT.

13.7.4 **Therapeutic assessment and follow-up**

Regular MRI of the pelvis is performed post-treatment to assess for local tumour recurrence, treatment-related complications, or to evaluate treatment.

13.7.5 **Summary**

MRI is the imaging modality of choice for local staging and assists in treatment planning.

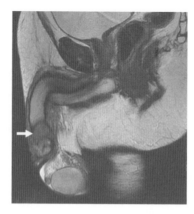

Fig. 13.12 Urethral carcinoma. Sagittal T2-weighted MR image of the penis showing locally-invasive squamous cell cancer of the urethra (arrow).

Table 13.8 TNM classification and group staging of urethral cancer

Primary tumour (T)

TX	Primary tumour cannot be assessed
T0	No evidence of primary tumour
Ta	Noninvasive papillary, polypoid, or verrucous carcinoma
Tis	Carcinoma *in situ*
T1	Tumour invades subepithelial connective tissue
T2	Tumour invades any of the following: corpus spongiosum, prostate, preiurethral muscle
T3	Tumour invades any of the following: corpus cavernosum, beyond prostatic capsule, anterior vagina, bladder neck
T4	Tumour invades other adjacent organs

Regional lymph nodes (N)

NX	Regional lymph nodes cannot be assessed
N0	No regional lymph node metastasis
N1	Metastasis in a single node ≤2cm in greatest dimension
N2	Metastasis in a single node >2cm in greatest dimension or in multiple nodes

Distant metastasis (M)

MX	Distant metastasis cannot be assessed
M0	No distant metastasis
M1	Distant metastasis

Group staging criteria

Stage 0a	Ta	N0	M0
Stage 0is	Tis	N0	M0
Stage I	T1	N0	M0
Stage II	T2	N0	M0
Stage III	T1	N1	M0
	T2	N1	M0
	T3	N0	M0
	T3	N1	M0
Stage IV	T4	N0	M0
	T4	N1	M0
	Any T	N2	M0
	Any T	Any N	M1

References

1. American Cancer Society. *Cancer Facts & Figures 2003*. Atlanta, GA: American Cancer Society, 2003.

2. Cancer Research UK. *Cancer Stats – Incidence & Mortality UK*. London: Cancer research UK, April 2003.

3. Lu-Yao GL, Greenberg ER. Changes in prostate cancer incidence and treatment in USA. *Lancet* 1994; **343**: 251–4.

4. Aus G, *et al.* Infection after transrectal core biopsies of the prostate – risk factors and antibiotic prophylaxis. *Br J Urol* 1996; **77**: 851–5.

5. Collins GN, *et al.* Multiple transrectal ultrasound-guided prostatic biopsies – true morbidity and patient acceptance. *Br J Urol* 1993; **71**: 460–3.

6. Smith JA, Jr. Transrectal ultrasonography for the detection and staging of carcinoma of the prostate. *J Clin Ultrasound* 1996; **24**: 455–61.

7. Shinohara K, Wheeler TM, Scardino PT. The appearance of prostate cancer on transrectal ultrasonography: correlation of imaging and pathological examinations. *J Urol* 1989; **142**: 76–82.

8. Zincke H, *et al.* Radical prostatectomy for clinically localized prostate cancer: long-term results of 1,143 patients from a single institution. *J Clin Oncol* 1994; **12**: 2254–63.

9. Smith JA, Jr., *et al.* Transrectal ultrasound versus digital rectal examination for the staging of carcinoma of the prostate: results of a prospective, multi-institutional trial. *J Urol* 1997; **157**: 902–6.

10. Platt JF, Bree RL, Schwab RE. The accuracy of CT in the staging of carcinoma of the prostate. *AJR Am J Roentgenol* 1987; **149**: 315–18.

11. Hricak H, *et al.* Carcinoma of the prostate gland: MR imaging with pelvic phased-array coils versus integrated endorectal–pelvic phased-array coils. *Radiology* 1994; **193**: 703–9.

12. Coakley FV, Hricak H. Radiologic anatomy of the prostate gland: a clinical approach. *Radiol Clin North Am* 2000; **38**: 15–30.

13. White S, *et al.* Prostate cancer: effect of postbiopsy hemorrhage on interpretation of MR images. *Radiology* 1995; **195**: 385–90.

14. Sonnad SS, Langlotz CP, Schwartz JS. Accuracy of MR imaging for staging prostate cancer: a meta-analysis to examine the effect of technologic change. *Acad Radiol* 2001; **8**: 149–57.

15. Engelbrecht MR, *et al.* Local staging of prostate cancer using magnetic resonance imaging: a meta-analysis. *Eur Radiol* 2002; **12**: 2294–302.

16. Husband JE, Sohaib SA. *Prostate cancer.* In: Husband JE, Reznek RH (eds). *Imaging in Oncology*, pp. 375–400. Oxford: ISIS Medical Media, 1998.

17. Kurhanewicz J, *et al.* The prostate: MR imaging and spectroscopy. Present and future. *Radiol Clin North Am* 2000; **38**: 115–38, viii–ix.

18. Oyen RH, *et al.* Lymph node staging of localized prostatic carcinoma with CT and CT-guided fine-needle aspiration biopsy: prospective study of 285 patients. *Radiology* 1994; **190**: 315–22.

19. Jager GJ, *et al.* Pelvic adenopathy in prostatic and urinary bladder carcinoma: MR imaging with a three-dimensional TI-weighted magnetization-prepared-rapid gradient-echo sequence. *AJR Am J Roentgenol* 1996; **167**: 1503–7.

20. Harisinghani MG, *et al.* Noninvasive detection of clinically occult lymph-node metastases in prostate cancer. *N Engl J Med* 2003; **348**: 2491–9.

21. Whitmore WF, Jr. Natural history and staging of prostate cancer. *Urol Clin North Am* 1984; **11**: 205–20.

22. O'Donoghue EP, *et al*. Bone scanning and plasma phosphatases in carcinoma of the prostate. *Br J Urol* 1978; **50**: 172–7.

23. Fujii Y, *et al*. Magnetic resonance imaging for the diagnosis of prostate cancer metastatic to bone. *Br J Urol* 1995; **75**: 54–8.

24. Khoo VS. Radiotherapeutic techniques for prostate cancer, dose escalation and brachytherapy. *Clin Oncol (R Coll Radiol)* 2005; **17**: 560–71.

25. Khoo VS. Magnetic resonance (MR) imaging in treatment planning. In: Mayles P, Nahum A, Rosenwald JC (eds). *Handbook of Radiotherapy Physics: Theory and Practice*, pp. 657–68 New York: Taylor and Francis, 2007.

26. Roach M, *et al*. Prostate volumes defined by magnetic resonance imaging and computerized tomographic scans for 3-dimensional conformal radiotherapy. *Int J Radiat Oncol Biol Phys* 1996; **35**: 1011–18.

27. Rasch C, *et al*. Definition of the prostate in CT and MRI: a multi-observer study. *Int J Radiat Oncol Biol Phys* 1999; **43**: 57–66.

28. Sannazzari GL, *et al*. CT-MRI image fusion for delineation of volumes in three-dimensional conformal radiation therapy in the treatment of localized prostate cancer. *Br J Radiol* 2002; **75**: 603–7.

29. Khoo VS, *et al*. Comparison of MRI with CT for the radiotherapy planning of prostate cancer: a feasibility study. *Br J Radiol* 1999; **72**: 590–7.

30. Khoo VS, Joon DL. New developments in MRI for target volume delineation in radiotherapy. *Br J Radiol* 2006; **79**(Suppl.1): 2–15.

31. Khoo VS, *et al*. Magnetic resonance imaging (MRI): considerations and applications in radiotherapy treatment planning. *Radiother Oncol* 1997; **42**: 1–15.

32. Finnigan DJ, *et al*. Distortion-corrected magnetic resonance images for pelvic radiotherapy treatment planning, in Quantitative Imaging. In: Faulkner K, *et al*. (eds). *Oncology*, pp. 72–6. London: British Institute of Radiology, 1997.

33. Tanner SF, *et al*. Radiotherapy planning of the pelvis using distortion corrected MR images: the removal of system distortions. *Phys Med Biol* 2000; **45**: 2117–32.

34. Khoo V. Utilization of portal imaging in positional control. *Oncologia* 2004; **27**: 23–7.

35. Khoo VS. 4D radiotherapy: On-line imaging on the linear accelerator. *RAD Magazine* 2005; 29–30.

36. Gregori A, *et al*. Comparison of ultrasound-guided biopsies and prostatectomy specimens: predictive accuracy of Gleason score and tumor site. *Urol Int* 2001; **66**: 66–71.

37. Oefelein MG, *et al*. The incidence of prostate cancer progression with undetectable serum prostate specific antigen in a series of 394 radical prostatectomies. *J Urol* 1995; **154**: 2128–31.

38. Leibman BD, *et al*. Distant metastasis after radical prostatectomy in patients without an elevated serum prostate specific antigen level. *Cancer* 1995; **76**: 2530–4.

39. Heidenreich A, Aus G, Abbou CC, *et* al. EAU Guidelines on Prostate Cancer. 2007. *Eur Urol* 2008; **53**: 68–80.

40. Heinisch M, *et al*. Positron emission tomography/computed tomography with F-18-fluorocholine for restaging of prostate cancer patients: meaningful at PSA < 5 ng/ml? *Mol Imaging Biol* 2006; **8**: 43–8.

41. Barentsz JO, Ruijs SH, Strijk SP. The role of MR imaging in carcinoma of the urinary bladder. *AJR Am J Roentgenol* 1993; **160**: 937–47.

42. Dershaw DD, Scher HI. Sonography in evaluation of carcinoma of bladder. *Urology* 1987; **29**: 454–7.

43. Watanabe H, Mishina T, Ohe H. Staging of bladder tumors by transrectal ultrasonotomography and U.I. Octoson. *Urol Radiol* 1983; **5**: 11–16.

44. Kim B, *et al*. Bladder tumor staging: comparison of contrast-enhanced CT, T1- and T2-weighted MR imaging, dynamic gadolinium-enhanced imaging, and late gadolinium-enhanced imaging. *Radiology* 1994; **193**: 239–45.

45. Husband JE, *et al*. Bladder cancer: staging with CT and MR imaging. *Radiology* 1989; **173**: 435–40.

46. Paik ML, *et al*. Limitations of computerized tomography in staging invasive bladder cancer before radical cystectomy. *J Urol* 2000; **163**: 1693–6.

47. Rholl KS, *et al*. Primary bladder carcinoma: evaluation with MR imaging. *Radiology* 1987; **163**: 117–21.

48. Amendola MA, *et al*. Staging of bladder carcinoma: MRI-CT-surgical correlation. *AJR Am J Roentgenol* 1986; **146**: 1179–83.

49. Barentsz JO, *et al*. MR imaging of the male pelvis. *Eur Radiol* 1999; **9**: 1722–36.

50. Davey P, *et al*. Bladder cancer: the value of routine bone scintigraphy. *Clin Radiol* 1985; **36**: 77–9.

51. Braendengen M, Winderen M, Fossa SD. Clinical significance of routine pre-cystectomy bone scans in patients with muscle-invasive bladder cancer. *Br J Urol* 1996; **77**: 36–40.

52. Turner SL, *et al*. Bladder movement during radiation therapy for bladder cancer: implications for treatment planning. *Int J Radiat Oncol Biol Phys* 1997; **39**: 355–60.

53. Mangar SA, Khoo VS. Radiotherapy for bladder cancer: improving clinical outcomes. *Brit J Cancer Manage* 2005; **1**: 4–7.

54. Mangar SA, *et al*. A feasibility study of using gold seeds as fiducial markers for bladder localization during radical radiotherapy. *Br J Radiol* 2007; **80**: 279–83.

55. Ellis JH, *et al*. Transitional cell carcinoma of the bladder: patterns of recurrence after cystectomy as determined by CT. *AJR Am J Roentgenol* 1991; **157**: 999–1002.

56. Koh DM, Husband JE. Patterns of recurrence of bladder carcinoma following radical cystectomy. *Cancer Imaging* 2003; **3**: 96–100.

57. Kellett MJ, *et al*. Computed tomography as an adjunct to bimanual examination for staging bladder tumours. *Br J Urol* 1980; **52**: 101–6.

58. Vock P, *et al*. Computed tomography in staging of carcinoma of the urinary bladder. *Br J Urol* 1982; **54**: 158–63.

59. Hawnaur JM, *et al*. Magnetic resonance imaging with Gadolinium-DTPA for assessment of bladder carcinoma and its response to treatment. *Clin Radiol* 1993; **47**: 302–10.

60. Dobson MJ, *et al*. The assessment of irradiated bladder carcinoma using dynamic contrast-enhanced MR imaging. *Clin Radiol* 2001; **56**: 94–8.

61. Yousem DM, *et al*. Synchronous and metachronous transitional cell carcinoma of the urinary tract: prevalence, incidence, and radiographic detection. *Radiology* 1988; **167**: 613–8.

62. Planz B, *et al*. Computed tomography for detection and staging of transitional cell carcinoma of the upper urinary tract. *Eur Urol* 1995; **27**: 146–50.

63. McCoy JG, *et al*. Computerized tomography for detection and staging of localized and pathologically defined upper tract urothelial tumors. *J Urol* 1991; **146**: 1500–3.

64. Richie JP. Neoplasms of the testis. In: Walsh PC, Retik AB, Stamey TA, *et al*. (eds). *Campbells Urology*, 7th edn, pp. 2411–52. Philadelphia, PA: W.B. Saunders, 1997.

65. Guthrie JA, Fowler RC. Ultrasound diagnosis of testicular tumours presenting as epididymal disease. *Clin Radiol* 1992; **46**: 397–400.

66. Schmoll HJ, *et al*. European consensus on diagnosis and treatment of germ cell cancer: a report of the European Germ Cell Cancer Consensus Group (EGCCCG). *Ann Oncol* 2004; **15**: 1377–99.

67. Husband JE, MacVicar D. Testicular germ cell tumours. In: Husband JE, Reznek RH (eds). *Imaging in Oncology*, pp. 259–76. Oxford: ISIS Medical Media, 1998.

68. Dalal PU, Sohaib SA, Huddart R. Imaging of testicular germ cell tumours. *Cancer Imaging* 2006; **6**: 124–34.

69. Fossa SD, *et al*. Optimal planning target volume for stage I testicular seminoma: A Medical Research Council randomized trial. Medical Research Council Testicular Tumor Working Group. *J Clin Oncol* 1999; **17**: 1146.

70. Martin J, Joon D, Ng N, *et al*. Towards individualised radiotherapy for stage I seminoma. *Radiother Oncol* 2005; **76**: 251–6.

71. Agrawal A, *et al*. Clinical and sonographic findings in carcinoma of the penis. *J Clin Ultrasound* 2000; **28**: 399–406.

72. Lont AP, *et al*. A comparison of physical examination and imaging in determining the extent of primary penile carcinoma. *BJU Int* 2003; **91**: 493–5.

73. Burgers JK, Badalament RA, Drago JR. Penile cancer. Clinical presentation, diagnosis, and staging. *Urol Clin North Am* 1992; **19**: 247–56.

74. Horenblas S, *et al*. Squamous cell carcinoma of the penis. III. Treatment of regional lymph nodes. *J Urol* 1993. **149**: 492–7.

75. Gerbaulet A, Lambin P. Radiation therapy of cancer of the penis. Indications, advantages, and pitfalls. *Urol Clin North Am* 1992; **19**: 325–32.

76. Aslam Sohaib SA, *et al*. Assessment of tumor invasion of the vena caval wall in renal cell carcinoma cases by magnetic resonance imaging. *J Urol* 2002; **167**: 1271–5.

77. Gez E, *et al*. Postoperative irradiation in localized renal cell carcinoma: the Rambam Medical Center experience. *Tumori* 2002; **88**: 500–2.

78. Fossa SD, Kjolseth I, Lund G. Radiotherapy of metastases from renal cancer. *Eur Urol* 1982; **8**: 340–2.

79. Rabinovitch RA, *et al*. Patterns of failure following surgical resection of renal cell carcinoma: implications for adjuvant local and systemic therapy. *J Clin Oncol* 1994; **12**: 206–12.

80. Hricak H, *et al*. Female urethra: MR imaging. *Radiology* 1991; **178**: 527–35.

81. Kawashima A, *et al*. Imaging of urethral disease: a pictorial review. *Radiographics* 2004; **24**(Suppl. 1): S195–216.

Chapter 14

Gynaecological cancers

Guy Burkill and Kate Lankester

Introduction

Ovarian, uterine, and cervical cancer account for only 5% of cancer cases in the UK. However, there has been an increasing incidence in older age groups, with the exception of invasive cervical carcinoma, which has been declining since 1990, and vaginal cancer which has remained stable[1]. Ovarian cancer accounts for more deaths from female malignancies than all the other gynaecological sites combined. Late presentation with advanced disease remains a challenge and screening is under investigation.

Imaging has become integrated into the management pathways for most patients with suspected gynaecological malignancy. They inform on treatment decisions, although evidence that they alter management in ways that impact on outcome measures, such as disease-free and overall survival, is still lacking. Combined functional and anatomical imaging modalities such as ^{18}F-fluorodeoxyglucose integrated positron emission tomography/computed tomography (FDG PET/CT) are becoming more accessible. Early studies of PET/CT in gynaecological cancer are encouraging but PET/CT and future imaging tests are likely to be subjected to more rigorous scrutiny than their predecessors before being adopted into patient care pathways.

14.1 Ovarian cancer

14.1.1 Clinical background

Carcinoma of the ovary is the most common gynaecological malignancy and the fourth most common malignancy amongst women in the UK, with an incidence of 22 per 100,000[1]. Tumours may arise from surface epithelium, germ cells, or stromal tissue. Almost 90% of ovarian tumours arise from surface epithelium, the most common pathological types being: serous (40%); endometrioid (20%); and mucinous (10%)[2]. Tumours can be benign, malignant, or of borderline malignant potential. Borderline tumours are characterized by cellular proliferation and nuclear atypia in the absence of stromal invasion[3]. The overall 5-year survival for ovarian epithelial cancer is 50%[4]. The majority of ovarian germ cell tumours are mature cystic teratomas (also known as dermoid cysts). Malignant germ cell tumours of the ovary are rare; whilst malignancy in association with a mature teratoma occurs in <2% of cases[2]. Granulosa cell tumours are the most common type of sex cord stromal tumour. Cancers of the fallopian tube are rare. They have a similar histology and behaviour to ovarian epithelial cancers and as such are essentially managed in the same way.

14.1.2 **Diagnosis and staging**

Staging is defined by the International Federation of Gynaecology and Obstetrics (FIGO) system (Table 14. 1).

14.1.2.1 Epithelial ovarian cancer

Ovarian cancer spreads locally by breaching the ovarian capsule. It disseminates transcoelomically through the abdominopelvic cavity typically up the right paracolic gutter and on to the under surface of the right hemidiaphragm. Late presentation is commonplace as non-specific symptoms are typical, such as lower abdominal or back pain, weight change, gastrointestinal upset, urinary frequency and/or urgency, and altered periods or postmenopausal bleeding.

Attention has turned to screening. Screening studies have focused on ultrasound (US) ± CA125 antigen measurement (elevated in >80% of epithelial ovarian cancers)[5]. Results from one screening study found a non-significant increase in stage I tumours in the screened compared to the control group[6]. Another study has shown that annual transvaginal ultrasound (TVUS) decreases disease stage at detection and reduces case-specific

Table 14.1 FIGO staging for carcinoma of the ovary

FIGO stages	
I	Tumour confined to ovaries
IA	Tumour limited to one ovary, capsule intact, no tumour on ovarian surface, no malignant cells in the ascites or peritoneal washings
IB	Tumour limited to both ovaries, capsules intact, no tumour on ovarian surface, no malignant cells in the ascites or peritoneal washings
IC	Tumour limited to one or both ovaries, with any of the following: capsule ruptured, tumour on ovarian surface, positive malignant cells in the ascites, or positive peritoneal washings
II	Tumour involves one or both ovaries with pelvic extension
IIA	Extension and/or implants in uterus and/or tubes, no malignant cells in the ascites or peritoneal washings
IIB	Extension to other pelvic organ, no malignant cells in the ascites or peritoneal washings
IIC	IIA/B with positive malignant cells in the ascites or positive peritoneal washings
III	Tumour involves one or both ovaries with microscopically confirmed peritoneal metastasis outside the pelvis and/or regional lymph nodes metastasis
IIIA	Microscopic peritoneal metastasis beyond the pelvis
IIIB	Macroscopic peritoneal metastasis beyond the pelvis, ≤2cm in greatest dimension
IIIC	Peritoneal metastasis beyond pelvis >2cm in greatest dimension and/or regional lymph nodes metastasis
IV	Distant metastasis beyond the peritoneal cavity

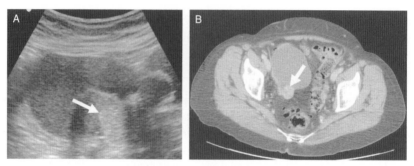

Fig. 14.1 Transvaginal ultrasound (A) and axial CT (B) of a complex ovarian cyst with solid nodule (arrow).

ovarian cancer mortality[7]. Screening strategies are being refined and are likely to rely on several serum markers in addition to CA125 coupled with TVUS[8,9].

The initial investigation for a suspected adnexal mass is pelvic US ± CA125. A transvaginal approach allows a higher frequency to be deployed, trading improved spatial resolution for a reduced field of view. US characteristics of an adnexal mass can help determine whether it is likely to be benign or malignant. A combination of greyscale features, colour Doppler, and Doppler flow indices improves sensitivity and specificity to >90%[10]. Greyscale features favouring malignancy are non-hyperechoic solid components (Fig. 14.1A), ≥3mm thick septations and free intraperitoneal fluid[11]. Ultrasonically borderline tumours tend to be large, multiloculated, predominantly cystic lesions with only small solid components and/or papillary projections[12]. Specific benign diagnoses can be made on US and, for most ovarian cysts, US provides all the diagnostic imaging information that is required to risk-stratify patients.

Computed tomography (CT) usually provides no additional information (Fig. 14.1B) regarding 'typical' cystic-solid lesions but is superior for assessing distant spread. Occasionally, CT and magnetic resonance imaging (MRI) may improve equivocal lesion characterization. CT and MRI are both sensitive and specific for the detection of intratumoural fat and MRI to the presence of blood and its breakdown products (Fig. 14.2). T1, T2, and fat suppression MRI sequences are required to distinguish fat from blood, whilst gadolinium-enhanced scans aid detection of septa, nodules, and metastases[13].

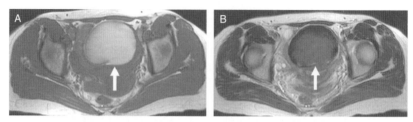

Fig. 14.2 MRI of an endometrioma (arrow) showing paramagnetic effect due to blood being (A) high signal on T1-weighted image; and mixed low and intermediate signal on (B) T2-weighted image.

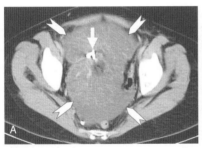
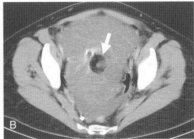

Fig. 14.3 Axial CT of a large soft tissue pelvic mass (large arrows)—a mature cystic teratoma containing a tooth (A) and fat (B) (arrows) surrounded by a mucinous adenocarcinoma.

Endometriosis can coexist with malignancy (particularly endometrioid and clear cell adenocarcinomas) and it is possible to have more than one pathology in a single ovary (Fig. 14.3). PET-CT is less accurate than MRI for ovarian tumour characterization. Whilst simple cysts usually do not show FDG avidity, problems arise due to physiological uptake (Fig. 14.4), uptake in benign cysts, dermoids, and endometriomas as well as false negative results in borderline tumours[14].

When an ovarian tumour is not clearly benign on TVUS, the ovarian risk of malignancy index (RMI) is calculated. This uses the TVUS findings, serum CA125 level, and menopausal status (Table 14.2) to aid decision-making[15]. The RMI has been modified (RMI 2) since its inception to place a greater emphasis on the US findings and menopausal status[16]. A value of >200 predicts malignancy with a sensitivity of 85% and specificity of 97%[15,16] and it remains a robust tool for cancer prediction[17].

The usual imaging features of disseminated ovarian malignancy include pelvic cystic-solid mass(es), ascites, omental and peritoneal nodules, and surface visceral deposits.

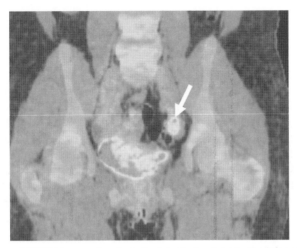

Fig. 14.4 Coronal PET/CT image showing physiological uptake in the left ovary (arrow). See colour section.

Table 14.2 RMI calculation original (RMI 1) and updated version (RMI 2)[15,16]

	RMI 1 score	RMI 2 score
Ultrasound feature:		
Multilocular cyst	None = 0	None = 0
Solid areas	One feature =1	One feature = 1
Bilateral disease	≥Two features = 3	≥Two features = 4
Ascites		
Intra-abdominal metastases		
Premenopausal	1	1
Postmenopausal	3	4
CA125	U/mL	U/mL

RMI = ultrasound × menopausal score × CA125

MRI is equivalent to CT in terms of accuracy, but MRI is a longer, more expensive examination, and more likely to be degraded by motion artefacts. Both techniques have a tendency to understage small peritoneal implants and early nodal spread[13,18]. PET/CT can upstage patients when compared with CT alone[19].

Whether neoadjuvant chemotherapy should be undertaken in preference to primary debulking surgery is influenced by individual surgical practice. Deposits often deemed difficult to resect include those in the falciform ligament, hepatic hilum, lesser sac, high diaphragm, pre-sacrum, and lymph node stations above the coeliac axis[13]. Studies examining the ability of CT to predict optimal surgical cytoreduction (defined as residual nodules measuring <1cm in maximum diameter[20]) have reported disappointing results[21,22]. Where de-bulking is felt likely to be suboptimal and primary chemotherapy is anticipated, cytological analysis of ascitic fluid or imaging-guided biopsy of the pelvic mass or metastatic disease such as in the omentum is usually successful at gaining a specific diagnosis[23].

14.1.2.2 Non-epithelial ovarian cancer

Non-epithelial tumours are imaged both incidentally and intentionally in the evaluation of a pelvic mass. Mature teratomas have complex imaging characteristics due to their varied tissue components which can be appreciated on US, CT, and MRI, allowing a specific diagnosis[24]. Thecomas typically have low signal on both T1- and T2-weighted MRI due to abundant fibrous tissue[25]. MRI is the most useful modality for investigating other hormone-producing ovarian tumours. The tumours are typically more solid than their epithelial counterparts (Fig.14.5) and hormonal influences on the uterus may be appreciated, such as uterine enlargement and endometrial thickening in premenarchal girls and postmenopausal women with oestrogen-producing tumours. Androgen-producing tumours such as Leydig cell tumours, gonadoblastomas, and Brenner tumours cause virilization. It should, however, be remembered that metastases to the ovaries can also have androgen-secreting stroma[25].

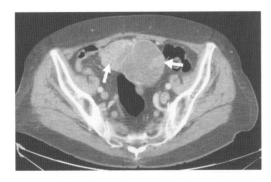

Fig. 14.5 Axial CT of a malignant ovarian germ cell tumour showing large solid components (arrows).

Primary peritoneal carcinoma has a similar clinical presentation in demographically similar women as advanced stage ovarian carcinoma, and comparable survival rates[26]. However, a personal history of breast cancer and a palpable pelvic mass are features more often absent in primary peritoneal carcinoma compared with ovarian carcinoma[26].

Fallopian tube carcinomas, usually adenocarcinoma, may be identified at an earlier stage compared with ovarian carcinoma due to more overt symptoms, which results in a better prognosis, although the actual diagnosis is usually made on pathological examination of the resected specimen[27]. Until more is known about tumour biological differences from ovarian carcinoma, if indeed they are significant, they will continue to be treated in a similar fashion, with cytoreductive surgery and chemotherapy[27].

14.1.3 Imaging for radiotherapy planning

Standard treatment of epithelial ovarian cancer is debulking surgery and chemotherapy. Radiotherapy has only a limited role, though there is some evidence to suggest that adjuvant radiotherapy in advanced disease increases disease-free survival[28]. A short course of palliative radiotherapy may be indicated for a recurrent pelvic mass.

14.1.4 Therapeutic assessment and follow-up

CT serves as a guide for interval debulking surgery either after initial suboptimal cytoreductive surgery or de novo following neoadjuvant chemotherapy. The best timing of surgery in relation to chemotherapy is currently being evaluated in the Chemotherapy or Upfront Surgery (CHORUS) trial. Potential limitations of CT in predicting the success or otherwise of interval surgery are similar to those experienced in the primary staging setting with the attendant difficulties of post-treatment fibrosis.

Once treatment is completed, further imaging is dictated by symptoms and signs or a rising CA125. Recurrence is typically with a pelvic mass, peritoneal tumour, and ascites. Visceral and lymph node metastases are a less frequent finding but can unusually be the dominant pattern of disease. CT is most frequently utilized for restaging. PET-CT appears more effective than anatomical imaging alone in detecting recurrence and should be considered when CT is non-contributory in the context of a rising tumour marker or clinical suspicion of disease relapse (Fig. 14.6)[29]. Due to the indolent nature of borderline tumours, the true risk of recurrence and impact on survival may not become apparent without long-term follow-up of 10–20 years[3].

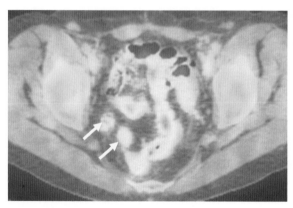

Fig. 14.6 PET/CT: Two metastatic deposits of granulosa cell carcinoma revealing low–moderate grade FDG uptake (arrows). See colour section.

14.2 **Uterine cancer**

14.2.1 **Clinical background**

Uterine cancer is the fifth most common malignancy in UK women with an incidence of 20 per 100,000[1]. The majority are adenocarcinomas arising from the endometrium. Most women (94%) are over the age of 50 years. Early stage presentation is the norm, reflected by an overall 5-year survival of 75%[1]. However, an improving survival rate has been offset by a rise in incidence of 24% (1993–2003). Other uterine tumours such as carcinosarcomas (malignant mixed mullerian tumours) and malignant myometrial tumours (leiomyosarcoma) are uncommon or rare.

14.2.2 **Diagnosis and staging**

Staging is defined by the FIGO system (Table 14.3). Endometrial cancer typically presents with postmenopausal bleeding (PMB), seen in 90%, resulting in early detection. Initial investigation often utilizes TVUS to establish the endometrial thickness. It has been shown to be a cost-effective means to determine the need for sampling, as a thickness of ≤4mm indicates a <1% risk of malignancy [30,31]. Although TVUS is able to locally stage endometrial tumours with an accuracy similar to MRI, it is common practice for patients to undergo MRI staging[32,33]. MRI is still recommended in patients in whom malignancy is not confirmed but who have a biopsy diagnosis of atypical hyperplasia, as there is a high prevalence of underlying invasive carcinoma[34].

The endometrium, junctional zone, and myometrium have high, low, and intermediate signal intensity respectively on T2-weighted MRI. This differential anatomy allows substaging of stage I tumours. Endometrial cancer initially penetrates the junctional zone to invade the myometrium which is depicted with an accuracy of 95% on MRI[35]. The tumour may grow caudally to invade the mucosa or stroma of the cervix (stage II) (Fig. 14.7). MRI is able to define cervical involvement with an accuracy of 88%[35]. The reduced accuracy for cervical invasion is due to a higher false negative rate[35]. Difficulties in tumour staging arise when the junctional zone is indistinct or abnormal (as in adenomyosis) and when the myometrium is thin.

Table 14.3 Carcinoma of the endometrium

Stage I*	Tumour confined to the corpus uteri
IA*	No or less than half myometrial invasion
IB*	Invasion equal to or more than half of the myometrium
Stage II*	Tumour invades cervical stroma, but does not extend beyond the uterus**
Stage III*	Local and/or regional spread of the tumour
IIIA*	Tumour invades the serosa of the corpus uteri and/or adnexae#
IIIB*	Vaginal and/or parametrial involvement#
IIIC*	Metastases to pelvic and/or para-aortic lymph nodes#
IIIC1*	Positive pelvic nodes
IIIC2*	Positive para-aortic lymph nodes with or without positive pelvic lymph nodes
Stage IV*	Tumour invades bladder and/or bowel mucosa, and/or distant metastases
IVA*	Tumour invasion of bladder and/or bowel mucosa
IVB*	Distant metastases, including intra-abdominal metastases and/or inguinal lymph nodes

* Either G1, G2, or G3.

** Endocervical glandular involvement only should be considered as stage I and no longer as stage II.

Positive cytology has to be reported separately without changing the stage.

Gadolinium enhancement can be of particular value in these cases as the tumour typically enhances less than the normal myometrium, improving tumour to muscle contrast.

Uterine carcinoma usually metastasizes initially to locoregional lymph nodes and the peritoneum. Anatomical imaging remains limited in its ability to stage nodal disease. However, primary tumour staging with MRI can be used to risk-stratify patients as the incidence of lymph node involvement rises from 3% with inner half myometrial invasion to 46% with the presence of outer half myometrial invasion[36]. A higher incidence of nodal invasion is also seen in endometrioid lower uterine segment tumours[37]. MRI is also effective where advanced disease is clinically suspected (Fig. 14.8).

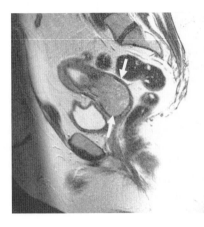

Fig. 14.7 Sagittal T2-weighted MRI of a large endometrial cancer (arrows) invading the cervical stroma—stage II.

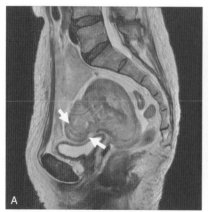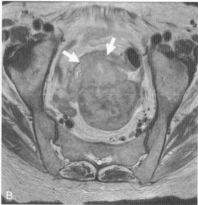

Fig. 14.8 Sagittal (A) and para-axial (B) T2-weighted MRI of an advanced endometrial cancer extending through the anterior uterine serosa to invade the sigmoid colon (arrows) confirmed on histology—stage IV.

Uterine sarcomas are rare tumours, comprising approximately 5% of all uterine malignancies[38]. They are subdivided into leiomyosarcomas, carcinosarcomas (malignant mixed müllerian tumours), and endometrial stromal tumours. The diagnosis is usually established histologically. Whilst nodularity and tumoral enhancement are seen more frequently in sarcoma, there is overlap of these features with the considerably more common endometrial adenocarcinoma[39]. Furthermore MRI is insufficiently specific for distinguishing degenerating fibroids from leiomyosarcoma[40,41]. However if such tumours are suspected on imaging or proven pathologically, a staging body CT is recommended as these tumours have a greater propensity for metastasizing to the lungs.

14.2.3 Imaging for radiotherapy planning

Surgery is the cornerstone of treatment which, given the often early presentation, comprises a total abdominal hysterectomy and bilateral salpingo-oophorectomy, as well as a lymphadenectomy in higher risk groups. Adjuvant radiotherapy to the pelvis is offered to patients with stage I disease with poor prognostic features (deep myometrial invasion, grade 3) and higher stages. Patients may be planned using a simulator and orthogonal films, but CT planning provides more accurate delineation of the planning target volume (see section 14.3.3).

14.2.4 Therapeutic assessment and follow-up

As uterine cancer is generally a surgically treated disease, post-treatment imaging is reserved for those patients who present with inoperable disease where palliative treatment (radiotherapy ± chemotherapy) and response monitoring is deemed appropriate. Relapse can affect many sites—the most frequent being lymph nodes, vaginal vault, peritoneum, and lung[42]. Patient education is an important part of post-treatment surveillance as the majority of relapses are symptomatic particularly those at the vaginal vault. If local recurrence is discovered, or disseminated disease clinically suspected, body imaging, usually with CT, is undertaken to establish the extent of disease for treatment planning. MRI and PET/CT may be useful where a radical surgical approach is proposed. A systematic review of 16 retrospective studies (in clinically disease-free patients following potentially curative treatment) found no evidence to support an intensive follow-up schedule[43].

14.3 Cervical cancer

14.3.1 Clinical background

The incidence of invasive cervical cancer is 10 per 100,000[1]. The majority are squamous cell carcinomas, though adenocarcinomas, adenosquamous, and undifferentiated carcinomas and other rare histological types may also occur[2].

14.3.2 Diagnosis and staging

Staging is defined by the FIGO system (Table 14. 4).

Table 14.4 Carcinoma of the cervix uteri

Stage I	The carcinoma is strictly confined to the cervix (extension to the corpus would be disregarded)
IA	Invasive carcinoma which can be diagnosed only by microscopy, with deepest invasion ≤5mm and largest extension ≥7mm
IA1	Measured stromal invasion of ≤3mm in depth and extension of ≤7mm
IA2	Measured stromal invasion of >3mm and not >5mm with an extension of not >7mm
IB	Clinically visible lesions limited to the cervix uteri or pre-clinical cancers greater than stage IA*
IB1	Clinically visible lesion ≤4cm in greatest dimension
IB2	Clinically visible lesion >4cm in greatest dimension
Stage II	Cervical carcinoma invades beyond the uterus, but not to the pelvic wall or to the lower third of the vagina
IIA	Without parametrial invasion
IIA1	Clinically visible lesion ≤4cm in greatest dimension
IIA2	Clinically visible lesion >4cm in greatest dimension
IIB	With obvious parametrial invasion
Stage III	The tumour extends to the pelvic wall and/or involves lower third of the vagina and/or causes hydronephrosis or non-functioning kidney**
IIIA	Tumour involves lower third of the vagina, with no extension to the pelvic wall
IIIB	Extension to the pelvic wall and/or hydronephrosis or non-functioning kidney
Stage IV	The carcinoma has extended beyond the true pelvis or has involved (biopsy proven) the mucosa of the bladder or rectum. A bullous oedema, as such, does not permit a case to be allotted to stage IV
IVA	Spread of the growth to adjacent organs
IVB	Spread to distant organs

* All macroscopically visible lesions—even with superficial invasion—are allotted to stage IB carcinomas. Invasion is limited to a measured stromal invasion with a maximal depth of 5mm and a horizontal extension of not >7mm. Depth of invasion should not be >5mm taken from the base of the epithelium of the original tissue—superficial or glandular. The depth of invasion should always be reported in mm, even in those cases with 'early (minimal) stromal invasion' (~1mm). The involvement of vascular/lymphatic spaces should not change the stage allotment.

**On rectal examination, there is no cancer-free space between the tumour and the pelvic wall. All cases with hydronephrosis or non-functioning kidney are included, unless they are known to be due to another cause.

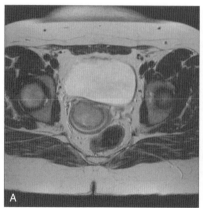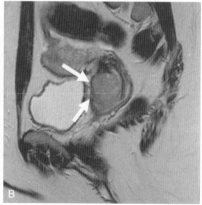

Fig. 14.9 Axial (A) and sagittal (B) T2-weighted MRI in the anterior lip of the cervix with a thin rim of intact low signal cervix (arrow)—stage Ib.

The majority of invasive cervical cancer presentations are those who have not participated in the programme rather than screening failures[44]. If not detected at screening, presentation with vaginal bleeding and discharge is usual. Gynaecological examination, colposcopy, and biopsy are used to establish the diagnosis. Although MRI is not part of the FIGO system for cervix cancer, it is adept at establishing tumour size (accuracy of 93%), which itself forms part of the clinical staging system and is of prognostic significance particularly when measured in the cranio-caudal plane[36,45]. MRI is also reliable in establishing if the disease is confined to the cervix, achieving a specificity of 96–99% when there is an intact low signal rim of cervix of at least 3mm around the tumour (Fig. 14.9)[45]. Overt parametrial invasion is also well demonstrated. Where MRI is less accurate is in differentiating stages IB from IIB (when there is full thickness stromal invasion but no parametrial mass)[45]. Imaging assessment for lymph node status, which is of great prognostic and treatment importance, remains a challenge. CT and MRI have sensitivities of just 57% and 73% respectively for lymph node metastases using size criteria. Attention is currently focusing on imaging techniques such as MRI with lymph node-specific contrast agents (ultrasmall superparamagnetic iron oxide (USPIO)) and FDG PET/CT, which are around 90% sensitive whilst maintaining high specificity[45]. The USPIO is phagocytosed by macrophages (which are abundant in normal lymph nodes but deficient in metastatic deposits) resulting in signal drop-out in normal nodes versus persistent high signal in metastatic nodes on a $T2^*$-weighted sequence.

Standard surgical management of cervical cancer is a radical hysterectomy plus pelvic lymphadenectomy. However, fertility-sparing surgery may be possible for small stage I tumours: a cone biopsy alone for a stage IA tumour or a radical trachelectomy (which removes the cervix and upper vagina, leaving the uterine body *in situ*) for a small IB tumour. Endovaginal MRI, although not widely available, may be useful in selecting patients for trachelectomy by improving accuracy in staging, particularly where early parametrial invasion is suspected on external coil imaging[46].

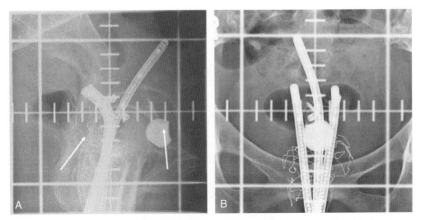

Fig. 14.10 Orthogonal lateral (A) and anterior (B) films with intra-uterine tube and vaginal ovoids *in situ*. Arrows show bladder catheter balloon filled with radio-opaque dye and vaginal packing.

14.3.3 **Imaging for radiotherapy planning**

If a cervical cancer is too advanced for surgery (a bulky stage IB or above), then radical radiotherapy with concomitant chemotherapy is recommended[47]. Radical radiotherapy comprises external beam radiotherapy followed by intrauterine brachytherapy. MRI enhanced with USPIO has been used to map the pelvic lymph nodes in relation to pelvic anatomy[48], in order to create an atlas of pelvic lymph node regions to aid three-dimensional (3D) target volume definition[49].

For brachytherapy, conventional planning uses orthogonal films to calculate dose to point A and rectal and bladder doses (Fig. 14.10). However, the advent of MRI- and CT-compatible applicators means that 3D treatment planning is now possible as cross-sectional imaging can be performed with the applicators *in situ*. Recommendations for the definition and delineation of the GTV and CTV have been published by the gynaecological GEC ESTRO working group[50,51]. 3D planning, particularly with T2-weighted MRI, allows tumour dose escalation while maintaining dose to bladder and rectum within tolerance levels[52]. MRI is superior to CT as, while organs at risk can be clearly identified on CT images, MRI provides more accurate tumour definition[53].

14.3.4 **Therapeutic assessment and follow-up**

Following chemoradiation, MRI is repeated to assess treatment response. If the cervix demonstrates uniform low signal, residual tumour is effectively excluded[45]. A residual mass is usually a sign of residual disease. However, persistent high signal in the cervix is more problematic for distinction between residual disease and radiation effect, usually resulting in multidisciplinary discussion as to whether follow-up imaging or biopsy is most appropriate.

MRI is frequently used for suspected recurrence as most occur within the pelvis and it is highly sensitive and certainly superior to CT[45]. However, MRI lacks specificity. Hence tumour suspected on imaging will usually lead to biopsy for clarification[54].

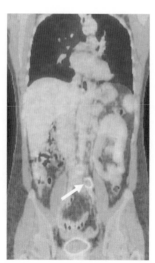

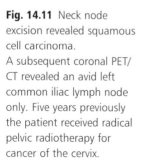

Fig. 14.11 Neck node excision revealed squamous cell carcinoma.
A subsequent coronal PET/CT revealed an avid left common iliac lymph node only. Five years previously the patient received radical pelvic radiotherapy for cancer of the cervix.

Depending on the results of MRI ± biopsy, CT may be utilized to evaluate potential distant sites. PET/CT is emerging as a useful adjunct or replacement to anatomical imaging as it has the potential to differentiate local recurrence from fibrosis, to more accurately detect distant metastases and to alter management in a significant proportion of patients[14,55,56]. PET/CT has been studied as a surveillance tool following definitive treatment. It is sensitive for the detection of both clinically suspected and occult recurrences (Fig. 14.11) but false negatives can occur, so follow-up imaging or biopsy if feasible and appropriate may be required[57]. Follow-up data is awaited to determine if there is a survival advantage to justify adoption of more intense functional imaging in this patient group.

14.4 Vaginal cancer

14.4.1 Clinical background

Vaginal cancers are rare, comprising <2% of gynaecological malignancies (incidence 0.8 per 100,000)[1] and the majority are squamous cell carcinomas, though rarely vaginal melanomas may occur. Five-year survival has improved across all age groups and stands close to 60% on average[1].

14.4.2 Diagnosis and staging

Staging is defined by the FIGO system (Table 14.5).

Clinical presentations include discharge, bleeding, itching, and dyspareunia. Initial investigation comprises an examination under anaesthetic and biopsy. MRI (Fig. 14.12) is able to depict the majority of tumours and in so doing can aid treatment planning and provide prognostic information[58]. PET is, not surprisingly, better than CT for primary tumour identification[59]. There is a paucity of published data comparing PET/CT and MRI in vaginal cancer staging, but based on cervical cancer practice, MRI will

Table 14.5 FIGO staging for vaginal cancer

FIGO stages	
I	Tumour confined to the vaginal wall
II	Tumour invades paravaginal tissues but does not extend to pelvic wall
III	Tumour extends to pelvic wall
IVA	Tumour invades mucosa of the bladder or rectum and/or extends beyond the true pelvis
IVB	Distant metastasis

be superior for defining the anatomical relationships of the primary tumour whilst PET/CT will be more accurate for detection of metastatic disease—which may have a particular bearing when local radical treatment is contemplated[59].

14.4.3 Imaging for radiotherapy planning

Radiotherapy is usually recommended for vaginal cancer, for organ preservation. Again 3D CT planning provides superior treatment planning.

14.4.4 Therapeutic assessment and follow-up

Once again, extrapolating cervical cancer practice to the rarer vaginal cancer group, MRI is likely to aid clinical assessment of treatment response and local recurrence with the attendant difficulties of distinguishing tumour from fibrosis where PET/CT and biopsy are likely to be useful adjuncts.

14.5 Vulval cancer

14.5.1 Clinical background

Vulval cancers are also rare, particularly amongst younger women (incidence 0.8 per 100,000)[1]. The vast majority are treated surgically. Overall 5-year survival is 58%[1].

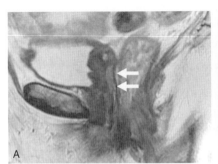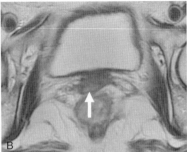

Fig. 14.12 Sagittal (A) and axial (B) T2-weighted MRI of a stage I vaginal cancer. Note the intact posterior vaginal wall (arrows). The patient has had a cervix sparing hysterectomy.

Table 14.6 Carcinoma of the vulva

Stage I	Tumour confined to the vulva
IA	Lesions ≤2cm in size, confined to the vulva or perineum and with stromal invasion ≤1.0mm*, no nodal metastasis
IB	Lesions >2cm in size or with stromal invasion >1.0mm*, confined to the vulva or perineum, with negative nodes
Stage II	Tumour of any size with extension to adjacent perineal structures (1/3 lower urethra, 1/3 lower vagina, anus) with negative nodes
Stage III	Tumour of any size with or without extension to adjacent perineal structures (1/3 lower urethra, 1/3 lower vagina, anus) with positive inguino-femoral lymph nodes
IIIA	(i) With 1 lymph node metastasis (≥5mm), or (ii) 1–2 lymph node metastasis(es) (<5mm)
IIIB	(i) With 2 or more lymph node metastases (≥5mm), or (ii) 3 or more lymph node metastases (<5mm)
IIIC	With positive nodes with extracapsular spread
Stage IV	Tumour invades other regional (2/3 upper urethra, 2/3 upper vagina), or distant structures
IVA	Tumour invades any of the following: (i) upper urethral and/or vaginal mucosa, bladder mucosa, rectal mucosa, or fixed to pelvic bone, or (ii) fixed or ulcerated inguino-femoral lymph nodes
IVB	Any distant metastasis including pelvic lymph nodes

* The depth of invasion is defined as the measurement of the tumour from the epithelialstromal junction of the adjacent most superficial dermal papilla to the deepest point of invasion.

14.5.2 **Diagnosis and staging**

Staging is defined by the FIGO system (Table 14.6).

90% of vulval cancers are squamous cell carcinomas. Presentation is typically with localized soreness, irritation, and a lump or ulcer. Tumours may also be detected

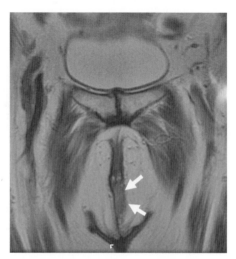

Fig. 14.13 Coronal T2-weighted MRI of a stage II vulval cancer (arrows).

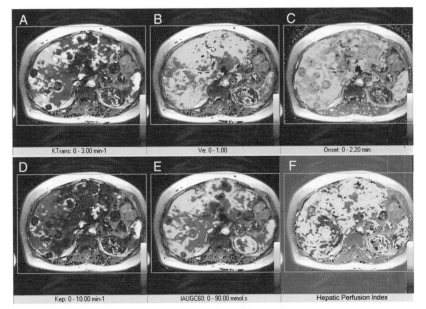

Fig. 2.6 Parametric images, all calculated from one DCE-MRI data set of 40 images: K^{trans}, (A), v_e, (B), onset time (C), k_{ep} (D), $IAUGC_{60}$ (E), and Hepatic Perfusion Index (F).

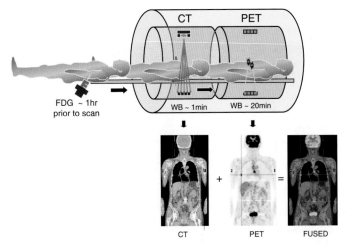

Fig. 2.9 Clinical PET/CT depicting transmission scanning in CT and emission scanning in PET leading to fused whole body images.

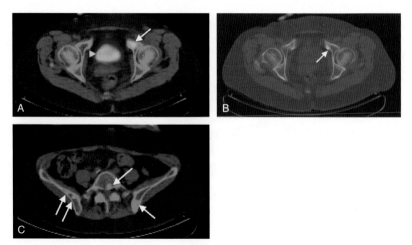

Fig. 3.4 PET/CT images of a 43-year-old woman with known metastatic breast cancer. (A) Fusion image shows abnormal uptake in the left superior pubic ramus (white arrow) and incidental physiological bladder FDG uptake (arrowhead). (B) Plain CT image does not show abnormality at this site, as a destructive lesion or sclerotic reaction has not yet formed. This was subsequently confirmed to be a new occult site of bone disease. (C) Other sites of known disease are not FDG avid on this fusion image (arrows), as they are inactive 'healed' metastases. Such bony response is not otherwise visible on any other cross-sectional imaging modality.

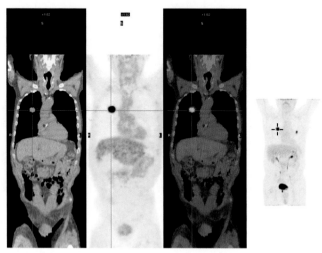

Fig. 4.1 Coronal images from a PET/CT study illustrating avid uptake of FDG in a right upper lobe nodule consistent with a bronchial carcinoma.

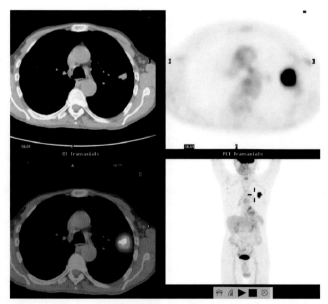

Fig. 4.4 Axial images from a PET/CT study showing avid uptake of FDG in a left upper lobe non-small cell bronchial carcinoma but no uptake in the enlarged left paratracheal lymph node; indicating that it is reactive rather than metastatic.

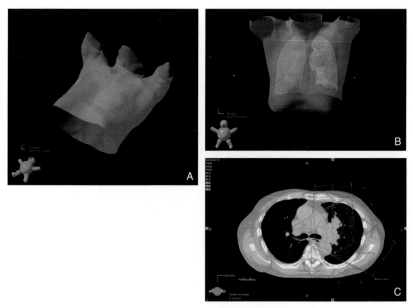

Fig. 4.5 Radiotherapy plan. (A) GTV marked in pink, surrounded by PTV in red on oblique view of body. (B) Anterior view of body with lungs marked on. (C) Transverse mid slice with field arrangement and isodose distribution marked.

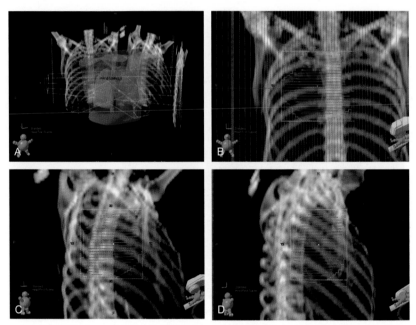

Fig. 4.6 Radiotherapy plan. (A) Three beam's eye view (BEV) images projected onto body showing orientation of fields. (B) Digitally reconstructed radiograph (DRR) of anterior field. PTV on each slice is marked in red. Blue lines show how multileaf collimator (MLC) conforms to target volume. (C) DRR for right anterior oblique field without MLC markings. (D) DRR for right posterior oblique filed without MLC markings.

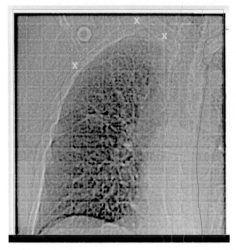

Fig. 4.11 Anterior portal image taken on treatment. Lungs outlined in green and orange. Spinal cord blue; pink GTV; red PTV. The image taken is larger than the field alone would be to allow use of reference marks (yellow X) for comparison against simulator and DRR images.

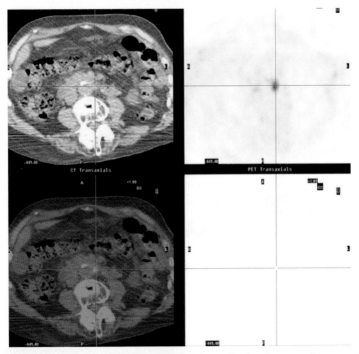

Fig. 5.5 FDG PET showing areas of increased FDG uptake despite normal para-aortic nodes on size criteria.

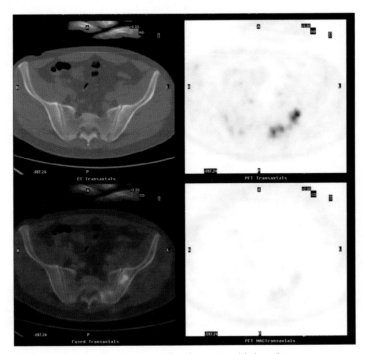

Fig. 5.6 FDG PET showing bone marrow involvement with lymphoma.

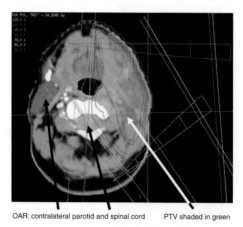

OAR: contralateral parotid and spinal cord   PTV shaded in green

Fig. 5.9 Planning CT images showing outlines for planning target volume (PTV) and organs at risk (OARs) and treatment beams with isodose contours.

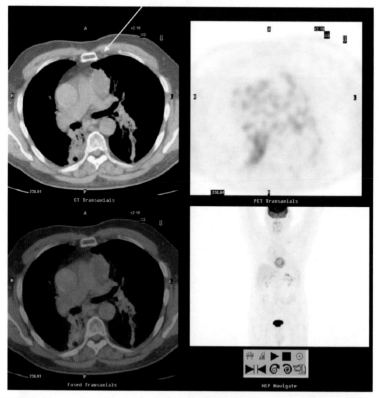

Fig. 5.10 Residual mediastinal mass on CT (arrowed) which is negative for uptake on the FDG PET image.

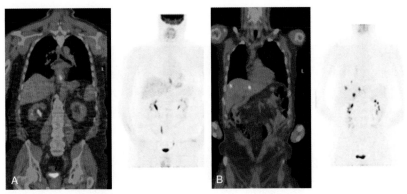

Fig. 6.4 63-year-old man with T3,N0,M0 adenocarcinoma of the lower oesophagus on baseline fused PET/CT and PET images (A). Following a complete response to neoadjuvant chemo-radiotherapy and subsequent surgery, disease has relapsed: 4 liver metastases now present (B).

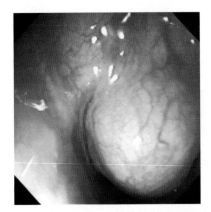

Fig. 10.1 Typical appearances of a submucosal bilobulated GIST in the stomach. Note the intact mucosa. Endoscopic biopsies were expectedly, unremarkable.

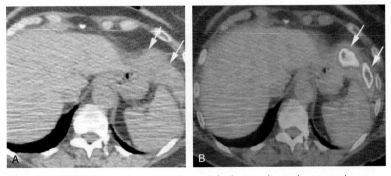

Fig. 11.5 FDG PET/CT image demonstrating uptake in a peritoneal metastasis.

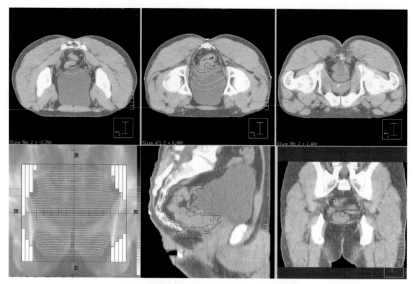

Fig. 11.6 Planning CT demonstrating definition of GTV, CTV expanded, CTV2, and PTV for a mid rectal cancer from its superior to inferior aspect.

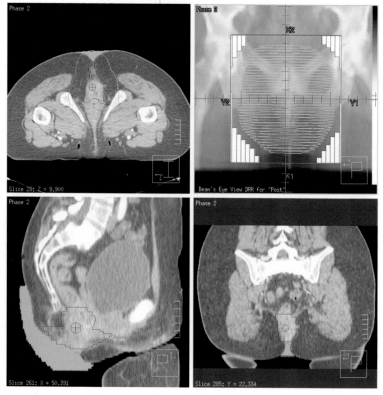

Fig. 12.3 Planning CT showing delineation of the GTV and treatment fields.

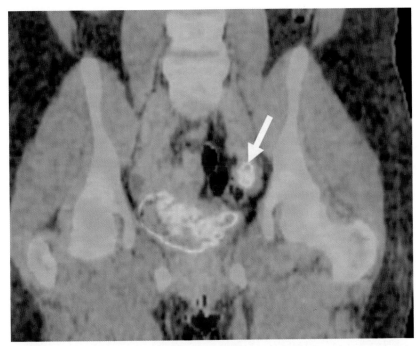

Fig. 14.4 Coronal PET/CT image showing physiological uptake in the left ovary (arrow).

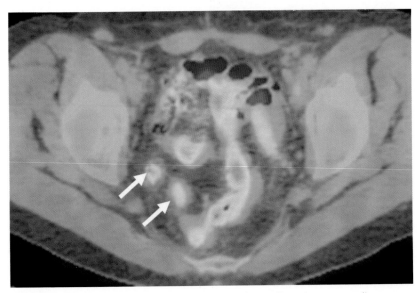

Fig. 14.6 PET/CT: Two metastatic deposits of granulosa cell carcinoma revealing low–moderate grade FDG uptake (arrows).

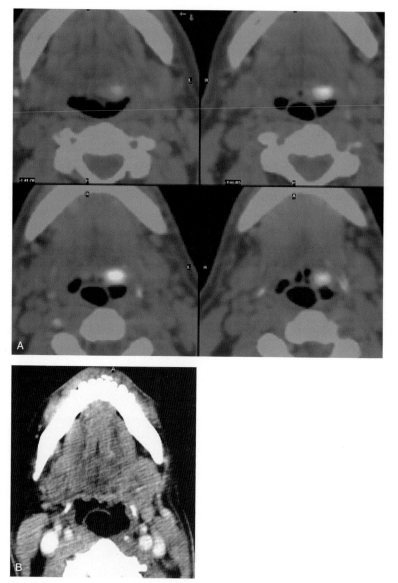

Fig. 15.1 Patient who presented with squamous cell carcinoma in left neck nodes. Full clinical assessment including flexible fibreoptic nasoendoscopy, CT, EUA, speculative biopsies, and ipsilateral tonsillectomy showed no primary site. (A) FDG PET/CT demonstrated a small focus in the base of tongue. Subsequent repeat biopsies of the base of tongue confirmed squamous cell carcinoma. (B) Even in retrospect, the primary site was difficult to identify on the diagnostic CT which was obtained just prior to FDG PET/CT.

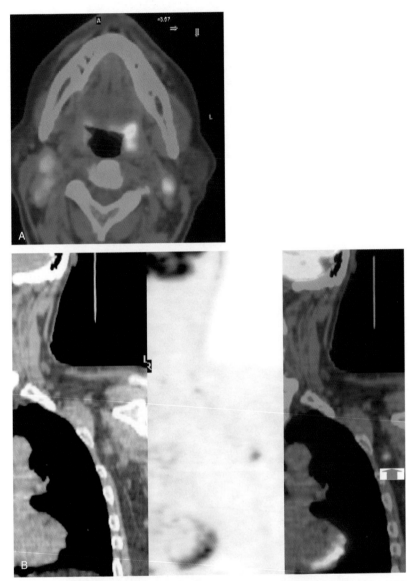

Fig. 15.2 Patient with a tonsil squamous cell carcinoma and bilateral neck nodes. FDG PET/CT showed uptake at the primary site and in the neck on both sides. It also showed unexpected uptake in a small left axillary node (arrow). Biopsy confirmed squamous cell carcinoma. RT treatment plan was modified as a result of the FDG PET/CT.

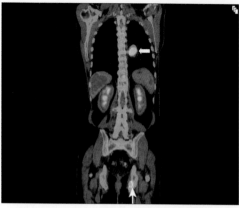

Fig. 17.6 Metastases. Fused FDG PET/CT coronal image of patient with lung (arrow) and left inferior pubic ramus (arrow) FDG avid metastases from a previously resected left shoulder high grade liposarcoma. The inferior pubic ramus lesion bone lesion was missed on conventional imaging (CT).

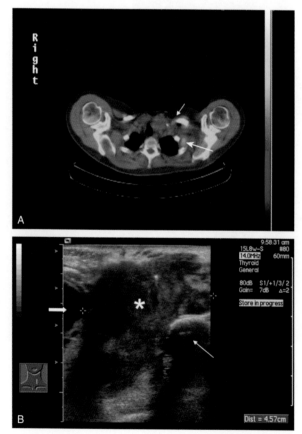

Fig. 17.7 Fused FDG PET/CT axial image (A) of a patient with locally recurrent MPST. A lesion seen adjacent to the left clavicle (arrow) with relatively low FDG uptake was misinterpreted as post treatment related change. A second FDG avid lesion seen between the left first and second ribs (large arrow) was interpreted correctly as recurrent disease. Longitudinal view from an USS (B) of the left supraclavicular fossa performed 2 weeks later confirmed a 4.5-cm solid echo poor mass (asterisk) superior to the clavicle (arrow) histologically confirmed as recurrent disease. An incidental thyroid cyst was also noted (large arrow).

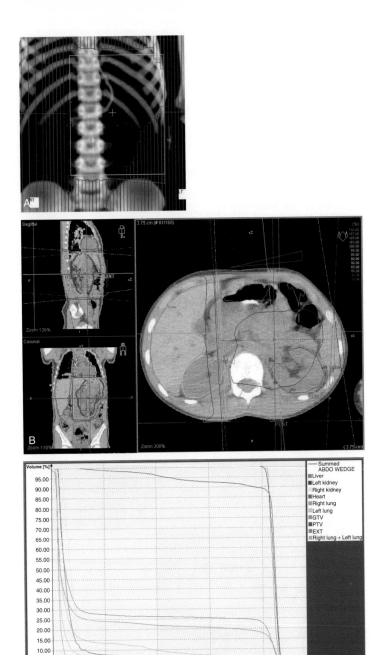

Fig. 20.8 Radiotherapy images. This patient had a left suprarenal tumour excised. Target volume definition was based on the post-chemotherapy, pre-surgical extent of the tumour. (A) Planning DRR to show anterior field. (B) Isodose plans in axial, coronal, and sagittal planes through the isocentre to show dose distribution to the target volume and organs at risk including the left kidney, right kidney, and liver. (C) Dose volume histograms demonstrating coverage of PTV and acceptable doses to organs at risk.

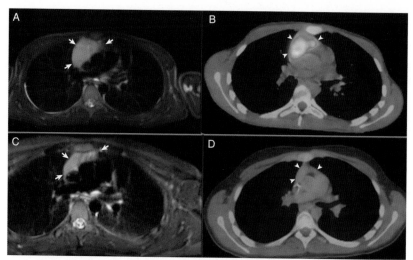

Fig. 20.9 Anterior mediastinal mass. (A) Staging axial MR image of anterior mediastinal mass (short arrows) with corresponding fused PET/CT (B) showing FDG avidity (arrowheads). Restaging following two cycles of chemotherapy. (C) MR image showing reduction in size, but persistant mediastinal disease. (D) Fused PET/CT image showing an excellent metabolic response to chemotherapy, with no residual FDG avidity.

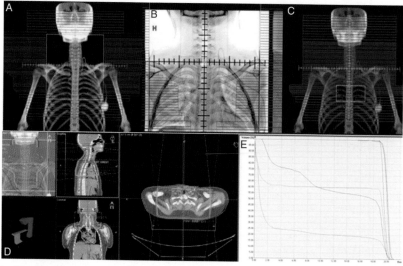

Fig. 20.10 Radiotherapy images. (A) Planning DRR to show complete anterior field covering neck, supraclavicular, and superior mediastinal nodal areas. (B) Simulator check film confirming correct field placement. (C) Planning DRR of anterior boost field used to achieve dose homogeneity. (D) Isodose plans showing dose distribution in axial, coronal, and sagittal planes. (E) Dose volume histograms confirming good coverage of target volumes and acceptable doses to organs at risk.

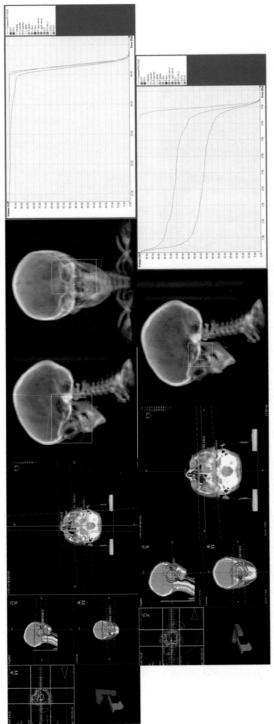

Fig. 20.14 Radiotherapy images. This patient had a parameningeal (nasopharyngeal) rhabdomyosarcoma, treated by a two phase technique. (A) Isodose distribution in axial, coronal, and sagittal planes showing coverage of the phase 1 PTV. (B) Planning DRR of the phase 1 lateral field. (C) Planning DRR of the phase 1 anterior field. (D) Dose volume histograms for phase 1. (E) Plan in three planes for the smaller phase 2 volume avoiding further dose to the eyes. (F) planning DRR of phase 2 field. (G) Dose volume histograms for phase 2.

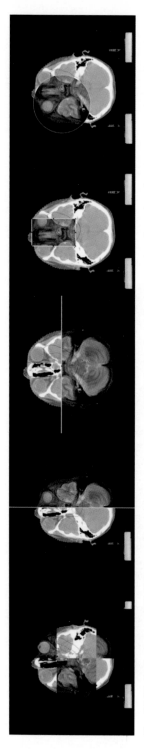

Fig. 20.15 Radiotherapy CT/MR fusion planning. Images to show MRI/CT fusion for radiotherapy planning. The planning CT scan images have been fused with the intial (pre-chemotherapy) diagnostic MRI scans. The target volumes have been drawn on the MRI and the planning is done on the CT images.

during surveillance of vulval intra-epithelial neoplasia (VIN) or lichen sclerosis. The primary tumour is assessed clinically with no specific role for cross-sectional imaging which is rarely utilized (Fig. 14.13)[60]. US combined with fine needle aspiration cytology has been used to select patients for lymphadenectomy, given the predictable spread of these tumours to the inguinal lymph nodes and the morbidity associated with inguinal nodal clearance[61]. Although more accurate than MRI, false negative cases occur so more recently attention has turned to sentinel lymph node sampling. However, larger series are required for validation of early promising results[62,63].

14.5.3 Imaging for radiotherapy planning

The majority of cancers are managed surgically. Adjuvant radiotherapy is recommended for close margin and lymph node-positive disease. Simulator films, using introital markers and wire markers for groin scars are used.

Inoperable locally advanced primary disease may be referred for radiotherapy. In these cases, an MRI scan of the pelvis will aid assessment of the extent of the primary tumour, and inguinal and pelvic lymph node involvement. CT planning may produce more accurate dosimetry and reduced normal toxicity.

14.5.4 Therapeutic assessment and follow-up

Pathological staging determines completion or otherwise of resection and hence the need for further surgery or radiotherapy. Recurrence is usually clinically apparent.

14.6 Summary

- Imaging is integral to the management of the majority of gynaecological cancer patients from diagnosis through treatment to follow-up.
- Functional imaging, using both MRI and PET/CT hardware, is set to play a greater role in all points of the patient care pathway, strengthening the case for ever closer collaboration between all members of the multidisciplinary team.

References

1. Cancerstats from Cancer Research UK. Available at: http://info.cancerresearchuk.org/cancerstats
2. Kumar V, Abbas AK, Fausto N (eds). Robbins and Cotran: *Pathologic Basis of Disease*, 7th edn. Philadelphia, PA: Elsevier Saunders, 2005.
3. Cadron I, Leunen K, Van Gorp T, *et al.* Management of borderline ovarian neoplasms. *J Clin Oncol* 2007; **25**: 2928–37.
4. Heintz APM, Odicino F, Maisonneuve P, *et al.* Carcinoma of the ovary. *Int J Gynecol Obstet* 2006; **95**: S161–S192.
5. Bast RC, Jr., Klug TL, St John E, *et al.* A radioimmunoassay using a monoclonal antibody to monitor the course of epithelial ovarian cancer. *NEJM* 1983; **309**: 883–7.
6. Kobayashi H, Yamada Y, Sado T, *et al.* A randomized study of screening for ovarian cancer: a multicenter study in Japan. *Int J Gynecol Cancer* 2008; **18**: 414–20.
7. van Nagell JR, Jr., DePriest PD, Ueland FR, *et al.* Ovarian cancer screening with annual transvaginal sonography: findings of 25,000 women screened. *Cancer* 2007; **109**: 1887–96.

8. Bast RC, Brewer M, Zou C, *et al.* Prevention and early detection of ovarian cancer: mission impossible? Recent Results. *Cancer Res* 2007; **174**: 91–100.

9. Ye B, Gagnon A, Mok SC. Recent technical strategies to identify diagnostic biomarkers for ovarian cancer. *Expert Rev Proteomics* 2007; **4**: 121–31.

10. Kinkel K, Hricak H, Lu Y, *et al.* US characterization of ovarian masses: a meta-analysis. *Radiology* 2000; **217**: 803–11.

11. Brown DL, Doubilet PM, Miller FH, *et al.* Benign and malignant ovarian masses: selection of the most discriminating gray-scale and Doppler sonographic features. *Radiology* 1998; **208**: 103–10.

12. Valentin L, Ameye L, Testa A, *et al.* Ultrasound characteristics of different types of adnexal malignancies. *Gynecol Oncol* 2006; **102**: 41–8.

13. Sohaib SA, Reznek RH. MR Imaging in ovarian cancer. *Cancer Imaging* 2007; **7**: S119–29.

14. Iyer RB, Balachandran A, Devine CE. PET/CT and cross sectional imaging of gynaecological malignancy. *Cancer Imaging* 2007; **7**: S130–8.

15. Jacobs I, Oram D, Fairbanks J, *et al.* A risk of malignancy index incorporating CA 125, ultrasound and menopausal status for the accurate preoperative diagnosis of ovarian cancer. *Br J Obstet Gynaecol* 1990; **97**: 922–9.

16. Tingulstad S, Hagen B, Skjeldestad FE, *et al.* Evaluation of a risk of malignancy index based on serum CA125, ultrasound findings and menopausal status in the pre-operative diagnosis of pelvic masses. *Br J Obstet Gynaecol* 1996; **103**: 826–31.

17. Bailey J, Tailor A, Naik R, *et al.* Risk of malignancy index for referral of ovarian cancer cases to a tertiary center: does it identify the correct cases? *Int J Gynecol Cancer* 2006; **16**: S30–4.

18. Tempany CM, Zou KH, Silverman SG, *et al.* Staging of advanced ovarian cancer: comparison of imaging modalities – report from the Radiological Diagnostic Oncology Group. *Radiology* 2000; **215**: 761–7.

19. Risum S, Høgdall C, Loft A, *et al.* The diagnostic value of PET/CT for primary ovarian cancer – a prospective study. *Gynecol Oncol* 2007; **105**: 145–9.

20. Fader AN, Rose PG. Role of surgery in ovarian carcinoma. *J Clin Oncol* 2007; **25**: 2873–83.

21. Bristow RE, Duska LR, Lambrou NC, *et al.* A model for predicting surgical outcome in patients with advanced ovarian carcinoma using computed tomography. *Cancer* 2000; **89**: 1532–40.

22. Axtell AE, Lee MH, Bristow RE, *et al.* Multi-institutional reciprocal validation study of computed tomography predictors of suboptimal primary cytoreduction in patients with advanced ovarian cancer. *J Clin Oncol* 2007; **25**: 384–9

23. Spencer JA, Swift SE, Wilkinson N, *et al.* Peritoneal carcinomatosis: image-guided peritoneal core biopsy for tumor type and patient care. *Radiology* 2001; **221**: 173–7.

24. Sheth S, Fishman EK, Buck JL, *et al.* The variable sonographic appearances of ovarian teratomas: correlation with CT. *AJR Am J Roentgenol* 1988; **151**: 331–4.

25. Tanaka YO, Tsunoda H, Kitagawa Y, *et al.* Functioning ovarian tumors: direct and indirect findings at MR imaging. *Radiographics* 2004; **24**(Suppl. 1): S147–66.

26. Barda G, Menczer J, Chetrit A, *et al.* National Israel Ovarian Cancer Group. Comparison between primary peritoneal and epithelial ovarian carcinoma: a population-based study. *Am J Obstet Gynecol* 2004; **190**: 1039–45.

27. Pectasides D, Pectasides E, Economopoulos T. Fallopian tube carcinoma: a review. *Oncologist* 2006; **11**: 902–12.

28. Einhorn N, Trope C, Ridderheim M, *et al.* A systematic overview of radiation therapy effects in ovarian cancer. *Acta Oncologia* 2003; **42**: 562–6.

29. Havrilesky LJ, Kulasingam SL, Matchar DB, *et al*. FDG-PET for management of cervical and ovarian cancer. *Gynecol Oncol* 2005; **97**: 183–91.

30. Epstein E, Valentin L. Managing women with post-menopausal bleeding. *Best Pract Res Clin Obstet Gynaecol* 2004; **18**: 125–43.

31. Clark TJ, Barton PM, Coomarasamy A, *et al*. Investigating postmenopausal bleeding for endometrial cancer: cost-effectiveness of initial diagnostic strategies. *BJOG* 2006; **113**: 502–10.

32. Yahata T, Aoki Y, Tanaka K. Prediction of myometrial invasion in patients with endometrial carcinoma: comparison of magnetic resonance imaging, transvaginal ultrasonography, and gross visual inspection. *Eur J Gynaecol Oncol* 2007; **28**: 193–5.

33. Royal College of Radiologists. *Imaging for Oncology: Collaboration between Clinical Radiologists and Clinical Oncologists in Diagnosis, Staging and Radiotherapy Planning.* London: Royal College of Radiologists, 2004.

34. Trimble CL, Kauderer J, Zaino R, *et al*. Concurrent endometrial carcinoma in women with a biopsy diagnosis of atypical endometrial hyperplasia: a Gynecologic Oncology Group study. *Cancer* 2006; **106**: 812–19.

35. Vasconcelos C, Felix A, Cunha TM. Preoperative assessment of deep myometrial and cervical invasion in endometrial carcinoma: comparison of magnetic resonance imaging and histopathologic evaluation. *J Obstet Gynaecol* 2007; **27**: 65–70.

36. Sala E, Wakely S, Senior E, *et al*. MRI of malignant neoplasms of the uterine corpus and cervix. *AJR Am J Roentgenol* 2007; **188**: 1577–87.

37. Madom LM, Brown AK, Lui F, *et al*. Lower uterine segment involvement as a predictor for lymph node spread in endometrial carcinoma. *Gynecol Oncol* 2007; **107**: 75–8.

38. Hensley ML. *Uterine sarcomas and carcinosarcomas: advances for advanced disease and updates on adjuvant therapy.* ASCO Educational book, 2006.

39. Ueda M, Otsuka M, Hatakenaka M, *et al*. MR imaging findings of uterine endometrial stromal sarcoma: differentiation from endometrial carcinoma. *Eur Radiol* 2001; **11**: 28–33.

40. Murase E, Siegelman ES, Outwater EK, *et al*. Uterine leiomyomas: histopathologic features, MR imaging findings, differential diagnosis, and treatment. *Radiographics* 1999; **19**: 1179–97.

41. Tanaka YO, Nishida M, Tsunoda H, *et al*. Smooth muscle tumors of uncertain malignant potential and leiomyosarcomas of the uterus: MR findings. *J Magn Reson Imaging* 2004; **20**: 998–1007.

42. Sohaib SA, Houghton SL, Meroni R, *et al*. Recurrent endometrial cancer: patterns of recurrent disease and assessment of prognosis. *Clin Radiol* 2007; **62**: 28–34.

43. Fung-Kee-Fung M, Dodge J, Elit L, *et al*. Follow-up after primary therapy for endometrial cancer: a systematic review. *Gynecol Oncol* 2006; **101**: 520–9.

44. Spayne J, Ackerman I, Milosevic M, *et al*. Invasive cervical cancer: a failure of screening. *Eur J Public Health* 2008; **18**: 162–5.

45. Zand KR, Reinhold C, Abe H, *et al*. Magnetic resonance imaging of the cervix. *Cancer Imaging* 2007; **7**: 69–76.

46. deSouza NM, Dina R, McIndoe GA, *et al*. Cervical cancer: value of an endovaginal coil magnetic resonance imaging technique in detecting small volume disease and assessing parametrial extension. *Gynecol Oncol* 2006; **102**: 80–5.

47. Green J, Kirwan J, Tierney J, *et al*. Concomitant chemotherapy and radiation therapy for cancer of the uterine cervix. *Cochrane Database Syst Rev* 2005; **3**: CD002225.

48. Taylor A, Rockall AG, Reznek RH, *et al*. Mapping pelvic lymph nodes: guidelines for delineation in intensity-modulated radiotherapy. *Int J Radiat Oncol Biol Phys* 2005; **63**: 1604–12.

49. Taylor A, Rockall AG, Powell MEB. An atlas of the pelvic lymph node regions to aid radiotherapy target volume definition. *Clin Oncol* 2007; **19**: 542–50.

50. Haie-Meder C, Pötter R, Van Limbergen E, *et al*. Recommendations from gynaecological (GYN) GEC ESTRO working group (I): Concepts and terms in 3D image based treatment planning in cervix cancer brachytherapy with emphasis on MRI assessment of GTV and CTV. *Radiother Oncol* 2005; **74**: 235–45.

51. Pötter R, Haie-Meder C, Van Limbergen E, *et al*. Recommendations from gynaecological (GYN) GEC ESTRO working group (II). Concepts and terms in 3D image based treatment planning in cervix cancer brachytherapy – 3D dose volume parameters and aspects of 3D image-based anatomy, radiation physics, radiobiology. *Radiother Oncol* 2006; **78**: 67–77.

52. Wachter-Gerstner N, Wachter S, Reinstadler E, *et al*. The impact of sectional imaging on dose escalation in endocavitary HDR-brachytherapy of cervical cancer: results of a prospective comparative trial. *Radiother Oncol* 2003; **68**: 51–9.

53. Viswanathan AN, Dimopoulos J, Kirisits C, *et al*. Computed tomography versus magnetic resonance imaging-based contouring in cervical cancer brachytherapy: results of a prospective trial and preliminary guidelines for standardized contours. *Int J Radiat Oncol Biol Phys* 2007; **68**: 491–8.

54. Weber TM, Sostman HD, Spritzer CE, *et al*. Cervical carcinoma: determination of recurrent tumor extent versus radiation changes with MR imaging *Radiology* 1995; **194**: 135–9.

55. Lin CT, Yen TC, Chang TC, *et al*. Role of [18F]fluoro-2-deoxy-D-glucose positron emission tomography in re-recurrent cervical cancer. *Int J Gynecol Cancer* 2006; **16**: 1994–2003.

56. Chung HH, Jo H, Kang WJ, *et al*. Clinical impact of integrated PET/CT on the management of suspected cervical cancer recurrence. *Gynecol Oncol* 2007; **104**: 529–34.

57. Chung HH, Kim SK, Kim TH, *et al*. Clinical impact of FDG-PET imaging in post-therapy surveillance of uterine cervical cancer: from diagnosis to prognosis. *Gynecol Oncol* 2006; **103**: 165–70.

58. Taylor MB, Dugar N, Davidson SE, *et al*. Magnetic resonance imaging of primary vaginal carcinoma. *Clin Radiol* 2007; **62**: 549–55.

59. Lamoreaux WT, Grigsby PW, Dehdashti F, *et al*. FDG-PET evaluation of vaginal carcinoma. *Int J Radiat Oncol Biol Phys* 2005; **62**: 733–7.

60. Land R, Herod J, Moskovic E, *et al*. Routine computerized tomography scanning, groin ultrasound with or without fine needle aspiration cytology in the surgical management of primary squamous cell carcinoma of the vulva. *Int J Gynecol Cancer* 2006; **16**: 312–17.

61. Hall TB, Barton DP, Trott PA, *et al*. The role of ultrasound-guided cytology of groin lymph nodes in the management of squamous cell carcinoma of the vulva: 5-year experience in 44 patients. *Clin Radiol* 2003; **58**: 367–71.

62. Bipat S, Fransen GA, Spijkerboer AM, *et al*. Is there a role for magnetic resonance imaging in the evaluation of inguinal lymph node metastases in patients with vulva carcinoma? *Gynecol Oncol* 2006; **103**: 1001–6.

63. Nyberg RH, Iivonen M, Parkkinen J, *et al*. Sentinel node and vulvar cancer: a series of 47 patients. *Acta Obstet Gynecol Scand* 2007; **86**: 615–19.

Chapter 15

Head and neck cancers

Wai-Lup Wong, Julian Kabala, and
Michele Saunders

15.1 Clinical background

Head and neck cancers are the sixth most common cancer worldwide with an
incidence of 500,000 cases per year (5325 in the UK) and a mortality of 270,000 cases
per year (1851 in the UK)[1].

15.2 Head and neck squamous cell carcinoma (HNSCC)

15.2.1 Diagnosis

A full clinical assessment which includes flexible fibreoptic nasoendoscopy will reveal
the primary site in the majority of HNSCC patients. In some patients, the primary site
will be only apparent on computed tomography (CT) or magnetic resonance imaging
(MRI). In a small number, examination under anaesthesia (EUA) will identify suspicious areas, and biopsy of these sites together with speculative biopsies of sites at high
risk of harbouring a primary site (including the posterolateral wall of the nasopharynx
and the base of tongue on the same side as neck metastases) will diagnose the primary
site; tonsillectomy on the same side as the nodal disease will establish the primary site in
a further percentage. ^{18}F-fluorodeoxyglucose (FDG) positron emission tomography
(PET), and now FDG PET/CT will detect a primary site in up to a further 30% of
patients[2–12] (Fig. 15.1). The effectiveness of FDG PET/CT depends to some extent on
the investigations prior to FDG PET/CT. There is debate as to the value of FDG PET/CT
in patients who have had tonsillectomies[13].

Locating the primary site in HNSCC can markedly alter the treatment plan from
irradiation of the whole head and neck including the nasopharynx, oropharynx, hypo-
pharynx, and larynx to directed treatment with a high dose to the primary cancer and
a lower dose to surrounding normal tissue so reducing morbidity.

The ultimate role of FDG PET/CT is to reduce the number of patients where a primary
site cannot be identified, achieved through increasing the biopsy yield by highlighting to
the head and neck surgeon the areas most likely to yield positive histology. PET/CT is best
performed before EUA to minimize false positive results. In addition to identifying the
primary site, FDG PET/CT may detect unexpected nodal disease in the contralateral neck,
undiagnosed nodal disease within the mediastinum, and synchronous second cancers
including cancers linked by a common aetiology such as head and neck, oesophageal,
lung cancer, and also other common cancers such as colorectal cancer[2,5–7,10,11].

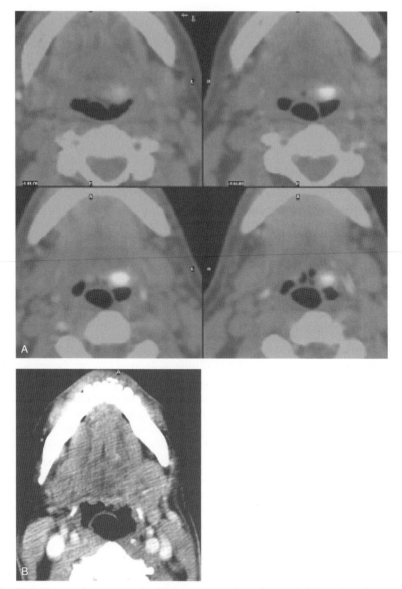

Fig. 15.1 Patient who presented with squamous cell carcinoma in left neck nodes. Full clinical assessment including flexible fibreoptic nasoendoscopy, CT, EUA, speculative biopsies, and ipsilateral tonsillectomy showed no primary site. (A) FDG PET/CT demonstrated a small focus in the base of tongue. Subsequent repeat biopsies of the base of tongue confirmed squamous cell carcinoma. (B) Even in retrospect, the primary site was difficult to identify on the diagnostic CT which was obtained just prior to FDG PET/CT. See colour section.

15.2.2 **Staging**

15.2.2.1 Primary site

In patients with the established diagnosis of HNSCC the main purpose of imaging is to determine the deep extent of local tumour involvement and the presence of nodal disease. Only very occasionally does imaging suggest an alternative or unexpected diagnosis.

Initial choice between CT and MRI as the main imaging tools will depend on a number of factors including availability and team preference. In many centres, MR is the preferred modality for imaging oral cavity and oropharyngeal tumours. However there is a body of experts who prefer high-resolution CT with intravenous contrast for patients with primary nasopharyngeal, hypopharyngeal, and laryngeal cancer and it will also have a role in patients with oral cavity and oropharyngeal cancers who are unable to tolerate MR.

The MRI protocol used will vary considerably, partly related to 1) time available on the scanner; 2) the preferences of the head and neck team; and 3) the make of the MRI scanner. In general, high-quality multi-planar data of the primary site, potential sites of direct invasion, and areas of predicted nodal drainage are included[14–16]. MR sequences typically performed include a coronal short tau inversion recovery (STIR) or fat-saturated T2-weighted (T2W) sequence which encompasses the primary tumour and neck, and coronal and/or axial T1-weighted (T1W) images specifically for primary tumour evaluation. Additional information is gained by using intravenous gadolinium, scanning in other planes, and additional sequences. Many centres include one or more of the following: post-gadolinium fat-saturated T1W sequence in the coronal and axial planes ± sagittal plane, fat-saturated T2W sequence in the sagittal ± axial ± coronal planes.

Presence or absence of cortical bone and marrow involvement is often of central importance for planning treatment. Initial assessment will be made at staging. In many patients it will clearly show no tumour involvement, or alternatively, definite tumour invasion, and no further assessment will be required. CT and MRI complement each other; if one is equivocal then the other can be performed.

Initial assessment of laryngeal cartilage invasion, as with cortical bone and marrow involvement will be made on the initial staging examination. Imaging will show clearly either no tumour involvement or alternatively definite invasion of tumour through laryngeal cartilage and CT and MRI complement each other. Laryngeal cartilage calcifies in an irregular manner and it can be particularly challenging to distinguish uncalcified cartilage from early cartilage destruction. The literature suggests that MRI is more sensitive but less specific, i.e. occurrence of false negatives is less with MRI compared with CT but false positives are higher with MRI compared with CT[16,17].

15.2.2.2 Neck

The presence of metastatic tumour within cervical nodes has a major influence on the treatment plan and determines the likely prognosis in patients with HNSCC. The neck is assessed routinely with the primary site on CT/MRI and they will diagnose neck disease in 20% of patients who are thought to have no disease on clinical assessment.

Imaging is particularly relevant in patients who are difficult to assess clinically, such as those with thick necks.

Ultrasound (US) with fine needle aspiration cytology (FNAC) is a useful adjunct to CT and MRI for detection of nodal disease[18,19]. In expert hands, an accuracy in excess of 90% can be achieved[19]. FDG PET/CT is generally reserved for patients with nodes not accessible to US, e.g. mediastinal and retropharyngeal nodes, and in cases where US does not provide the diagnosis.

15.2.2.3 Distant metastases

In patients with no suspicion of disseminated disease, further imaging other than a chest radiograph is usually not considered. General opinion is that routine use of whole body CT and radionuclide bone scan is not cost effective and should be discouraged. The value of including a CT of the chest in HNSCC patients remains a topic of debate.

In patients with a high risk of distant metastases, such as locally advanced disease (T3/4, N2/3) and tumours arising from subsites which have a particular predilection to metastasize, e.g. nasopharyngeal cancer, FDG PET/CT potentially provides a single whole body investigation which is cost-effective[20,21] (Fig. 15.2).

15.2.3 Radiotherapy planning

Localization of tumour volume and delineation of normal structures is based on CT complemented by MRI. The inclusion of FDG PET/CT may result in substantial change in CTV definition compared to conventional CT [22–26] alone leading to more accurately targeted radiotherapy fields. There is also evidence that FDG PET/CT improves consistency in volume definition between different operators. There is, however, at present a paucity of evidence to show that this translates into improvements in local control or toxicity

Tumour edge definition using FDG PET/CT has not yet been standardized[25]. Segmentation based on a fixed threshold of radioactivity is most commonly used but there is no standardization; 30%, 40%, 50%, and even 60% of maximum SUV of the tumour is taken as the cut-off. More elaborate methods are being developed such as those based on signal-to-noise ratios to refine delineation of tumour margins[26]. In the future, functional imaging with MR and PET/CT may be used to provide information on the biological status of regions within HNSCC and to identify radio-resistant subregions that could be targeted for higher doses of radiation using intensity modulated radiotherapy (IMRT).

15.2.4 Therapeutic assessment and follow-up

On CT and MRI the features which highly suggest residual and recurrence include the presence of one or more soft tissue masses which is enlarging on sequential scans and especially if associated with bone or cartilage destruction. Other features, although less specific, that raise the suspicion of recurrence include focal soft tissue swelling >1cm, that cannot be readily explained by post-surgical appearances, such as those due to a reconstruction flap and any abnormal soft tissue which shows enhancement with intravenous contrast 6 weeks or more after surgery and 12 weeks or more after radiotherapy.

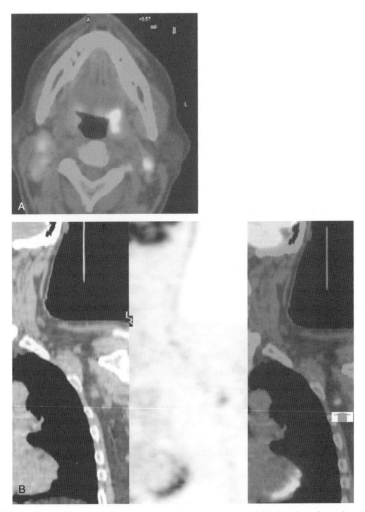

Fig. 15.2 Patient with a tonsil squamous cell carcinoma and bilateral neck nodes. FDG PET/CT showed uptake at the primary site and in the neck on both sides. It also showed unexpected uptake in a small left axillary node (arrow). Biopsy confirmed squamous cell carcinoma. RT treatment plan was modified as a result of the FDG PET/CT. See colour section.

Because many changes that follow intervention may be confused with or mask tumour recurrence, many experts recommend a baseline CT or MRI during the interval when most alterations due to treatment have resolved and there is only little chance of tumour recurrence. Four to 8 weeks post-treatment seems to be the best compromise. Nevertheless, even with a baseline scan in many patients the early diagnosis of recurrent disease while it is still amenable to treatment remains a challenge.

A survey of the literature shows that FDG PET/CT is accurate at diagnosing recurrent HNSCC and has an advantage over CT and MRI[27]. In addition to more accurate assessment of the post-treatment head and neck, FDG PET/CT detects unexpected distant metastases and will from time to time diagnose synchronous cancers. Assessment of the postchemoRT (CRT) neck deserves special consideration. Currently there are no reliable non-invasive methods of predicting complete pathological response of nodal disease to CRT. This means that, presently, a significant number of patients have unnecessary neck dissection with associated morbidity and others have suboptimal treatment of the neck. Preliminary FDG PET results are promising; when performed 8 weeks or more following CRT, FDG PET is has a negative predictive value of 97–100%. The positive predictive value is much more variable ranging from 33–100%[28–31].

15.2.5 Surveillance

Preliminary studies show FDG PET can detect sub-clinical recurrent disease. In a study of 30 patients with no clinical suspicion of recurrence, where FDG PET was done 21 months ± 14 months post-treatment, all 31 patients with negative FDG PET were disease free at 6 months. Of the nine patients with positive FDG PETs, there was local recurrence in four, local recurrence and lung metastases in two, lung metastases in one and local recurrence and nodal metastases in one. There was only one false negative result and this was at the primary site[32]. In a study of 30 patients with stage III/IV HNSCC and no clinical suspicion of recurrence, FDG PET at 2 and 10 months post treatment was conclusively more accurate than usual methods of assessment[33]. A study of 189 patients confirms the results of the other smaller studies and found FDG PET more accurate than usual methods for detecting recurrence in asymptomatic patients[34]. Further work needs to be done to clarify the role of FDG PET/CT in the surveillance of HNSCC patients, including the optimal time points when FDG PET/CT should be considered and especially in those with a high risk of relapse.

15.3 Salivary gland tumours

US is the usual initial investigation for patients with suspected tumours of the salivary glands; it is quick, cheap, and often no further imaging will be required. This is especially the case when the mass is small, clinically benign, easily localized, and delineated, as with the classic and common pleomorphic adenoma lying superficially in the parotid gland. US will determine the location of the lesion, particularly whether or not it lies within a major salivary gland or outside it (e.g. a lymph node or asymmetric masseteric muscle hypertrophy). It will also often provide a confident diagnosis of the nature of the lesion based on its US anatomy, echogenicity, and marginal definition[35]. The main limitation of US is its inability to accurately assess the extent of disease deep to the parotid gland, beyond the stylomandibular canal and CT and MRI are indicated for this, MRI having the additional benefit of more accurate assessment of skull base invasion.

As a general rule, the vast majority of benign tumours are well-defined on all modalities whereas salivary gland malignancies show a broad spectrum of appearances from relatively well-defined benign appearing masses to ill-defined clearly invasive lesions[36]. The commonest salivary gland malignancy encountered is the mucoepidermoid carcinoma. These lesions show a variable degree of malignancy. Low-grade tumours appear similar to benign lesions, showing well-defined margins and a signal intensity on

MRI similar to pleomorphic adenomas. They may be associated with cystic areas which may be complicated by rupture and inflammation, necrosis, and haemorrhage. In keeping with cystic lesions anywhere in the body these processes can alter the appearances on MRI to almost anything. However, generally the presence of blood or a significant amount of protein/mucin will produce high signal on both T1W and T2W sequences. There may be a layering effect with blood products and debris settling posteriorly. High-grade carcinomas are ill defined and more cellular, appearing more homogeneous and with a lower signal intensity on the T2W sequence[37–40]. FDG PET/CT is of limited value for distinguishing between benign and malignant salivary gland tumours as both can be intensely avid for FDG.

Adenocystic carcinomas, in common with other malignancies in the head and neck may show some variable reduction in signal on the T2W sequence and there is some evidence that the degree of reduction correlates with increased cellularity and a higher grade of malignancy[41]. Regardless of site of origin (major salivary gland or ectopic salivary gland tissue) this tumour shows a predilection for perineural invasion and classically extends into skull base foramina and then intracranially. Where extension is gross, CT may demonstrate tumour along the cranial nerves and widened foramina. More subtle perineural/neural invasion is better seen with MRI following intravenous gadolinium.

Diagnosis of recurrent adenocystic carcinoma can be a challenge on imaging including FDG PET/CT. In this situation a positive scan is useful but a negative scan cannot exclude recurrent disease. Perineural invasion cannot be reliably diagnosed on FDG PET/CT and perhaps MR with gadolinium is superior.

Adenocarcinoma within the parotid typically has ill-defined margins and is locally invasive. It can be a primary tumour of the gland or a metastatic deposit within lymph nodes in the salivary gland. Consequently, imaging should be extended to search for possible primary sites with CT chest (for carcinoma of the bronchus), abdomen, and pelvis (for gastrointestinal, pancreatic, and renal carcinomas), and, where appropriate, clinical or mammographic assessment of the breasts.

Squamous cell carcinoma within the parotid with its typically similar imaging appearance to adenocarcinoma is more likely to be metastatic. It is most often due to spread from a local primary site such as the scalp and external auditory canal. However, if the primary site is not obvious clinically, then CT of the chest should be considered as likely primary sites include the bronchus and thoracic oesophagus.

15.4 **Thyroid cancer**

15.4.1 **Background**

Thyroid cancer is a relatively uncommon condition but most countries have shown a significant increase in thyroid cancer over the last 30 years to around 7 cases per 100,000[42].

15.4.2 **Diagnosis**

The vast majority of thyroid cancer is differentiated and will present with a mass or swelling in the neck. US is the key imaging modality for diagnosis, usually combined

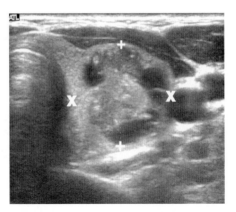

Fig. 15.3 Patient with a papillary carcinoma. Transverse US image through the left lobe of thyroid shows an ill defined predominantly echo poor mass with areas of punctuate calcification and cystic change.

with fine needle aspiration or core biopsy[43]. Features suggestive of papillary carcinoma, the commonest cancer, include ill-defined margins, reduced echogenicity, punctate calcific areas (25–40%), and, in up to 30% of cases, cystic areas (Fig. 15.3).

Follicular carcinoma is notoriously non-specific in appearance at US, usually appearing well defined and similar to a benign adenoma (Fig. 15.4). Colour flow Doppler of a thyroid nodule may be of some assistance. Chaotic intranodal vascular flow suggests a malignant lesion while benign nodules typically have absent or only peripheral flow. The diagnosis often depends on examination of the histological specimen obtained at surgery, the decision to operate being made on the basis of a solitary (or dominant) thyroid mass >3cm.

For more overtly invasive carcinomas of all types (including the rare undifferentiated carcinomas) US features are more obviously malignant with the tumour being ill defined and invasive both within the thyroid gland and extending into adjacent structures.

15.4.3 **Staging**

Most patients will undergo CT of the chest to look for pulmonary metastases following thyroidectomy. A minority, however, will have clinically (or ultrasonographically)

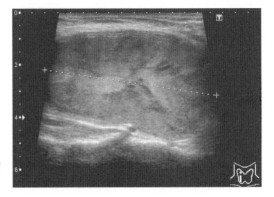

Fig. 15.4 Patient with a follicular carcinoma. Longitudinal US image through the right lobe of thyroid shows relatively well-defined margins, lack of cystic change or calcification, fairly typical of this pathology.

Table 15.1 TNM classification of thyroid cancer[44]

Primary tumour (T)	
pT1	Intrathyroidal tumour ≤1cm in greatest dimension
pT2	Intrathyroidal tumour 1–4cm in greatest dimension
pT3	Intrathyroidal tumour >4cm in greatest dimension
pT4	Tumour (any size) extending beyond the thyroid capsule
pTX	Primary tumour cannot be assessed
Regional lymph nodes (N)—cervical and upper mediastinal	
N0	No nodes involved
N1	Regional lymph nodes involved:
	N1a: ipsilateral cervical nodes
	N1b: bilateral, midline or contralateral cervical nodes or mediastinal nodes
NX	Nodes cannot be assessed
Distant metastases (M)	
M0	No distant metastases
M1	Distant metastases
MX	Distant metastases cannot be assessed

locally advanced tumour at initial presentation. In these circumstances, preoperative staging is indicated, either in those cases for whom thyroidectomy is likely to be unfeasible or inappropriate (advanced undifferentiated carcinoma) or to guide the surgery (Tables 15.1 and 15.2). In these situations imaging is required to describe as accurately as possible the local invasion. Tumour may extend into adjacent critical structures (trachea, larynx, pharynx, oesophagus, and the carotid arteries) and inferiorly into the mediastinum.

Either MRI or CT may be used to assess the neck (Fig. 15.5). The protocols based on the recommendations of the UK Royal College of Radiologists[45] are shown in Table 15.3

Table 15.2 Staging protocol for thyroid cancer[44]

Papillary or follicular carcinoma	Under 45 years	45 years and older		
Stage I	Any T, Any N, M0	T1	N0	M0
Stage II	Any T, Any N, M1	T2	N0	M0
		T3	N0	M0
Stage III		T4	N0	M0
		Any T	N1	M0
Stage IV		Any T	Any N	M1
Anaplastic or undifferentiated carcinoma	All stage IV	All stage IV		

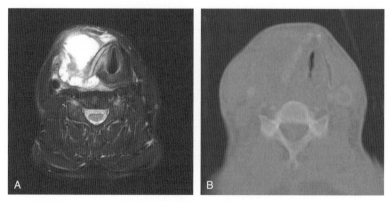

Fig. 15.5 MRI (A) transverse fat-saturated T2-weighted image, demonstrating a large right-sided anaplastic thyroid cancer involving the right thyroid lamina and extending around the posterior margin of the cartilage towards the larynx. CT (B; bone windows) on the same patient demonstrates the markedly abnormal involved right thyroid lamina with ill definition, permeative destruction, and reactive sclerosis.

Intravenous iodine containing contrast media interferes with radioactive iodine uptake by the thyroid for several weeks. It is therefore important to establish with the referring clinician if this is planned before using intravenous contrast.

MRI has a reported accuracy of 86–94% in predicting significant local extension. The following appear to be reliable signs of invasion[46–49];

- Encasement of the organ in excess of:
  - 90° for thyroid cartilage or oesophagus;
  - 135–180° for the trachea; and
  - 225° for the carotid artery.
- Soft tissue within the trachea.

Table 15.3 MRI and CT sequences performed (based on the UK Royal College of Radiologists' recommendations for cross-sectional imaging in cancer management, 2006)[45]

MRI sequences
Coronal T1W and fat-saturated T2W or STIR
Transverse fat-saturated T2W
Post-gadolinium coronal, sagittal and transverse (5mm) fat-saturated T1W
Small field of view, 3-mm slices except where indicated
CT sequences
Neck and chest
Thin slice acquisition: 1.2–2.5mm
Indication from the clinician with reference to the use of iodine containing contrast medium

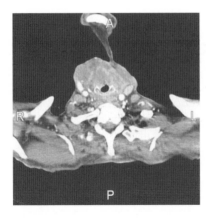

Fig. 15.6 CT scan demonstrating a large anaplastic thyroid carcinoma invading posteriorly, destroying the thyroid cartilage and extending into the larynx.

- Effacement of fat in the tracheo-oesophageal groove or between the laryngeal cartilage and hypopharyngeal wall on multiple slices has an accuracy of 88% in predicting of recurrent laryngeal nerve invasion.

CT may produce better quality images than MRI when patients have respiratory distress and have difficulty lying flat due to compromise of the airway by tumour invasion (Fig. 15.6). CT is also quicker and superior for the detection of pulmonary metastases.

Lymphatic drainage from the thyroid gland is extensive and includes deep and superficial cervical, para- and pretracheal, paraoesophageal, paralaryngeal, supraclavicular, submandibular, and anterior mediastinal lymph nodes. The lymph node groups at highest risk of metastases are the central compartment (level VI, pre- and paratracheal), lower deep cervical (levels III and IV), and the lower half of the posterior triangle (level Vb)[50]. Papillary carcinoma has the highest rate of lymph node metastases, in excess of 75% of cases at presentation[51]. The rate of early lymph node spread is also high with both anaplastic and medullary carcinoma, >50%[52,53], whereas the rate is low with follicular carcinoma, <20%[54].

Papillary carcinoma lymph node metastases may show multiple discrete foci of calcification on CT and areas of reduced (cystic or necrotic change) or increased (intranodal haemorrhage or areas of high thyroglobulin concentration) density[55] (Fig. 15.7).

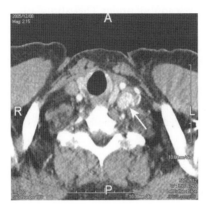

Fig. 15.7 CT scan demonstrating an enlarged left-sided lymph node (arrow) with multiple punctuate calcific foci characteristic of papillary carcinoma metastasis.

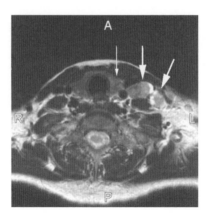

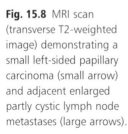

Fig. 15.8 MRI scan (transverse T2-weighted image) demonstrating a small left-sided papillary carcinoma (small arrow) and adjacent enlarged partly cystic lymph node metastases (large arrows).

On MR these changes may appear as high signal on the T2W and low, intermediate, or high signal on T1W sequences (Fig. 15.8). Papillary carcinoma may present with abnormal lymph nodes without a primary thyroid lesion demonstrable on imaging[55].

Lymph node metastases from medullary and anaplastic carcinoma also often show necrotic changes[52,56]. Consequently MRI and CT are reasonably accurate in the detection of involved lymph nodes both at the time of presentation and in recurrent disease, an accuracy of 82–93% being reported[57–59]. This, however, falls to 67% for follicular carcinoma, due to the lower incidence of morphological changes in the affected lymph nodes.

15.4.4 **Therapeutic assessment and follow-up**

The commonest site of recurrence is cervical lymph nodes; recurrence outside the neck is most often in the chest, usually in the form of pulmonary metastases which are often multiple tiny metastases with a relatively indolent course. The only other common metastases are skeletal.

One-third of recurrences occur >10 years after treatment[59] therefore long-term follow-up is required based on clinical examination, thyroid stimulating hormone (TSH) monitoring to ensure adequate suppression, and serum thyroglobulin measurement (calcitonin levels for medullary thyroid cancer)[58]. If the thyroglobulin level rises then iodine-131 (^{131}I) whole body scanning under TSH stimulation (with thyroxine withdrawn or after recombinant TSH stimulation) and US of the neck (with biopsy if appropriate) are indicated[60]. MRI or CT may then be further used to evaluate positive findings in the neck (Fig. 15.9). CT may also be indicated to assess the chest for metastases, especially deposits too small to be reliably detected with radionuclide studies.

In patients where the ^{131}I whole body scan is negative but there is persistently elevated thyroglobulin (or calcitonin), PET/CT scanning is indicated and has been shown to identify lesions undetected on other modalities[61,62].

15.5 **Summary**

- MRI and CT offer good demonstration of the local extent of head and neck tumours; MRI offers better delineation of soft tissue invasion. MRI is the modality of choice for assessing skull base invasion.

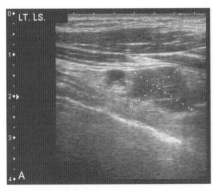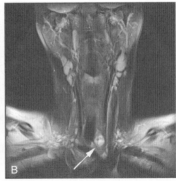

Fig. 15.9 Longitudinal US (A) through the left thyroid bed demonstrating an ill-defined echo-poor deposit of recurrent papillary carcinoma. MRI scan (B; coronal fat saturated T2W image) demonstrating the same deposit as a slightly heterogenous high signal lesion between the trachea and left internal jugular vein (arrow).

♦ FDG PET may improve detection of occult primary tumours, is a cost-effective single staging investigation in tumours at high risk of metastases, and superior to MRI and CT for detection of recurrent disease.

♦ Superficial salivary tumours and thyroid tumours are best assessed initially with ultrasound.

References

1. CancerStats from Cancer Research UK. Available at: http://info.cancerresearchuk.org/cancerstats
2. Wong WL, Saunders M. The impact of FDG PET on the management of occult primary head and neck tumour. *Clin Oncol* 2003; **15**: 461–6.
3. Wong WL, Saunders M. Role of FDG PET in the management of head and neck squamous cell cancer. *Clin Oncol* 1998; **10**: 361–6.
4. Johansen J, Eigtved A, Buchwald C, *et al*. Implication of 18F-fluoro-2-deoxy-D-glucose positron emission tomography on management of carcinoma of unknown primary in the head and neck: a Danish cohort study. *Laryngoscope* 2002; **112**: 2009–14.
5. Jungehulsing M, Klemens S, Damm M, *et al*. FDG PET is a sensitive tool for the detection of occult primary cancer (cancer of unknown primary syndrome) with head and neck lymph node manifestation. *Otolaryngol Head Neck Surg* 2000; **123**: 294–301.
6. Schipper JH, Schrade M, Artweiler D, *et al*. PET to locate primary tumour in patients with cervical lymph node metastases from an occult tumor. *HNO* 1996; **44**: 254–7.
7. Bohusavizki KH, Klutman S, Sonnemann U, *et al*. F-18 FDG PET zur detection des okkulten Primartumors bei Patienten mit Lymphnotenmetastasen der Halsregion. *Laryngo-Rhino-Otol* 1999; **78**: 445–9.
8. Braams JW, Prium J, Kole AC, *et al*. Detection of unknown primary head and neck tumors by PET. *Int J Oral Maxillofac Surg* 1997; **26**: 112–15.
9. Safa AA, Tran LM, Rege S, *et al*. The role of PET in occult primary head and neck cancers. *Cancer J Sci Am* 1999; **5**: 214–18.
10. Regelink G, Brouwer J, deBree R, *et al*. Detection of unknown primary tumours and distant metastases in patients with cervical nodes: value of FDG PET versus conventional studies. *Eur J Nucl Med* 2002; **29**: 1024–30.

11. Fogarty GB, Peters LJ, Stewart J, *et al*. The usefulness of fluorine 18-labelled deoxyglucose PET in the investigation of patients with cervical lymphadenopathy from an unknown primary tumour. *Head Neck* 2003: **25**: 138–45.

12. Stoeckli SJ, Mosna-Firlejczyk K, Goerres GW. Lymph node metastases of SCC from an unknown primary: impact of PET. *Eur J Nucl Med* 2003; **30**: 411–16.

13. Gutzeit A, Antoch G, Kulh H, *et al*. Unknown primary tumors: detection with dual PET/CT- initial experience. *Radiology* 2005; **234**: 227–34.

14. Campbell RSD, Baker E, Chippindale AJ, *et al*. MRI T staging of squamous cell carcinoma of the oral cavity: radiological–pathological correlation. *Clinical Radiology* 1995; **50**: 533–40.

15. Sigal R, Zagdanski A, Schwaab G, *et al*. CT and MR imaging of squamous cell carcinoma of the tongue and floor of the mouth. *Radiographics* 1996; **16**: 787–810.

16. Held P, Breit A. MRI and CT of tumours of the pharynx: comparison of the two imaging procedures including fast and ultrafast MR sequences. *Eur J Radiol* 1994; **18**: 81–91.

17. Becker M, Zbaren P, Laeng H, *et al*. Neoplastic invasion of the laryngeal cartilage: comparision of MR imaging and CT with histological correlation *Radiology* 1995; **194**: 661–9.

18. Takes RD, Kregt P, Manni JJ, *et al*. Regional metastasis in head and neck squamous cell carcinoma: revised value of US with US-guided FNAB. *Radiology* 1996; **198**: 819–23.

19. Van den Brekel MWM. *Assessment of lymph node metastases in the neck*. Academic thesis, Free University of Amsterdam, 1992.

20. Fleming AJ, Smith Jr S, Paul CM, *et al*. Impact of FDG PET CT on previously untreated head and neck cancer patients. *Layngoscope* 2007; **117**: 1173–9.

21. Basu D, Siegel BA, McDonald DJ, *et al*. Detection of occult bone metastases from head and neck squamous cell cancer. *Arch Otoloaryngol Head Neck Surg* 2007; **113**: 801–5.

22. Koshy M, Paulino AC, Howell R, *et al*. FDG PET CT fusion in radiotherapy treatment for head and neck cancer. *Head Neck* 2005; **27**: 494–502.

23. Ciernik IF, Dizendorf E, Baumert BG, *et al*. Radiation treatment planning with integrated PET and CT (PET/CT): a feasibility study. *Int J Radiat Oncol Biol Phys* 2003; **57**: 853–63.

24. Scarfone C, Lavely WC, Cmelak AJ, *et al*. Prospective feasibility trial of radiotherapy target definition for head and neck cancer using 3 dimensional PET and CT imaging. *J Nucl Med* 2004; **43**: 543–52.

25. Gregoire V. Is there any future in radiotherapy planning without the use of PET: unraveling the myth. *Radiother Oncol* 2004; **73**: 261–3.

26. Daisne JF, Sibomana M, Bol A, *et al*. Tri-dimensional automatic segmentation of PET volumes based on measured source to background ratios: influence of reconstruction algorithms. *Radiother Oncol* 2003; **69**: 247–50.

27. Klabbers BM, Lammertsma AA, Slotman BJ. The value of positron emission tomography for monitoring response to radiotherapy in head and neck cancer *Mol Imaging and Biol* 2003; **5**: 257–70.

28. Yao M, Smith RB, Graham MM, *et al* The role of post-radiation therapy FDG PET in prediction of necessity for post-radiation therapy neck dissection in locally advanced head and neck squamous cell carcinoma. *Int J Radiation Oncology Biol Phys* 2005; **63**: 991–9.

29. Porceddu SV, Jarmolowski E, Hicks RJ, *et al*. Utility of PET for the detection of disease in residual neck nodes after (chemo) radiotherapy in head and neck cancer. *Head Neck* 2005; **27**: 175–81.

30. McCullom DA, Burrell SC, Haddad RI, *et al*. PET with 18F-FDG to predict pathological response after induction chemotherapy and definitive chemoradiotherapy in head and neck cancer. *Head Neck* 2004; **26**: 890–6.

31. Rogers JW, Greven KM, McGuirt FW, *et al.* Can post RT neck dissection be omitted for patients with head and neck cancer who have a negative PET scan after definitive radiation therapy? *Int J Radiation Oncology Biol Phys* 2004; **58**: 694–7.

32. Saluan PY, Abgral R, Querellou S, *et al.* Does 18fluoro-fluorodeoxyglucose positron emission tomography improve recurrence detection in patients treated for head and neck squamous cell carcinoma with negative clinical follow-up? *Head Neck* 2007; **29**: 1115–20.

33. Lowe VJ, Boyd JH, Dunphy FR, *et al.* Surveillance for recurrent head and neck cancer using positron emission tomography. *J Clin Oncol* 2000; **18**: 651–8.

34. Lee JC, Kim JS, Lee JH, *et al.* F-18 FDG-PET as a routine surveillance tool for the detection of recurrent head and neck squamous cell carcinoma. *Oral Oncol* 2007; **43**: 686–92.

35. Carter BL. Sonography of the large salivary glands. In: Valvassori GE, Magfe MF, Carter BL (eds). *Imaging of the Head and Neck*. New York: Thieme, 1995.

36. Howlett DC. High resolution ultrasound assessment of the parotid gland. *Br J Radiol* 2003; **76**: 271–7.

37. Silvers AR, Som PM. Salivary glands. *Radiol Clin North Am* 1998; **36**: 941–66.

38. Som PM, Biller HF. High grade malignancies of the parotid gland: identification with MR imaging. *Radiology* 1989; **173**: 823–6.

39. Teresi LM, Lufkin RB, Wortham DG, *et al.* Parotid masses: MR imaging. *Radiology* 1987; **163**: 405–9.

40. Casselman JW, Mancuso AA. Major salivary gland masses: comparison of MR imaging and CT. *Radiology* 1987; **165**: 183–9.

41. Sigal R, Monnet O, de Baere T, *et al.* Adenoid cystic carcinoma of the head and neck: evaluation with MR imaging and clinical–pathologic correlation in 27 patients. *Radiology* 1992; **184**: 95–101

42. Mazzaferri EL. An overview of the management of thyroid cancer. In: Mazzaferri EL, Harmer, C, Mallick UK (eds). *Practical Management of Thyroid Cancer*, pp. 1–28. London: Springer, 2006.

43. King AD, Ahuja AT, To EW, *et al.* Staging papillary carcinoma of the thyroid: magnetic resonance imaging vs ultrasound of the neck. *Clin Radiol* 2000; **55**: 222–6.

44. British Thyroid Association. *Guidelines for the management of thyroid cancer (second edition)*. London: Royal College of Physicians; 2007.

45. Royal College of Radiologists. *Recommendations for Cross-Sectional Imaging in Cancer Management*. London: RCR, 2006.

46. Takashima S, Takayama F, Wang Q, *et al.* Differentiated thyroid carcinomas. Prediction of tumor invasion with MR imaging. *Acta Radiol* 2000; **41**: 377–83.

47. Wang J, Takashima S, Matsushita T, *et al.* Esophageal invasion by thyroid carcinomas: prediction using magnetic resonance imaging. *J Comput Assist Tomogr* 2003; **27**: 18–25.

48. Wang J, Takashima S, Takayama F, *et al.* Tracheal invasion by thyroid carcinoma: prediction using MR imaging. *AJR Am J Roentgenol* 2001; **177**: 929–36.

49. Takashima S, Takayama F, Wang J, *et al.* Using MR imaging to predict invasion of the recurrent laryngeal nerve by thyroid carcinoma. *AJR Am J Roentgenol* 2003; **180**: 837–42.

50. Watkinson J. Management of cervical lymph nodes. In: Mazzaferri EL, Harmer, C, Mallick UK (eds). *Practical Management of Thyroid Cancer*, pp. 149–63. London: Springer, 2006.

51. Cady B. Papillary carcinoma of the thyroid. *Semin Surg Oncol* 1991; **7**: 81–6.

52. Yousem DM, Sceff AM. Thyroid and parathyroid. In: Som PM, Curtin HD, (eds). *Head and Neck Imaging*, 3rd edn, pp. 952–75. St Louis, MO: Mosby, 1996.

53. Ukkat J, Gimm O, Brauckhoff M, *et al*. Single centre experience in primary surgery for medullary thyroid carcinoma. *World J Surg* 2003; **28**: 1271–4.

54. Grebe SKG, Hay ID. Thyroid cancer nodal metastases: biologic significance and therapeutic considerations. *Surg Oncol Clin N Am* 1996; **5**: 43–63.

55. Som PM, Brandwein M, Lidov M, *et al*. The varied presentations of papillary thyroid carcinoma cervical nodal disease: CT and MR findings. *AJNR Am J Neuroradiol* 1994; **15**: 1123–8.

56. Wang Q, Takashima S, Fukuda H, *et al*. Detection of medullary thyroid carcinoma and regional lymph node metastases by magnetic resonance imaging. *Arch Otolaryngol Head Neck Surg* 1999; **125**: 842–8.

57. Gross ND, Weissman JL, Talbot JM, *et al*. MRI detection of cervical metastasis from differentiated thyroid carcinoma. *Laryngoscope* 2001; **111**: 1905–9.

58. Takashima S, Sone S, Takayam F, *et al*. Papillary thyroid carcinoma: MR diagnosis of lymph node metastasis. *Am J Neuroradiol* 1998; **3**: 509–13.

59. Keston Jones M. Management of papillary and follicular thyroid cancer. *J of the RSM* 2002; **95**: 325–6.

60. Pacini F. Follow-up of differentiated thyroid cancer. *Eur J Nucl Med Mol Imaging* 2002; **29**(Suppl. 2): S492–6.

61. Conti PS, Durski JM, Bacqai F, *et al*. Imaging of locally recurrent and metastatic thyroid cancer with positron emission tomography. *Thyroid* 1999; **9**: 797–804.

62. Chung JK, So Y, Lee JS. Value of FDG PET in papillary thyroid carcinoma with negative ^{131}I whole-body scan. *J Nucl Med* 1999; **40**: 486–92.

Chapter 16

Central nervous system

Sara C. Erridge, Rod Gibson, and
David Summers

Introduction

The purpose of imaging is to try to predict the nature and histological type of an
intracranial lesion (solitary or multiple; intraparenchymal or extra-axial; benign or
aggressive) and to demonstrate the size and extent of the lesion. Demonstration of the
relationship between the lesion and adjacent neuroanatomy allows more precise surgical planning and accurate targeting of radiotherapy treatment volumes. Multidetector
computed tomography (CT) and magnetic resonance imaging (MRI) permit detailed
analysis of masses deep within the brain and spine. Modern developments in imaging
such as MR spectroscopy, CT and MR perfusion and diffusion imaging are also providing further insights into lesion pathology and spread. Unfortunately none of the
current imaging tools can predict the histological tumour type with sufficient cer-
tainty, and pathological confirmation is needed in most cases. Conversely a small
biopsy of a heterogeneous lesion may yield appearances consistent with low-grade
tumour, when the imaging suggests a more aggressive lesion. Best practice requires the
correlation of imaging and pathological findings, usually in the context of a multidisciplinary meeting.

Which imaging modality to use in the assessment of a probable tumour depends
greatly on the issues which imaging is being asked to resolve. Both CT and MRI have
strengths and weaknesses. MRI provides the best tissue contrast, displaying excellent
definition of intracerebral structures, and showing subtle contrast enhancement not
visible on CT. The panoply of modern MR techniques such as perfusion and diffusion
imaging, spectroscopy, and functional studies may provide useful additional
information beyond the pure macroscopic structure of an abnormality. Unfortunately
these sequences are more time-consuming and sometimes less well-tolerated by the
patient. MRI is usually the preferred modality in most circumstances.

Nevertheless CT is often the first examination performed as multidetector CT is
accessible and fast, and allows multiplanar image reconstruction akin to MR. However,
the tissue contrast and the distinction between normal brain and tumour remains
inferior. CT may be all that is required, e.g. in planning the resection of a skull vault
meningioma, and CT has advantages in the skull base where the quality of bone
imaging is considerably better. CT will also demonstrate lesion calcification that may
not be visible on MRI. The two modalities are often complementary, e.g. in the

assessment of a skull base tumour where high-resolution CT provides bone detail and MRI shows the extent of soft tissue involvement.

16.1 How to look at imaging of the central nervous system (CNS)

The first and most important consideration, whether reviewing CT or MR, is to decide on the anatomical location of the lesion, in particular, is it *intraparenchymal* (within the substance of the brain) or *extra-axial* (outside the brain itself, and arising from vault, dura or other meninges)?

16.1.1 Intraparenchymal lesions

A solitary intraparenchymal lesion may be either a primary tumour of the CNS, most commonly a glioma, or a metastasis. The relative likelihood depends upon the patient's age and the lesion site; e.g. a solitary posterior fossa lesion in a middle-aged adult is most likely to be a solitary metastasis.

Intraparenchymal lesions expand the cortical gyri, narrowing the subarachnoid and extra-axial spaces. The outer margins of the lesion may be distinct and sharp (as in a metastasis) or ill defined and spiculated (as in a primary aggressive glioma). As a generalization, more aggressive lesions enhance more avidly, and the absence of central enhancement raises the possibility of necrosis or tumour cyst. Intraparenchymal tumours provoke varying degrees of surrounding white-matter change. This is demonstrated as high signal on T2 and FLAIR imaging and may be due to vasogenic tumour oedema, tumour infiltration, or both. This is a particular problem for intraparenchymal primary tumours, where definition of the tumour margin is important for planning radiotherapy. Studies examining stereotactic biopsies have demonstrated glioblastoma cells as much as 6cm away from the enhancing lesion[1]; however, the majority of tumours recur within 2–3cm of the enhancing margin[2,3]. Metastases often have more sharply-defined enhancing margins, and also provoke disproportionately large areas of vasogenic oedema relative to the size of the lesion.

16.1.2 Extra-axial lesions

Extra-axial masses are commonly benign. Meningiomas form the largest group. Typical features include a sharp cleft of cerebrospinal fluid (CSF) between the lesion and the cortical surface, and a broad base on the dura or the skull. Other lesions include bone and dural metastases, and tumours of nerves such as vestibular schwannomas. This latter group is usually easily identifiable by their anatomical location. The presence of a tail of enhancement along the dura is a feature of extra-axial lesions, but is not specific to meningioma.

16.1.3 Other features

In addition to location, other features such as the degree of enhancement following the injection of contrast media can help differentiate between types of lesions. Tumour enhancement, whether on MRI or CT, reflects either disruption of the normal blood–brain barrier, or significantly increased vascularity of a lesion. Assessment of contrast enhancement characteristics is an essential part of the diagnostic study—only patients with a known allergic reaction to contrast media or significantly impaired renal function should not receive contrast. The enhancement characteristics do not directly correlate with tumour grade. For example, meningiomas usually enhance uniformly and avidly, whilst some moderately aggressive gliomas demonstrate only minor enhancement. Many intracranial gliomas are heterogeneous in both imaging and histological features, containing areas of low- and high-grade tumour.

16.2 **Treatment planning**

Three-dimensional (3D) imaging now plays a vital role in the planning of surgery and radiotherapy for all CNS lesions. Prior to surgery most patients will have a volumetric MRI scan performed, which can be used in conjunction with a neural navigation system to direct surgery. This enables the surgeon to perform stereotactic biopsies, guiding them to a specific area on a scan using a 3D coordinate system. A similar system may be used during a resection to establish the extent of tumour tissue to be removed. Some larger neurosurgical centres have intraoperative MRI scanners, which are used to perform a scan with the cranium open to assess the degree of resection already performed and to plan the next phase of the surgery. When the tumour is close to an eloquent area of brain, a functional MRI (fMRI) can be performed to assess the potential impact of a resection. This is often used in conjunction with an 'awake craniotomy'. For example, if the lesion is close to the language centre the patient can be instructed to perform naming tasks during the operation[4].

When treating CNS lesions, CT-planned conformal radiotherapy is now standard in all but the most palliative of situations. Although CT images can provide information on tumour location and enable 3D dose calculations, the inferior tissue contrast makes the images less suitable for target delineation than MRI. Therefore, when planning radiotherapy for most tumours, MR images should also be used. Studies have shown that these should be fused with the planning CT scan to provide the most accurate target definition[5]. Most planning systems now have integral fusion software, although they vary significantly in their accuracy and speed of alignment.

16.3 **New imaging techniques**

Over the last decade there has been a large amount of research investigating the role of new MRI and nuclear medicine techniques to improve the accuracy of initial radiological diagnosis, guide biopsies, and also to identify the extent of tumour spread.

16.3.1 **MRI techniques**

MRI spectroscopy examines the chemical content of tissues and in brain tumours has been used to examine the levels of N-acetylasparate (NAA), creatine, choline, and lactate. The ratio of these compounds, for example NAA to choline, may help different normal brain from tumour infiltration[6,7]. However, at present the low spatial resolution (6–10mm) limits the use in target definition[8].

Diffusion-weighted imaging (DWI) measures the ability of fluid to move in the extra cellular space, and may become restricted in higher grade and very cellular tumours.

Diffusion tensor imaging (DTI) examines the white matter tracts and their integrity, and these may be disrupted by tumour before macroscopic lesions are visible on standard MR sequences[9].This may be useful in the planning of radiotherapy[10] but whilst DWI is now part of standard brain tumour imaging protocols, DTI still requires considerable image processing time to perform well, and its availability is limited in most clinical settings.

Perfusion MRI attempts to measure the degree of angiogenesis and capillary permeability. The role of perfusion imaging has yet to be established though it may be helpful in determining grade of astrocytic (not oligodendroglial) lesions and may help assess the response to antiangiogenesis agents[11].

16.3.2 Nuclear medicine techniques

Single photon emission tomography (SPECT) and, more recently, positron emission tomography (PET) scanning examine functional parameters rather than structure and have been extensively investigated in brain tumours. SPECT scanning uses a number of different radioisotope tracers, e.g. ^{99m}Tc-HMPAO (technesium-hexamethylpropylene amine oxime) to examine brain blood flow or ^{201}thallium chloride to identify areas of increased metabolism. These tracers generally have a long half-life and are more readily available so SPECT can be performed in most hospitals with a gamma camera, but the spatial resolution is inferior to PET/CT which has largely superseded SPECT as metabolic imaging of choice for brain lesions.

^{18}F-fluorodeoxyglucose (FDG) PET scanning can be used in the evaluation of brain tumours with the degree of uptake correlating with tumour grade and survival, but the high level of glucose metabolism in normal grey matter makes differentiation from tumour difficult. Other tracers, which identify increased amino acid uptake or increased protein or DNA synthesis, have also been developed. The most commonly used tracer in brain imaging is carbon-11 (^{11}C) methionine (MET) and has been shown to be useful in assessing tumour grade, guidance of biopsies and radiotherapy target delineation[8], but the very short half-life of ^{11}C makes this tracer difficult to use. Other tracers using fluoride-18 have been developed, principally fluorothymidine-18 (FLT), which measures cell proliferation rates and more recently fluoroethyl-L-tyrosine-18 (FET) that assesses amino acid uptake. FLT is good at grading tumours and predicting prognosis and FET may also prove useful in differentiating normal brain from tumour. In a biopsy study MRI-alone had a specificity of only 53% compared with 94% for combined FET-PET and MRI[12].

Although these techniques appear promising in helping in the differentiation of tumour and normal brain, whether or not these studies will prove useful and cost-effective in the routine planning of radiotherapy requires prospective, ideally randomized studies.

16.4 Intraparenchymal tumours

16.4.1 Gliomas

These intraparenchymal tumours arise from a glial precursor cell[13] and consist of two main groups: 1) the astrocytomas and 2) the oligodendrogliomas, though mixed lesions occur. The World Health Organization categorizes intracranial tumours into four grades ranging from I (most benign) to IV (most aggressive) according to the degree of nuclear atypia (grade II), mitotic activity (grade III), endothelial proliferation, and necrosis (grade IV).

16.4.1.1 Astrocytomas

16.4.1.1.1 **Glioblastoma (grade IV) (GBM)**   This is the commonest of all CNS tumours accounting for around 15% of all lesions and 60% of astrocytomas. In one series of nearly 1000 adult patients, 31% occurred principally in temporal lobes, 24% parietal, 23% frontal, and 16% occipital. Frequently more than one region is affected. Infiltrative growth is characteristic with spread along white matter tracts, e.g. across the corpus callosum, the internal capsule, fornix, or anterior commissure. Multifocal lesions occasionally occur and have a worse prognosis. Spread via the CSF is relatively rare and extraneural metastases are even rarer, but are occasionally observed in long-term survivors.

Imaging features (Fig. 16.1):

- Complex-looking tumour.
- Cystic or necrotic centre.
- Irregular thick enhancing walls on T1 following gadolinium (Gd).
- Usually significant mass effect.
- Moderate surrounding white-matter high signal on T2/FLAIR.
- May cross corpus callosum.
- Haemorrhage unusual.
- Calcification rare.

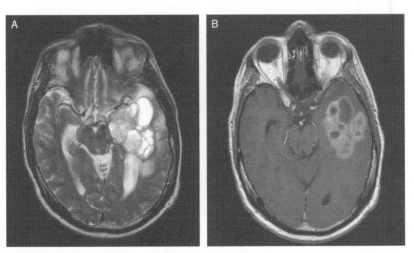

Fig. 16.1 Glioblastoma. T2 (A) and T1 post-gadolinium (B) axial MR image shows a heterogeneous solid/necrotic mass in the left temporal lobe typical of glioblastoma with internal enhancement following gadolinium administration.

Target definition: Ideally, a postoperative MRI fused with a contrast-enhanced planning CT scan should be used for planning. There is controversy over the margin required to cover microscopic spread and whether it is necessary to encompass the whole of the region at risk. Opinions vary as to whether or not to use a two-phase technique encompassing the entire region of peritumoural oedema followed by a boost to the macroscopic tumour (defined by area enhancement/tumour bed) or simply a single-phase technique confining the CTV to the macroscopic tumour with a margin of 2–2.5cm.

When defining this volume it is important to take into account the anatomy of the brain and the tendency of glioblastoma cells to spread along white matter tracts but not to invade other structures such as the tentorium cerebelli, the falx cerebri, or the ventricles.

16.4.1.1.2 **Anaplastic astrocytoma (grade III)**   These lesions, representing around 20% of astrocytomas, occur at a slightly younger age than glioblastomas. They are diffuse lesions with marked cellular atypia and mitotic activity but without frank necrosis. There may be evidence of progression from a grade II diffuse astrocytoma. They have similar growth pattern to GBMs

Imaging features (Fig. 16.2):

- Infiltrative mass, predominantly along white matter tracts.
- Uniformly high signal on T2-weighted sequences.
- Often of considerable size with local mass effect.
- Typically does not enhance, but small focal areas of enhancement may occur.

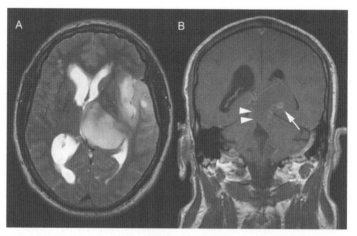

Fig. 16.2 Anaplastic astrocytoma. T2 axial MR image (A) shows a diffusely infiltrating high-signal mass in the left hemisphere and basal ganglia. There is moderate shift of the midline structures to the right and hydrocephalus due to mass effect. T1 coronal MR post-gadolinium (B) shows small focus of enhancement (arrow) and infiltration of non-enhancing tumour into cerebral peduncle (arrowheads).

Target definition: Due to their propensity to progress to GBM similar targets are used. The current global trial (EORTC 26053/BR14) recommends the T2 abnormality is encompassed with a 1.5–2.0cm margin to make a CTV.

16.4.1.1.3 **Diffuse astrocytoma (grade II)**   These lesions represent around 15% of all astrocytomas and are diagnosed most frequently in early adulthood. They can occur anywhere in the brain with the temporal and frontal lobes commonly affected. Certain features suggest a more aggressive clinical course:

◆ Size >6cm.

◆ Crossing mid-line.

◆ Age >40 years.

◆ Localizing clinical signs.

Imaging features (Fig. 16.3):

◆ Bland homogeneous lesions, usually in frontal or parietal lobes.

◆ Usually uniform T2 high signal.

◆ Infiltrate along white matter tracts.

◆ Contrast enhancement absent or minimal.

◆ Often less mass effect than expected for lesion size.

◆ May be indistinguishable from anaplastic astrocytoma.

Target definition: Randomized clinical trials have shown no difference in the overall survival following either immediate or deferred radiotherapy[14] therefore most neuro-oncologists recommend withholding radiotherapy until symptomatic progression, unless two or more of the previously noted poor prognostic features are present[15]. When defining the target for a low-grade astrocytoma it is particularly important to use fused MR images as the lesion is often difficult to identify on CT scans. A margin of 1.5–3cm is usually added to the hyperintense region on T2 MRI, but spectroscopy studies suggest that it might be possible to reduce this margin[16].

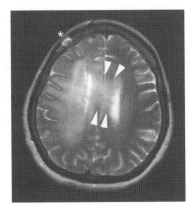

Fig. 16.3 Diffuse astrocytoma. T2 axial MR reveals diffuse white matter high signal with very little mass effect, infiltrating through the body of corpus callosum (arrowheads). The asterisk marks the site of previous biopsy.

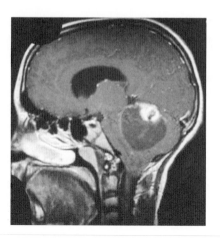

Fig. 16.4 Pilocytic astrocytoma. T1 sagittal MR post-gadolinium demonstrates a large cyst within the cerebellum, lying lateral to the midline, with avidly-enhancing nodule superiorly. This is a typical appearance of posterior fossa pilocytic astrocytoma.

16.4.1.1.4 **Pilocytic astrocytoma (grade I)**   These well-circumscribed, slow growing tumours usually occur in children and young adults. They can occur anywhere throughout the neuraxis but frequently occur in the cerebellar hemispheres (60%) ('cerebellar astrocytoma'), optic pathway (30%) ('optic nerve glioma', particularly seen in patients with neurofibromatosis type 1 (NF1)), third ventricle and hypothalamus (also associated with NF1).

Imaging features (Fig. 16.4):

♦ Avid enhancement of mural nodule.

♦ Rounded cyst or cysts.

♦ Variable size of cyst(s), usually without enhancement in cyst wall.

♦ Sharply-defined margins with normal brain.

Target definition: Most pilocytic astrocytomas can be successfully treated with resection, requiring no additional therapy. However, occasionally a lesion grows or recurs locally or even seeds along the neural axis. When local radiotherapy is required, the enhancing tumour nodule and cyst should be treated with a small margin, e.g. 1–1.5cm to account for microscopic spread and set-up errors.

16.4.1.2 Oligodendrogliomas

16.4.1.2.1 **Oligodendrogliomas (grade II)**   These are slow-growing infiltrative gliomas usually occurring supra-tentorially. They are typically located peripherally in the frontal lobe. One of the pathognomonic features is the presence of dense foci of calcification.

Imaging features (Fig. 16.5):

♦ Peripheral location.

♦ Most commonly frontal.

♦ Nodular calcification in 80%+, best seen on CT.

♦ Margins often relatively well defined.

♦ May contain cystic areas.

- Variable enhancement, usually heterogeneous within tumour.
- Haemorrhage in 20%.
- Skull vault may be scalloped.

Target definition: As with diffuse astrocytoma these patients are often managed with deferred treatment, waiting for tumour progression before commencing treatment. Although initial radiotherapy is currently considered the standard of care comparison with chemotherapy is under investigation in a global clinical trial. The margins added to an oligodendroglioma are similar to those for other grade II gliomas with 1.5–3cm added to the hyperintense lesion on the T2-weighted MRI.

16.4.1.2.2 **Anaplastic oligodendroglioma (grade III)** These lesions usually occur on the background of a grade II lesion and are diagnosed at a slightly older age. The features of a grade II oligodendroglioma are present along with marked nuclear atypia, high mitotic activity and sometimes the presence of vascular proliferation and necrosis.

Imaging features (Fig. 16.6):

- Similar to grade II oligodendroglioma but more aggressive features include
- Avid enhancement, or new areas of enhancement.
- Increasing mass effect.
- Extensive cystic change.

Target definition: There are few data on which to base recommendations but most neuro-oncologists add the same margin as for other high-grade glioma, namely 2–3cm around the enhancing lesion.

16.4.1.3 Mixed gliomas

Oligoastrocytomas and anaplastic oligoastrocytomas are well-recognized entities. In order to be defined as such, a tumour must have two distinct neoplastic cells types present. The prognosis is usually shorter than a pure oligodendroglial lesion so they are managed as astrocytomas with similar radiotherapy margins.

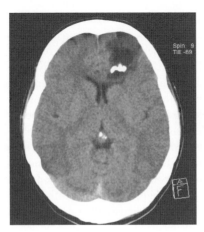

Fig. 16.5 Oligodendroglioma. Axial contrast-enhanced CT shows a left frontal mass, with minor mass effect on the frontal horn of the left ventricle, containing both cystic and calcified elements.

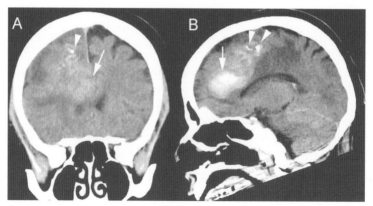

Fig. 16.6 Anaplastic oligodendroglioma. Coronal reformat of contrast-enhanced CT (A) show a diffusely enhancing mass with more marked mass effect than Fig.16.5, containing calcification (arrowhead) and crossing the corpus callosum (arrow). In the sagittal plane (B) calcification (arrowheads) and focal high density consistent with acute haemorrhage into the lesion (arrow).

16.4.1.4 Gliomatosis cerebri

These are rare diffuse glial lesions that affect more than two lobes of the brain and are often bilateral. They are usually graded as III but some lesions behave more like a grade IV lesion[17]. Because of the diffuse nature of the lesion the whole brain is usually included in the radiotherapy volume.

16.4.1.5 Therapeutic assessment and follow-up for glioma

The interpretation of images acquired following surgery or radiotherapy can be difficult. Immediate postoperative MRI should be performed within 72 hours of surgery, as enhancement due to surgical granulation tissue will not be present until after this time. Imaging may however be confounded by postsurgical haematoma and mass effect. Alternatively imaging after several weeks may be performed[9]. Following radiotherapy there are marked changes, particularly in the white matter which can take a number of months to resolve. The appreciation of these changes is particularly important following concurrent chemoradiation as they can be falsely interpreted as tumour progression[18]. Radiation necrosis is unusual, but when it occurs there is often mass effect, irregular peripheral enhancement, and necrosis, and is difficult to distinguish from recurrent high-grade tumour on structural imaging. MR perfusion demonstrates considerably reduced cerebral blood volume in areas of radiation necrosis (as compared with increased blood volume in recurrent tumour), and MR spectroscopy shows decrease in all metabolites in radiation necrosis, unlike recurrent tumour. Other modalities such as PET/CT will also demonstrate the hypometabolism of radiation necrosis.

The optimal follow-up schedule for high-grade glioma has not been established and depends on the patient's fitness for treatment at progression and departmental philosophy. Some centres perform imaging every 3–4 months in order to detect small recurrences amenable to re-resection, whereas other neuro-oncologists feel that the early detection of asymptomatic recurrence is unlikely to be beneficial. There are no studies investigating which approach results in the best patient outcome. For patients with low-grade lesions, especially where there are more treatment options, patients are usually followed with routine MRI scanning, initially every 3–6 months to assess growth characteristics and then annually.

16.4.2 Ependymoma

Ependymomas commonly develop in the posterior fossa, spinal cord, or lateral ventricles. They can spread along the CNS axis so whole brain and spine imaging should be performed. They may be either grade I, II, or III (anaplastic). CSF spread has been documented, but is rare.

Imaging features of grade II and III lesions:

◆ Typically arise from the floor of the fourth ventricle.

◆ Conform to shape of ventricle.

◆ Extend through foramina of Luschka and Magendie.

◆ Enhancement variable, often mild and heterogeneous.

◆ 'Drop metastases' into spine and CSF spaces are common.

Spinal cord myxopapillary ependymoma are grade I lesions, which principally occur in the conus and cauda equina, growing very slowly over years.

Target definition: Historically the whole cranial axis was treated for all grade II and III ependymoma but retrospective studies have shown that the risk of out-of-field relapse is low, particularly for grade II lesions, so most neuro-oncologists recommend local treatment only for these lesions, encompassing gross tumour with a margin of 1–2cm. Grade III lesions, particularly of the posterior fossa, have an increased propensity to spread in the CSF so there is a 'lower threshold' to treat the whole cranial spinal axis.

Imaging features of myxopapillary ependymoma:

◆ Well-demarcated mass centred on conus or cauda equina.

◆ Haemorrhage common.

◆ Enhancement typical.

◆ Bony canal may be expanded.

Target definition: As complete surgical resection is difficult often a combination of subtotal resection and radiotherapy is used and has very good long-term control rates. The target should encompass the whole spinal canal from 2–3cm above the lesion to the thecal sac.

16.4.2.1 Therapeutic assessment and follow-up of ependymal lesions

These patients usually undergo MRI scanning every 3–6 months, particularly if focal radiotherapy only has been used.

16.4.3 Embryonal tumours

This group of undifferentiated round-cell tumours occur principally in children and young adults. Medulloblastomas, which occur in the cerebellar region, are the most common followed by supratentorial primitive neuroectodermal tumours (PNET). Both are classified as grade IV lesions.

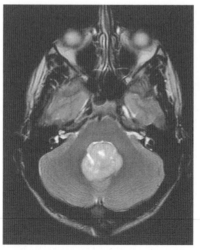

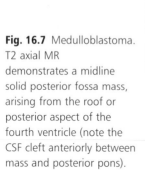

Fig. 16.7 Medulloblastoma. T2 axial MR demonstrates a midline solid posterior fossa mass, arising from the roof or posterior aspect of the fourth ventricle (note the CSF cleft anteriorly between mass and posterior pons).

Medulloblastomas are typically midline tumours arising from the *roof* of the fourth ventricle posteriorly (unlike fourth ventricular ependymoma), growing to occupy the ventricle. In older age groups the lesion may arise laterally in the cerebellar hemispheres.

Imaging features (Fig. 16.7):

- Usually solid, rounded, slightly heterogeneous mass.
- Small intralesional cysts common, large tumour cyst rare.
- Well-defined margins, little oedema.
- Do not grow through foramina of fourth ventricle (unlike ependymoma).
- Heterogeneous enhancement in 80%+.
- Early leptomeningeal spread so post-contrast imaging of the whole of the brain and spine is required for complete staging.

Target definition: Because of their tendency to disseminate throughout the whole CNS axis, patients with medulloblastoma should be treated with craniospinal irradiation encompassing the whole of the meninges. Particular attention should be paid to the cribriform plate, the optic nerve reflection, the temporal lobe reflection, and any post-surgical meningocoele[19,20]. The inferior limit of the thecal sac should be defined individually using the MRI of the spine. The boost usually consists of the whole of the posterior fossa defined using fused MRI scan with the inferior border at C2/3 junction.

16.4.3.1 Therapeutic assessment and follow-up of embryonal tumours

Most patients are followed up by routine post-contrast MRI of the CNS axis every 3–6 months for at least 5 years.

16.4.4 Primary CNS lymphoma (PCNSL)

These are usually B-cell lymphomas though T-cell lesions occur. The usual site is the supratentorial white matter, typically in periventricular regions or in the deep grey

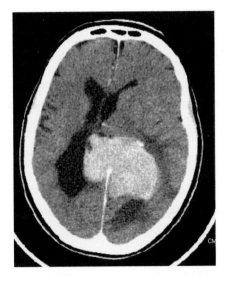

Fig. 16.8 Primary CNS lymphoma. T1 axial post-gadolinium MR shows a typical appearance of primary intracerebral lymphoma—an evenly enhancing lobulated mass in a periventricular location. There is moderate shift of the midline structures to the right and hydrocephalus due to mass effect.

matter nuclei. They may cross the corpus callosum, extending along ventricular ependyma, and may be multifocal. Though normally occurring in older patients PCNSL also occurs in patients with immunosuppression either from HIV-AIDS or post-transplantation.

Imaging features (Fig. 16.8):

- Usually enhances avidly.
- Necrosis or cyst formation rare.
- High density on pre-contrast CT, and restricted diffusion on DWI MR—reflects tumour cellularity.
- Minor oedema for lesion size.
- Calcification rare pre-treatment.
- In immunocompromised patients the appearances are very different—often appearing as ring-enhancing lesions.

Target definition: The role of post-surgical chemotherapy/radiotherapy, particularly in older patients, is controversial because of concerns about late neurocognitive toxicity. However, when radiotherapy is delivered, the whole of the cranial meninges encompassing the optic nerve reflection, base of temporal lobes, and taking the inferior border to the C2/3 junction should be treated and any residual disease boosted with a margin of 1–2cm.

16.4.4.1 Therapeutic assessment and follow-up for PCNSL

This is highly dependant on the clinical condition of the patient and if radiotherapy has been used. If it has been decided to defer radiotherapy then routine imaging every 3–6 months is usually performed to detect any recurrence at an early stage when radiotherapy maybe more effective.

16.4.5 **Pineal lesions**

Lesions in this region can either arise from the pineal parenchyma itself: 1) pineoblastoma—embryonal lesions which can disseminate through the CNS axis, or pineocytoma—relatively benign slow growing lesions; or 2) germ cell lesions (germinoma (akin to seminoma of testes), teratoma, yolk sac tumours, embryonal carcinoma or choriocarcinoma) The pineal gland is the commonest site of intracranial germ cell tumours, though they can occur anywhere, most often in the midline.

Imaging features:

Pineocytoma:

- Well defined.
- Homogeneous signal.
- Avid homogeneous enhancement.
- May be cystic.
- Obstructive hydrocephalus rare.
- Pineal calcification pushed peripherally.

Pineoblastoma:

- Aggressive, heterogeneous appearance.
- Enhancement often only moderate.
- Multicystic/necrotic change.
- Obstructive hydrocephalus common.
- Pineal calcification pushed peripherally.

Germ cell tumours (Fig. 16.9):

- Germinoma—homogeneous and often low T2 signal with avid homogeneous enhancement.
- Calcification often remains central within tumour mass.
- 'Mature' teratoma may show differentiation into fat and dense calcification.

Target definition: As pineoblastoma and germ cell lesions disseminate throughout the CSF they have been classically treated with craniospinal irradiation with a boost to

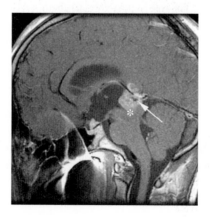

Fig. 16.9 Germinoma. T1 sagittal post-gadolinium MR shows a vividly enhancing mass surrounding the small low signal pineal gland (white arrow). Note the obstruction of the cerebral aqueduct (star) due to tumour infiltration.

the local tumour with a 1–2-cm margin. When treating germinomas some authors advocate chemotherapy followed by localized radiotherapy to minimize late toxicity[21].

16.4.5.1 Therapeutic assessment and follow-up for pineal lesions

Most patients undergo craniospinal axis imaging every 3–6 months to detect recurrences which could be treated with chemotherapy.

16.4.6 Brain metastases

Secondary spread to the brain is common with some autopsy series finding up to a quarter of cancer patients have intracranial spread. Classically the commonest primary tumours to spread to the brain are lung, renal, melanoma, and breast cancers.

Imaging features (Fig. 16.10):

◆ Well-defined lesions, sharp interface with brain parenchyma.

◆ Usually located peripherally at grey–white junction.

◆ Posterior fossa lesions common.

◆ May be cystic, solid, or mixed.

◆ Often provoke marked adjacent white matter oedema for lesion size.

Target definition: For most patients, whole-brain radiotherapy is used to treat sites of known macroscopic and potential microscopic disease. However, some fit patients with up to three lesions may be suitable for stereotactic radiosurgery[22] when treatment planning is based on MRI fused to the planning CT scan.

16.5 Extra-axial tumours

16.5.1 Meningioma

These are the commonest extra-axial lesions, accounting for around 20% of all CNS tumours. Most intracerebral meningiomas are associated with the falx cerebri or dura

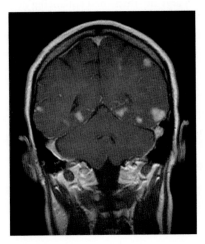

Fig. 16.10 Metastases. T1 coronal post-gadolinium MR shows multiple variably size nodules in both cerebral hemispheres. The typical location for metastases is at the grey–white matter junction.

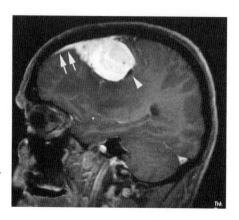

Fig. 16.11 Meningioma. T1 sagittal post-gadolinium MR shows an evenly enhancing mass applied to the inner table of the skull with an anterior dural 'tail' (arrows). Small arachnoid cysts on the tumour surface (arrowhead) are a common finding.

over the cerebral convexity, but they also occur around the orbit and base of skull. Spinal meningiomas are most common in the thoracic region.

Imaging features (Fig. 16.11):

+ Well defined extra axial mass.

+ Broad dural base.

+ CSF cleft between lesion and brain.

+ Uniform avid enhancement.

+ Adjacent bony hyperostosis.

+ Parenchymal vasogenic oedema/white matter gliosis.

+ A 'tail' of enhancement may extend along the adjacent dura (non-specific).

Target definition: There are few data on which to base any recommendation, but the current European Organisation of Research and Treatment in Cancer (EORTC) protocol suggests that the radiotherapy target should be defined on a fused MRI scan and a post-contrast planning CT scan[23]. The GTV should consist of the enhancing tumour on T1 MRI and any thickened enhancing dural tails and hyperostotic bone. A margin of 5–10mm is then added to this for microscopic spread, especially along the dura. If there is no visible disease on postoperative imaging it maybe useful to fuse the preoperative scan to help with target definition. The whole of the meningioma tumour bed is treated as the lesion may recur at any point.

16.5.1.1 Therapeutic assessment and follow-up imaging

Most patients undergo MRI every 6–12 months for at least 5 years to detect recurrences which might be amenable to further surgery.

16.5.2 Tumours of the sellar region

There are three principal lesions which occur at this location; pituitary adenomas, craniopharyngiomas, and meningiomas.

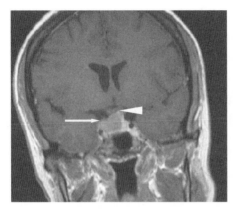

Fig. 16.12 Pituitary macroadenoma with cavernous sinus invasion. T1 coronal post-gadolinium MR shows a poorly-enhancing mass arising from the pituitary fossa encroaching on the optic chiasm (arrowhead) and invading the cavernous sinus (arrow).

16.5.2.1 Pituitary adenomas

These benign lesions present either with hormonal effects or local symptoms such as visual disturbance. They are defined as either microadenomas (<1cm) or macroadenomas (>1cm).

Imaging features (Fig. 16.12):

Pituitary microadenoma:

- Intrapituitary mass.
- Enhance less rapidly than normal pituitary (i.e. hypointense on post-Gd imaging).
- Distortion of superior border of gland.
- May be difficult or impossible to see despite biochemical abnormality.

Pituitary macroadenoma:

- Large sellar mass with suprasellar extension.
- 'Cottage loaf' or 'snowman' appearance.
- Usually enhance avidly.
- May contain cysts or haemorrhage.
- May invade cavernous sinuses, pituitary fossa floor.

Target definition: Radiotherapy is usually offered to patients with residual postoperative disease or recurrence. The treatment should be planned using recent MRI scan and preoperative images. Ideally these should be fused with the planning CT scan. The target should include the whole of the pituitary fossa paying particular attention to any areas of cavernous sinus invasion, and to the roof of the sphenoid sinus following transphenoidal surgery.

16.5.2.2 Craniopharyngiomas

These occur mainly in children but they may also be diagnosed in adulthood. Patients present commonly with visual disturbance or hormonal problems but children may present with a non-specific cognitive changes.

Imaging features:

- Mixed cystic and solid mass centred on suprasellar cistern.
- Enhancement of solid components and cyst walls.
- Calcification occurs in 90%, best seen on CT.
- The pituitary may be visible separate from the mass.

Target definition: The radiotherapy should be planned using a postoperative T1 MRI fused with the planning CT scan. Any residual solid tumour and cyst should be encompassed with a small margin to account for setup accuracy.

16.5.2.2.1 **Therapeutic assessment and follow-up imaging** These patients undergo annual MRI scanning to detect recurrences which might be amenable to further surgery.

16.5.3 **Benign nerve sheath tumours of the CNS**

Schwannomas are the most common lesion occurring on the cranial nerves, particularly the vestibulocochlear nerve ('vestibular schwannoma', also called acoustic neuroma) or the spinal nerves. There are seen more frequently in patients with neurofibromatosis 2 (NF2). Neurofibromas can occur on the spinal nerve roots but do not occur on the cranial nerves. These are connected with NF1.

Imaging features:

- Extraaxial mass centred on internal auditory canal (IAC).
- May be intracanalicular or extend into cerebellopontine angle cistern.
- May expand IAC.
- Avid uniform enhancement.
- 'Ice cream cone' appearance typical.

Target definition: Radiotherapy, delivered either as radiosurgery or a fractionated course is often used to treat schwannomas not amenable to surgical resection. The target should be defined on a T1 contrast-enhanced MRI scan treating the lesion with a margin to account for setup errors.

16.5.3.1 Therapeutic assessment and follow-up imaging

These patients undergo annual MRI scanning to detect recurrences which might be amenable to surgery. On follow-up imaging following stereotactic radiotherapy, lesions may be slow to reduce in size, but often become cyst-like with loss of enhancement.

References

1. Kelly PJ, Daumas-Duport C, Scheithauer BW, *et al*. Stereotactic histologic correlations of computed tomography- and magnetic resonance imaging-defined abnormalities in patients with glial neoplasms. *Mayo Clin Proc* 1987; **62**: 450–9.
2. Chang EL, Akyurek S, Avalos T, *et al*. Evaluation of peritumoral edema in the delineation of radiotherapy clinical target volumes for glioblastoma. *Int J Radiat Oncol Biol Phys* 2007; **68**: 144–50.

3. Lee SW, Fraass BA, Marsh LH, *et al.* Patterns of failure following high-dose 3-D conformal radiotherapy for high-grade astrocytomas: a quantitative dosimetric study. *Int J Radiat Oncol Biol Phys* 1999; **43**: 79–88.

4. Duffau H. Lessons from brain mapping in surgery for low-grade glioma: insights into associations between tumour and brain plasticity. *Lancet Neurol* 2005; **4**: 476–86.

5. Lattanzi JP, Fein DA, McNeeley SW, *et al.* Computed tomography-magnetic resonance image fusion: a clinical evaluation of an innovative approach for improved tumor localization in primary central nervous system lesions. *Radiat Oncol Investig* 1997; **5**: 195–205.

6. Herholz K, Coope D, Jackson A. Metabolic and molecular imaging in neuro-oncology. *Lancet Neurol* 2007; **6**: 711–24.

7. Croteau D, Scarpace L, Hearshen D, *et al.* Correlation between magnetic resonance spectroscopy imaging and image-guided biopsies: semi-quantitative and qualitative histopathological analyses of patients with untreated glioma. *Neurosurgery* 2001; **49**: 823–9.

8. Jacobs AH, Kracht LW, Gossmann A, *et al.* Imaging in neuro-oncology. *NeuroRx* 2005; **2**: 333–47.

9. Cha S. Update on brain tumor imaging: from anatomy to physiology. *AJNR Am J Neuroradiol* 2006; **27**: 475–87.

10. Jena R, Price SJ, Baker C, *et al.* Diffusion tensor imaging: possible implications for radiotherapy treatment planning of patients with high-grade glioma. *Clin Oncol (R Coll Radiol)* 2005; **17**: 581–90.

11. Jenkinson MD, Plessis DG, Walker C, *et al.* Advanced MRI in the management of adult gliomas. *Br J Neurosurg* 2007; **21**: 550–61.

12. Pauleit D, Floeth F, Hamacher K, *et al.* O-(2-[18F]fluoroethyl)-L-tyrosine PET combined with magnetic resonance imaging improves the assessment of cerebral gliomas *Brain* 2005; **128**: 678–87.

13. Vescozi AL, Galli R, Reynolds BA. Brain tumour stem cells. *Nat Rev Cancer* 2006; **6**: 425–36.

14. van den Bent MJ, Afra D, de Witte O, *et al.* EORTC Radiotherapy and Brain Tumor Groups and the UK Medical Research Council. Long-term efficacy of early versus delayed radiotherapy for low-grade astrocytoma and oligodendroglioma in adults: the EORTC 22845 randomised trial. *Lancet* 2005; **366**: 985–90.

15. Pignatti F, van den Bent M, Curran D, *et al.* European Organization for Research and Treatment of Cancer Brain Tumor Cooperative Group; European Organization for Research and Treatment of Cancer Radiotherapy Cooperative Group. Prognostic factors for survival in adult patients with cerebral low-grade glioma. *J Clin Oncol* 2002; **20**: 2076–84.

16. Pirzkall A, Nelson SJ, McKnight TR, *et al.* Metabolic imaging of low-grade gliomas with three-dimensional magnetic resonance spectroscopy. *Int J Radiat Oncol Biol Phys* 2002; **53**: 1254–64.

17. Taillibert S, Chodkiewicz C, Laigle-Donadey F, *et al.* Gliomatosis cerebri: a review of 296 cases from the ANOCEF database and the literature. *J Neurooncol* 2006; **76**: 201–5.

18. Mason WP, Maestro RD, Eisenstat D, *et al.* For the Canadian GBM Recommendations Committee. Canadian recommendations for the treatment of glioblastoma multiforme. *Curr Oncol* 2007; **14**: 110–17.

19. Taylor RE, Bailey CC, Robinson KJ, *et al.* United Kingdom Children's Cancer Study Group Brain Tumour Committee; International Society of Paediatric Oncology. Impact of radiotherapy parameters on outcome in the International Society of Paediatric

Oncology/United Kingdom Children's Cancer Study Group PNET-3 study of preradiotherapy chemotherapy for M0-M1 medulloblastoma. *Int J Radiat Oncol Biol Phys* 2004; **58**: 1184–93.

20. Merchant TE, Kun LE, Krasin MJ, *et al.* Multi-Institution Prospective Trial of Reduced-Dose Craniospinal Irradiation (23.4 Gy) Followed by Conformal Posterior Fossa (36 Gy) and Primary Site Irradiation (55.8 Gy) and Dose-Intensive Chemotherapy for Average-Risk Medulloblastoma. *Int J Radiat Oncol Biol Phys* 2008; **70**: 782–7.

21. Bouffet E, Baranzelli MC, Patte C, *et al.* Combined treatment modality for intracranial germinomas: results of a Multicentre SFOP experience. Société Française d'Oncologie Pédiatrique. *Br J Cancer* 1999; **79**:1199–204.

22. Andrews DW, Scott CB, Sperduto PW, *et al.* Whole brain radiation therapy with or without stereotactic radiosurgery boost for patients with one to three brain metastases: phase III results of the RTOG 9508 randomised trial. *Lancet* 2004; **363**: 1665–72.

23. Khoo VS, Adams EJ, Saran F, *et al.* Comparison of clinical target volumes determined by CT and MRI for the radiotherapy planning of base of skull meningiomas. *Int J Radiat Oncol Biol Phys* 2000; **46**: 1309–17.

Chapter 17

Connective tissue (soft tissue sarcoma)

Derek Svasti-Salee, Eleanor Moskovic, and Frank Saran

17.1 Clinical background

Sarcomas are rare tumours accounting for approximately 1% of all tumours[1]. Despite the variety of different histological subtypes many of the soft tissue sarcomas (STSs) behave in a similar clinical and pathological pattern primarily determined by anatomical location, grade, and size at the time of diagnosis. The dominant pattern of metastases is via a haematogenous route. Lymphatic spread is rare (approximately 3–5%) and associated with a limited number of histological subtypes (e.g. synovial sarcomas, rhabdomyosarcomas, and epithelioid sarcomas[2,3]).

17.2 Diagnosis and staging

17.2.1 Diagnosis

The role of radiology in diagnosing STS has changed remarkably over the last 20 years. In the past a plain radiograph and ultrasound were the main imaging modalities available. Although this provided some useful information the contribution to primarily diagnosing and staging of a STS was limited. The advent of computed tomography (CT) allowed detailed knowledge of the cross-sectional anatomy and better characterization of a suspicious mass lesion and increased the potential to identify sites of metastatic spread. More recently magnetic resonance imaging (MRI) has offered even further improved contrast resolution and multiplanar reconstruction of a mass in question.

The optimal management strategy for a patient with a STS is defined on the knowledge of location, resection margin status, size, and grade. The initial hope that differentiating benign from malignant lesions would eventually be possible with this modality has not yet been met with success. Nevertheless, at present MRI remains the imaging modality of choice for many clinicians, particularly for STSs arising in the limbs, limb girdle, and head and neck. There is growing evidence that ^{18}F-flurodeoxyglucose positron emission tomography (FDG PET) has a potential role in grading, staging and follow-up of patients with primary STSs.

17.2.1.1 Plain film

Although there have been tremendous technological advances in the area of imaging, the plain radiograph remains a frequent form of imaging when assessing a soft tissue lesion.

A plain radiograph can detect the extent of a soft tissue mass by determining the degree of distortion of soft tissue/fat and soft tissue/bone interface. A plain radiograph is also useful at detecting and characterizing calcification which, when present, can be quite specific—e.g. phleboliths in haemangiomas (Fig. 17.1)—or determine any bony erosion/invasion.

17.2.1.2 Sonography

Ultrasound remains an important technique in the initial assessment of a soft tissue swelling. The advantages of ultrasound over both CT and MRI are its low cost and wide availability. Due to its superior spatial resolution it is a particularly useful tool for assessing tumours of wrist, fingers, and skin. However, the features seen on ultrasound are not sufficiently specific to differentiate benign from malignant lesions.

The principle role of ultrasound is to confirm the presence of a lesion, determine its size, and provide clues to the internal structures. Ultrasound is often used as a problem-solving tool, for instance in confirming that a myxoid lesion seen on MRI is solid rather than cystic and demonstrating blood flow in venous haemangiomas.

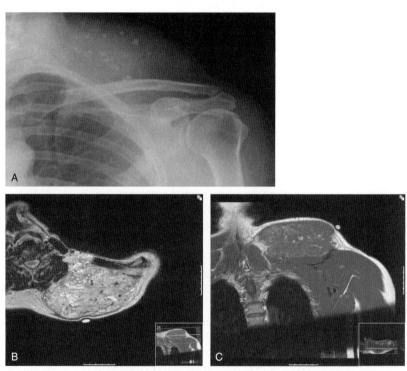

Fig. 17.1 Haemangioma. Plain radiograph (A) demonstrating multiple calcified phleboliths projected superior to the left clavicle characteristic of an haemangioma. The same lesion is depicted on axial T2-weighted MRI (B) as being predominantly high signal with punctuate areas of low signal corresponding to calcified pheloboliths. (C) shows the same lesion on a coronal T1-weighted post contrast MRI demonstrating generalised increased enhancement.

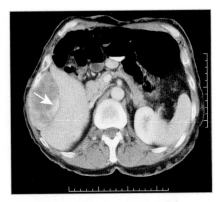

Fig. 17.2 Malignant peripheral nerve sheath tumour. Axial contrast-enhanced CT image through the upper abdomen depicts an enhancing low density extrahepatic mass (white arrow) confirmed as a malignant peripheral nerve sheath tumour. Note numerous subcutaneous nodules in this patient with neurofibromatosis type 1.

17.2.1.3 CT

The use of CT in characterizing the nature of lesions is of limited value. Only in a minority of cases are there sufficient imaging characteristics to accurately predict a correct histological subtype, namely lipoma, haemangioma[4], or elastofibroma. CT is the preferred tool if patients are intolerant of MRI and there is no doubt that CT is more sensitive at detecting and characterizing calcification or ossification within a lesion compared to MRI. The patient's size or the location of a lesion may, however, also dictate the preferred use of CT. In particular, lesions involving the anterior abdomen or chest where motion artefact can degrade image quality on other forms of imaging (Figs. 17.2–17.4). It is important to note that there are currently no data examining the

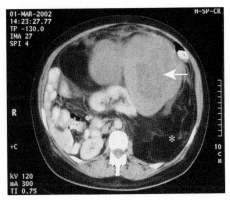

Fig. 17.3 Malignant liposarcoma. Axial contrast-enhanced abdominal CT demonstrating a large retroperioneal fatty lesion (asterisk). The lesion arises from behind the left kidney and displaces it to the right. This finding differentiates it from an intraperitoneal lesion. A more solid area, seen anteriorly (arrow), represents a dedifferentiated component typical for a malignant liposarcoma.

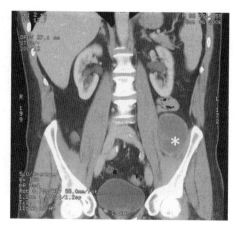

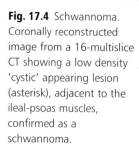

Fig. 17.4 Schwannoma. Coronally reconstructed image from a 16-multislice CT showing a low density 'cystic' appearing lesion (asterisk), adjacent to the ileal-psoas muscles, confirmed as a schwannoma.

merits of multidetector row computed tomography (MDCT) and MRI. The advent of MDCT with superior spatial resolution and isotropic acquisition may negate some of the benefits traditionally achieved with MRI.

17.2.1.4 MRI

The sequences required and their relative merits are discussed in more detail in Chapter 2. Due to their reproducibility and clinicians' familiarity with T1 and T2 spin-echo sequences, these sequences in two orthogonal planes should be included in any study. Additional images are carried out depending on primary location. As a general rule, sagittal sequences should be included with lesions that are orientated anteriorly–posteriorly and coronal in medial or lateral lesions. Fast scanning techniques should be considered to reduce motion artefact and increase compliance in those patients unable to tolerate prolonged scanning times. Gradient echo, short T1 inversion recovery, fluid attenuated inversion recovery, and use of chemical shift artefact are additional sequences that can be used to further characterize a lesion.

17.2.1.5 Differential diagnosis

The ability of MRI to characterize lesions has been shown to be of limited value[5,6]. A correct histological diagnosis being reached solely on imaging characteristics is seen in only 25–35% of cases[5,6]. Characterization of a lesion is usually based on clinical parameters, signal intensity, pattern of growth, location, and associated 'signs' (e.g. 'flow void' seen with haemangiopericytoma[17] and 'bowl of fruit' sign seen with malignant fibrous histiocytoma and synovial sarcoma[7]).

Using exclusively imaging characteristics such as size, lesion margin, signal, neurovascular or bone involvement, it is possible to differentiate a benign from a malignant lesion with variable success[5,6,8,9]. Traditionally features such as smooth, well-defined outline and homogeneous signal characteristics are considered to be more common with benign lesions. However many malignant lesions can share the same radiological characteristics. Even more 'aggressive' characteristics such as bone invasion and neurovascular encasement, although relatively uncommon in STSs, are not reliable indicators for malignancy[5]. However, when using a combination of features malignancy was predicted with the highest sensitivity when a lesion is >33mm, has an inhomogeneous signal on T1-weighted images, and had high signal on T2-weighted images. Signs which had the greatest specificity for malignancy includes the presence of tumours necrosis, bone, or neurovascular involvement and a mean diameter of >66mm[10].

MRI is able to provide certain clues as to the histological component of a lesion which can then be used to narrow the differential and thus potentially guide the surgical diagnostic approach. The presence of a myxoid component can be seen with neurogenic tumours and myxoid liposarcomas. Myxoid lesions characteristically appear high signal on T2- and low on T1-weighted images. They often show mild enhancement and can often be misinterpreted as cysts. Collagen fibres are commonly low on both T1- and T2-weighted images and characteristically exhibit delayed enhancement. Fibrosarcoma, malignant fibrous histiocytoma, and retroperitoneal fibrosis are examples of lesions containing a predominant fibrous component[11,12]. Fat within a lesion can be reliably detected on MRI depending on whether the fat is intra- or extracellular. Extracellular fat is commonly seen in lipomas, myolipomas, and well-differentiated liposarcomas. Extracellular fat is characteristically high signal on both T1- and T2-weighted images and can be confirmed to be low signal on fat-saturated sequences. Calcification can also be depicted on MRI although not with such great sensitivity as CT. Calcification can be seen in neuroblastomas, haemangiomas, and osteosarcomas.

The use of contrast has been proposed to be of value in differentiating benign from malignant lesions. The pattern of enhancement is thought to reflect tissue vascularity and perfusion with malignant lesions generally showing greater degree of enhancement as well as a greater rate of enhancement than benign lesions[13–16]. More specifically, malignant lesions show increased neovascularity at their periphery and show characteristic 'rim to centre' enhancement patterns (Fig. 17.5)[17]. The pattern, rate, and degree of enhancement are by no means diagnostic. In addition, sampling errors will occur with large tumours that have a heterogeneous pattern of enhancement. The degree of

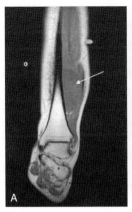
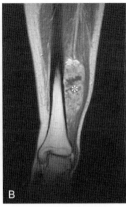

Fig. 17.5 T1-weighted MRI prior (A) and following (B) intravenous gadolinium showing lacking of contrast uptake centrally (asterisk). This corresponds to the area of faint high signal (arrow) on the unenhanced image. This area was confirmed as an area of necrosis on biopsy.

overlap between benign and malignant lesions is so great that gadolinium was found not to contribute to the care or diagnosis of 89% of patients when used to evaluate a suspected STS[18]. The use of contrast is reserved for detecting a small tumour nodule which would otherwise not have been apparent, it can be used to differentiate solid from cystic/necrotic component and be useful as a guide for biopsy.

There are a number of new approaches utilizing MRI spectroscopy and diffusion-weighted imaging under investigation[19]. MRI spectroscopy shows potential in differentiating benign from malignant lesions[20] and in evaluating tumour necrosis[21] but these techniques are not yet widely practised.

17.2.1.6 PET

There is growing evidence that FDG PET can be used to image and stage STS. There are several studies[22,23] and meta-analyses[24,25] suggesting a correlation between FDG PET and tumour grade. There are a number of parameters used to assess the metabolic rate of a lesion including qualitative visualization, standard uptake value (SUV), and metabolic rate of glucose (MRG). There appears to be no major differences in performance when using either one of these parameters[24].

Pooled sensitivities, specificity and accuracy for tumour detection by FDG PET has been reported as 0.91, 0.85, and 0.88 respectively[25]. Tumours with high SUVs appear to be associated with higher histopathological grades[24]. The relationship between FDG uptake and tumour grade is promising as a preoperative prognostic tool and suggests that tumours with low FDG uptake may potentially confer a better prognosis[26,27]. There is, however, considerable overlap with low-grade and high-grade sarcomas. Whereas 93% of lesions with an SUV of >7.5 are high-grade sarcomas, only 43% of high-grade sarcomas have an SUV of this level[28]. False positives may result from scar tissue and inflammatory lesions[23,29]. The main cause for false negatives is finding that low-grade tumours have low SUVs due to low FDG uptake[30] and can be mistaken for benign or inflammatory lesions. Therefore the value of FDG PET has to be interpreted in a wider clinical context and does *not* at present replace the need for a histological confirmation.

17.2.1.7 The role of imaging in biopsy

This is of increasing importance as a significant number of patients are being offered preoperative treatment based on the findings at biopsy. Given the primary size of many STS (>10cm) samples from limited tru-cut biopsies may not reflect the true malignant capacity of a lesion[31]. Both CT and ultrasound-guided biopsies are well-established methods for directing biopsies to improve the diagnostic yield in assessing soft tissue masses particularly in locations not amenable to direct clinical palpation[28,29].

FDG PET is proven to be of use in recognizing intratumoural heterogeneity (seen as areas of high and low SUV). In this setting FDG PET has been shown to be useful for targeting biopsy[32,33] to the area of highest biological activity. In a similar way MRI can differentiate solid from cystic lesions[34], differentiate necrosis from tumour[35], and contrast-enhanced MRI can be useful in differentiating tumour from haemorrhage[36].

17.2.2 **Staging systems**

Commonly used staging systems include the Enneking system[37], frequently used in peripheral musculoskeletal tumours, and the American Joint Committee for Cancer (AJCC) classification[38]. Both these systems incorporate a pathological grade into the traditional TNM (tumour, node, metastasis) system most frequently used in Europe to stage STSs (Table 17.1). The pathological grading system offers the strongest prognostic factor for STS[39,40].

17.2.2.1 **T stage**

Local staging (T) is used to plan the optimal approach to biopsy and identify the choice of definitive surgical treatment as well as advice on non-surgical treatment modalities (radiotherapy and chemotherapy). The principal role of imaging in this

Table 17.1 AJCC classification and staging of soft tissue sarcoma[38]

T stage			
Tx	Primary tumour can not be treated		
T0	No evidence of primary tumour		
T1	Tumour ≤5cm: ◆ T1a: superficial tumours ◆ T1b: deep tumours		
T2	Tumour >5cm: ◆ T2a: superficial tumours ◆ T2b: deep tumours		
N stage			
N0	No regional lymph node metastases		
N1	Regional lymph node metastases		
M stage			
M0	No distant metastases		
M1	Distant metastases		
Histological stage			
G1	Well differentiated		
G2	Moderately differentiated		
G3	Poorly differentiated		
G4	Undifferentiated		
Stage groupings			
Stage I	T1a,1b,2a,2b	N0	M0	G1–2
Stage II	T1a,1b,2a	N0	M0	G3–4
Stage III	T2b	N0	M0	G3–4
Stage IV	Any T	N0	M1	Any G

setting is to provide an accurate assessment of lesion size, contiguity to adjacent visceral structures, and neurovascular land marks. The type of imaging required will therefore depend on the site of primary lesion.

MRI is the preferred imaging modality for extremity STS given the superior contrast resolution over other modalities. MRI is also the preferred modality in imaging the soft tissue component of head and neck STS. MRI will provide information on tumour size, involvement of neurovascular structures, and demonstrate bone involvement. The strengths of CT lie in its speed of image acquisition and the ability to concurrently image the abdominal viscera and chest. In addition, CT provides the highest contrast resolution within the lung and the advent of MDCT means that it is now possible to acquire isotropic imaging for image reconstruction. In this regard CT is the preferred modality for imaging the abdominal[41] and thoracic STSs. The detailed anatomy of the skull base is best appreciated on CT and should also be considered when imaging of head and neck STS.

Several authors have performed small comparative studies examining the relative merits of CT vs. MRI. Issues such as tumour size, invasion of adjacent structures, and compartment involvement have shown that MRI is superior to CT[42,43]. In the only large multi-institutional trial by the Radiologic Diagnostic Oncology Group which compared the two modalities using histological and intraoperative findings found no difference between the two in assessing tumour involvement of bone, muscle, joint, or neurovascular structures[44]. The accuracy of CT for local staging ranges from 81% (periosteal involvement) to 98% (intra-articular extension) and similarly with MRI 83% (periosteal involvement) to 97% (intra-articular extension).

The use of FDG PET to asses the T stage is limited. Tateishi and colleagues compared the performance of FDG PET and FDG PET/CT to conventional imaging (i.e. whole body CT, MRI of primary site, ^{99m}Tc bone scintigraphy and chest X-ray). They concluded that the accuracy of conventional staging was 94%, FDG PET staging 84%, FDG PET/CT staging 96%, and the combination of FDG PET/CT and conventional imaging 99%[45].

17.2.2.2 N stage

Lymphatic spread is generally rare[2,3] and as a consequence evidence for the role of imaging in this setting is limited. Beyond using size measurement to predict lymph node involvement there are no specific features in the assessment of STS when an assessment is made with MRI of CT. However sensitivities of 53%, specificity of 97% and an accuracy of 91% have been quoted for conventional imaging (CT and MRI) compared to 72%, 96% and 93% for FDG PET and 88%, 97% and 96% for FDG PET/CT respectively[45].

17.2.2.3 M stage

Metastases are detected in 7–25% of cases at presentation. In addition metastases may develop in up to 30% these patients within the first year[46–47]. It is estimated that isolated metastases to the lungs, the commonest site of metastatic spread, will occur in 70% of patients who develop metastatic disease[48]. A plain chest radiograph is recognized as a first screening tool for determining the presence of a pulmonary metastasis.

The availability and low radiation dose means that it should be considered in all patients. It is the recommendation of the AJCC that tumours >5cm or with moderate to poor differentiation should undergo a CT scan of the chest as part of staging. The roles of CT, FDG PET, and FDG PET/CT in assessing for a pulmonary metastasis are well established for many tumours but there is little available data to fully assess the efficacy of each of these tests in the context of STSs. Despite the additional benefit of functionality provided by FDG PET, high-resolution CT (particularly when using MDCT) appears superior to FDG PET in assessing for lung metastases[49]. There are currently no data examining the value of FDG PET/CT.

17.3 Imaging during radiotherapy planning and treatment

It is mandatory that all preoperative and, if applicable, postoperative imaging is made available for radiotherapy planning at the time of target volume definition. The CTV definition for recurrent tumours has to take into account the extent of disease at the time of primary diagnosis and at relapse. Unfortunately in a substantial number of cases no adequate imaging of the primary tumour is available as the primary surgeon was not suspicious of an underlying malignancy at the time of presentation of the mass lesion. Thus clinical target volume (CTV)/planning target volume (PTV) definitions rely on correct interpretation of postoperative changes on diagnostic imaging and the planning CT in collaboration with a radiologist experienced in the interpretation of imaging for STS. In a small number of highly selected cases CT/MRI/FDG PET fusion can be helpful to guide appropriate target volume and organ at-risk definition.

Routine diagnostic imaging is only indicated during radiotherapy in a select number of cases undergoing neoadjuvant radiotherapy when tumours are considered to be of borderline resectability at diagnosis. Repeat MRI/ CT of the primary tumour are performed after 45–50Gy to inform the definitive surgical procedure. Should the tumour be deemed inoperable by the surgical team planning to perform the definitive procedure then the radiotherapy to a reduced target volume can be continued until a radical therapeutic dose (usually 66–70Gy) is reached.

17.4 Therapeutic assessment and follow-up

The overall rate of local recurrence with STS after surgery alone remains between 40–60%. The majority, approximately two-thirds, will recur within 2 years. Following current standards of care, including radiotherapy for high-risk patients, local recurrence is reduced to between 10–15%. It is noteworthy that the development of local recurrence does not appear to increase the likelihood of developing metastatic spread[8,50].

A successful follow-up strategy should provide early detection but avoid excessive testing. The type and frequency of follow-up is adjusted for the likelihood of developing a recurrence either local or systemic. Postoperative surveillance is based on the assumption that early intervention will provide improved long-term survival. There is some evidence that aggressive resection of recurrent disease with or without other therapeutic techniques may provide improved long-term survival[51–53]. There are well established (Table 17.2) guidelines available for the follow-up of patients treated for STS[54].

Table 17.2 Follow-up guidelines of soft tissue sarcoma (based on the NCCN recommendations[54]) for resectable peripheral STS and resectable retroperitoneal sarcomas

Stage	Follow-up recommendation: resectable peripheral sarcomas
I and II	History and physical examination every 2–3 months
	Consider periodic imaging of local site based on estimated risk of local recurrence
	Consider baseline imaging after primary therapy
	Consider chest X-ray every 6–12 months
II and III	History and physical examination and chest imaging (chest X-ray or CT) every 3–6 months for 2 years then every 6 months for 2 years then annually
	Consider periodic imaging of local site based on estimated risk of local recurrence (MRI, CT, and ultrasound)
	Consider baseline imaging after primary therapy
Stage	**Follow-up recommendation: resectable retroperitoneal sarcoma**
Low	History and physical examination with imaging (CT abdomen and pelvis) every 3–6 months for 2–3 years, then annually
	Consider chest imaging

17.4.1 The assessment of local regional recurrence

There is limited data available on the most effective surveillance strategy for local recurrence[55]. Clinical examination in experienced hands is an excellent tool in assessing for local recurrence following treatment for superficial tumours. CT and MRI will provide more information for deep seated tumours or those who have received adjuvant therapy. MRI is a well-established tool for assessing post-treatment recurrence[56].

Table 17.3 Identified translocation and fusion genes of primary soft tissue sarcomas

Synovial sarcoma	t(X;18)	SSX1,2,4	SS18
DFSP/GCF	t(17;22)	COL1A1	PDGFB
Congenital fibrosa	t(12;15)	ETV6	NTRK3
E/S myx chondrosa	t(9;22)	CHN	EWS
	t(9;17)	CHN	RBP56
MRC liposa	t(12;16)	CHOP	FUS
	t(12;22)	CHOP	EWS
LG fibromyxoid sarcoma	t(7;16)	CREB3L	FUS
Alveolar SPS	t(X;17)	TFE3	ASPL
Clear cell sarcoma	t(12;22)	ATF-1	EWS
Angiomatoid FH	t(12;22)	ATF-1	EWS
	t(12;16)	ATF-1	FUS

Distinguishing post-therapeutic change from tumour can prove difficult[57–58]. Following surgery and radiotherapy, scar tissue is seen to be low signal on both T1- and T2-weighted sequences and can show variable enhancement with contrast. However, if an enhancing lesion is seen within the post-treatment field which is high on T2- and low on T1-weighted imaging then recurrence is strongly suspected[59]. When assessing for local recurrence of superficial lesions ultrasound and MRI have both been shown to be of equal value[60]. There is some evidence that ultrasound may be superior to CT in this setting[61].

Radiation induced inflammation and scar tissue will accumulate FDG but this is lower in inflammatory tissue than highly active tumour. Inflammatory tissue can be distinguished from recurrent disease in lung and oesophageal cancers[62,63] but this has not been fully validated in soft tissue sarcomas. There is, however, growing evidence that FDG PET provides additional information in patients with equivocal imaging features in the detection of local recurrence and at the same time examine the entire body for additional metastases[64] (Fig. 17.6). False negatives have been demonstrated in low-grade liposarcomas and chondrosarcomas[30].

More often than not either the patient or the physician will detect the presence of a local recurrence[56,65]. Local site imaging is considered to have a low yield and high cost. It is generally reserved for confirming a suspected recurrence and routine assessment of difficult cases. Baseline post-treatment imaging is invaluable in this context and FDG PET is reserved for difficult and equivocal cases (Fig. 17.7).

17.4.2 Assessment for metastasis

The lungs are the commonest site for metastases and should be included in any post-treatment surveillance. In low-grade extremity STS, CT confers little benefit over a plain radiograph in detecting pulmonary metastases[56,66]. With the increased risk, seen in large high-grade tumours, CT of the chest and abdomen may be more useful enabling early detection of further sites of metastases. With time, as the risk of metastases falls, there should be a reduction in imaging frequency.

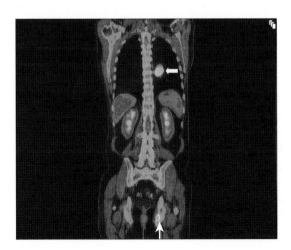

Fig. 17.6 Metastases. Fused FDG PET/CT coronal image of patient with lung (arrow) and left inferior pubic ramus (arrow) FDG avid metastases from a previously resected left shoulder high grade liposarcoma. The inferior pubic ramus lesion bone lesion was missed on conventional imaging (CT). See colour section.

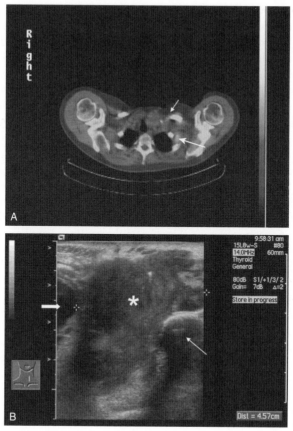

Fig. 17.7 Fused FDG PET/CT axial image (A) of a patient with locally recurrent MPST. A lesion seen adjacent to the left clavicle (arrow) with relatively low FDG uptake was misinterpreted as post treatment related change. A second FDG avid lesion seen between the left first and second ribs (large arrow) was interpreted correctly as recurrent disease. Longitudinal view from an USS (B) of the left supraclavicular fossa performed 2 weeks later confirmed a 4.5-cm solid echo poor mass (asterisk) superior to the clavicle (arrow) histologically confirmed as recurrent disease. An incidental thyroid cyst was also noted (large arrow). See colour section.

17.4.3 Monitoring treatment response

The role of imaging in the assessment of response of neoadjuvant treatment is limited. Its role in the setting of radiotherapy is discussed above. There are several studies which have shown that the assessment of tumour size in response to neoadjuvant radiotherapy[67] and neoadjuvant radiotherapy plus chemotherapy[68] and neoadjuvant chemotherapy alone[69] for STSs is imperfect. There is no consensus amongst studies that radiological response assessment can predict survival[70] but some evidence exists that radiological response may predict local relapse[71]. FDG PET and FDG PET/CT, has been shown to predict histological response[72] and survival[73].

17.5 Summary

- The best local imaging modality for the assessment of lesions suspicious of STS depends on the primary tumour site. MRI is the preferred modality for extremity, limb girdle, and head and neck primaries while contrast-enhanced CT is preferential for chest and abdominal masses.

- Imaging is a vital tool in directing the diagnostic surgical approach to target the most appropriate area for representative tissue sampling and gives vital information when deciding on the definitive procedure.

- Primary systemic staging includes a CT scan of the chest and other imaging techniques only when clinically indicated.

- When using neoadjuvant therapies, assessment of response based on RECIST (Response Evaluation Criteria In Solid Tumors) criteria can be made accurately with CT, MRI, or ultrasound depending on primary tumour site. Correlation with outcome and histological response is limited but FDG PET may predict outcome.

- When amenable to manual examination assessment for local recurrences is accurately made by physical examination. Imaging is reserved for the confirmation or evaluation of equivocal clinical findings as well as intrathoracic or intraabdominal primaries. MRI and FDG PET can be useful in differentiating recurrence from post-treatment related change.

- The commonest site of metastatic spread during follow-up is the lung. This should be routinely imaged with a chest X-ray.

- The frequency and type of imaging in follow-up depends on the primary tumour location, size, tumour grade, and surgical resection margins as these predict most accurately the risk of local and systemic relapse.

References

1. Rydholm A. Improving the management of soft tissue sarcoma. Diagnosis and treatment should be given in specialist centres. *Brit Med J* 1998; **317**: 93–4.

2. Fong Y, Coit DG, Woodruff JM, *et al.* Lymph node metastasis from soft tissue sarcoma in adults. Analysis of data from a prospective database of 1772 sarcoma patients. *Ann Surg* 1993; **217**: 72–7.

3. Zagars GK, Ballo MT, Pisters PW, *et al.* Prognostic factors for patients with localized soft-tissue sarcoma treated with conservation surgery and radiation therapy: an analysis of 225 patients. *Cancer* 2003; **97**: 2530–43.

4. Weekes RG, McLeod RA, Reiman HM, *et al.* CT of soft-tissue neoplasms. *AJR Am J Roentgenol* 1985; **144**: 355–60.

5. Crim JR, Seeger LL, Yao L, *et al.* Diagnosis of soft-tissue masses with MR imaging: can benign masses be differentiated from malignant ones? *Radiology* 1992; **185**: 581–6.

6. Berquist TH, Ehman RL, King BF, *et al.* Value of MR imaging in differentiating benign from malignant soft-tissue masses: study of 95 lesions. *AJR Am J Roentgenol* 1990; **155**: 1251–5.

7. Nishimura H, Zhang Y, Ohkuma K, *et al.* MR imaging of soft-tissue masses of the extraperitoneal spaces. *Radiographics* 2001; **21**: 1141–54.

8. Wetzel LH, Levine E. Soft-tissue tumors of the foot: value of MR imaging for specific diagnosis. *AJR Am J Roentgenol* 1990; **155**: 1025–30.

9. Sundaram M, McGuire MH, Herbold DR. Magnetic resonance imaging of soft tissue masses: an evaluation of fifty-three histologically proven tumors. *Magn Reson Imaging* 1988; **6**: 237–48.

10. De Schepper AM, De Beuckeleer L, Vandevenne J, *et al*. Magnetic resonance imaging of soft tissue tumors. *Eur Radiol* 2000; **10**: 213–23.

11. Arrive L, Hricak H, Tavares NJ, *et al*. Malignant versus nonmalignant retroperitoneal fibrosis: differentiation with MR imaging. *Radiology* 1989; **172**: 139–43.

12. Miller TT, Hermann G, Abdelwahab IF, *et al*. MRI of malignant fibrous histiocytoma of soft tissue: analysis of 13 cases with pathologic correlation. *Skeletal Radiol* 1994; **23**: 271–5.

13. Erlemann R, Reiser MF, Peters PE, *et al*. Musculoskeletal neoplasms: static and dynamic Gd-DTPA – enhanced MR imaging. *Radiology* 1989; **171**: 767–73.

14. Verstraete KL, Dierick A, De Deene Y, *et al*. First-pass images of musculoskeletal lesions: a new and useful diagnostic application of dynamic contrast-enhanced MRI. *Magn Reson Imaging* 1994; **12**: 687–702.

15. Verstraete KL, De Deene Y, Roels H, *et al*. Benign and malignant musculoskeletal lesions: dynamic contrast-enhanced MR imaging – parametric 'first-pass' images depict tissue vascularization and perfusion. *Radiology* 1994; **192**: 835–43.

16. van der Woude HJ, Verstraete KL, Hogendoorn PC, *et al*. Musculoskeletal tumors: does fast dynamic contrast-enhanced subtraction MR imaging contribute to the characterization? *Radiology* 1998; **208**: 821–8.

17. Ma LD, Frassica FJ, McCarthy EF, *et al*. Benign and malignant musculoskeletal masses: MR imaging differentiation with rim-to-center differential enhancement ratios. *Radiology* 1997; **202**: 739–44.

18. May DA, Good RB, Smith DK, *et al*. MR imaging of musculoskeletal tumors and tumor mimickers with intravenous gadolinium: experience with 242 patients. *Skeletal Radiol* 1997; **26**: 2–15.

19. Einarsdottir H, Karlsson M, Wejde J, *et al*. Diffusion-weighted MRI of soft tissue tumours. *Eur Radiol* 2004; **14**: 959–63.

20. Wang CK, Li CW, Hsieh TJ, *et al*. Characterization of bone and soft-tissue tumors with in vivo 1H MR spectroscopy: initial results. *Radiology* 2004; **232**: 599–605.

21. Sostman HD, Prescott DM, Dewhirst MW, *et al*. MR imaging and spectroscopy for prognostic evaluation in soft-tissue sarcomas. *Radiology* 1994; **190**: 269–75.

22. Adler LP, Blair HF, Williams RP, *et al*. Grading liposarcomas with PET using [18F]FDG. *J Comput Assist Tomogr* 1990; **14**: 960–2.

23. Kern KA, Brunetti A, Norton JA, *et al*. Metabolic imaging of human extremity musculoskeletal tumors by PET. *J Nucl Med* 1988; **29**: 181–6.

24. Ioannidis JP, Lau J. 18F-FDG PET for the diagnosis and grading of soft-tissue sarcoma: a meta-analysis. *J Nucl Med* 2003; **44**: 717–24.

25. Bastiaannet E, Groen H, Jager PL, *et al*. The value of FDG-PET in the detection, grading and response to therapy of soft tissue and bone sarcomas; a systematic review and meta-analysis. *Cancer Treat Rev* 2004; **30**: 83–101.

26. Eary JF, O'Sullivan F, Powitan Y, *et al*. Sarcoma tumor FDG uptake measured by PET and patient outcome: a retrospective analysis. *Eur J Nucl Med Mol Imaging* 2002; **29**: 1149–54.

27. Schwarzbach MH, Hinz U, Mitrakopoulou-Strauss A, *et al*. Prognostic significance of preoperative [18-F] fluorodeoxyglucose (FDG) positron emission tomography (PET) imaging in patients with resectable soft tissue sarcomas. *Ann Surg* 2005; **241**: 286–94.

28. Folpe AL, Lyles RH, Sprouse JT, *et al.* (F-18) fluorodeoxyglucose positron emission tomography as a predictor of pathologic grade and other prognostic variables in bone and soft tissue sarcoma. *Clin Cancer Res* 2000; **6**: 1279–87.

29. Strauss LG. Fluorine-18 deoxyglucose and false-positive results: a major problem in the diagnostics of oncological patients. *Eur J Nucl Med* 1996; **23**: 1409–15.

30. Schwarzbach MH, Mitrakopoulou-Strauss A, Willeke F, *et al.* Clinical value of [18-F]] fluorodeoxyglucose positron emission tomography imaging in soft tissue sarcomas. *Ann Surg* 2000; **231**: 380–6.

31. Jones C, Liu K, Hirschowitz S, *et al.* Concordance of histopathologic and cytologic grading in musculoskeletal sarcomas: can grades obtained from analysis of the fine-needle aspirates serve as the basis for therapeutic decisions? *Cancer* 2002; **96**: 83–91.

32. Schulte M, Brecht-Krauss D, Heymer B, *et al.* Grading of tumors and tumorlike lesions of bone: evaluation by FDG PET. *J Nucl Med* 2000; **41**: 1695–701.

33. Hain SF, O'Doherty MJ, Bingham J, *et al.* Can FDG PET be used to successfully direct preoperative biopsy of soft tissue tumours? *Nucl Med Commun* 2003; **24**: 1139–43.

34. Beltran J, Chandnani V, McGhee RA, Jr., *et al.* Gadopentetate dimeglumine-enhanced MR imaging of the musculoskeletal system. *AJR Am J Roentgenol* 1991; **156**: 457–66.

35. Erlemann R, Reiser MF, Peters PE, *et al.* Musculoskeletal neoplasms: static and dynamic Gd-DTPA–enhanced MR imaging. *Radiology* 1989; **171**: 767–73.

36. Seeger LL, Widoff BE, Bassett LW, *et al.* Preoperative evaluation of osteosarcoma: value of gadopentetate dimeglumine-enhanced MR imaging. *AJR Am J Roentgenol* 1991; **157**: 347–51.

37. Enneking WF. A system of staging musculoskeletal neoplasms. *Clin Orthop Relat Res* 1986; **204**: 9–24.

38. Greene FL, Page DL, Flemming FD, *et al. American Joint Committee on Cancer: Cancer Staging Manual*, 6th edn. New York: Springer, 2002.

39. Markhede G, Angervall L, Stener B. A multivariate analysis of the prognosis after surgical treatment of malignant soft-tissue tumors. *Cancer* 1982; **49**: 1721–33.

40. Costa J, Wesley RA, Glatstein E, *et al.* The grading of soft tissue sarcomas. Results of a clinicohistopathologic correlation in a series of 163 cases. *Cancer* 1984; **53**: 530–41.

41. Heslin MJ, Smith JK. Imaging of soft tissue sarcomas. *Surg Oncol Clin N Am* 1999; **8**: 91–107.

42. Demas BE, Heelan RT, Lane J, *et al.* Soft-tissue sarcomas of the extremities: comparison of MR and CT in determining the extent of disease. *AJR Am J Roentgenol* 1988; **150**: 615–20.

43. Tehranzadeh J, Mnaymneh W, Ghavam C, *et al.* Comparison of CT and MR imaging in musculoskeletal neoplasms. *J Comput Assist Tomogr* 1989; **13**: 466–72.

44. Panicek DM, Gatsonis C, Rosenthal DI, *et al.* CT and MR imaging in the local staging of primary malignant musculoskeletal neoplasms: Report of the Radiology Diagnostic Oncology Group. *Radiology* 1997; **202**: 237–46.

45. Tateishi U, Yamaguchi U, Seki K, *et al.* Bone and soft-tissue sarcoma: preoperative staging with fluorine 18 fluorodeoxyglucose PET/CT and conventional imaging. *Radiology* 2007; **245**: 839–47.

46. Nijhuis PH, Schaapveld M, Otter R, *et al.* Epidemiological aspects of soft tissue sarcomas (STS) – consequences for the design of clinical STS trials. *Eur J Cancer* 1999; **35**: 1705–10.

47. Torosian MH, Friedrich C, Godbold J, *et al.* Soft-tissue sarcoma: initial characteristics and prognostic factors in patients with and without metastatic disease. *Semin Surg Oncol* 1988; **4**: 13–19.

48. Gadd MA, Casper ES, Woodruff JM, *et al.* Development and treatment of pulmonary metastases in adult patients with extremity soft tissue sarcoma. *Ann Surg* 1993; **218**: 705–12.

49. Iagaru A, Chawla S, Menendez L, *et al.* 18F-FDG PET and PET/CT for detection of pulmonary metastases from musculoskeletal sarcomas. *Nucl Med Commun* 2006; **27**: 795–802.

50. Mccarter MD, Jaques DP, Brennan MF. Randomized clinical trials in soft tissue sarcoma. *Surg Oncol Clin N Am* 2002; **11**: 11–22.

51. Putnam JB, Jr., Roth JA, Wesley MN, *et al.* Survival following aggressive resection of pulmonary metastases from osteogenic sarcoma: analysis of prognostic factors. *Ann Thorac Surg* 1983; **36**: 516–23.

52. Casson AG, Putnam JB, Natarajan G, *et al.* Five-year survival after pulmonary metastasectomy for adult soft tissue sarcoma. *Cancer* 1992; **69**: 662–8.

53. Singer S, Antman K, Corson JM, *et al.* Long-term salvageability for patients with locally recurrent soft-tissue sarcomas. *Arch Surg* 1992; **127**: 548–53.

54. Demetri GD, Pollock R, Baker L, *et al.* NCCN sarcoma practice guidelines. National Comprehensive Cancer Network. *Oncology (Williston Park)* 1998; **12**: 183–218.

55. Whooley BP, Gibbs JF, Mooney MM, *et al.* Primary extremity sarcoma: what is the appropriate follow-up? *Ann Surg Oncol* 2000; **7**: 9–14.

56. Vanel D, Shapeero LG, Tardivon A, *et al.* Dynamic contrast-enhanced MRI with subtraction of aggressive soft tissue tumors after resection. *Skeletal Radiol* 1998; **27**: 505–10.

57. Fletcher BD. Effects of pediatric cancer therapy on the musculoskeletal system. *Pediatr Radiol* 1997; **27**: 623–36.

58. Verstraete KL, Lang P. Post-therapeutic magnetic resonance imaging of bone tumors. *Top Magn Reson Imaging* 1999; **10**: 237–46.

59. Vanel D, Shapeero LG, De Baert T, *et al.* MR imaging in the follow-up of malignant and aggressive soft-tissue tumors: results of 511 examinations. *Radiology* 1994; **190**: 263–8.

60. Choi H, Varma DG, Fornage BD, *et al.* Soft-tissue sarcoma: MR imaging vs sonography for detection of local recurrence after surgery. *AJR Am J Roentgenol* 1991; **157**: 353–8.

61. Pino G, Conzi GF, Murolo C, *et al.* Sonographic evaluation of local recurrences of soft tissue sarcomas. *J Ultrasound Med* 1993; **12**: 23–6.

62. Hicks RJ, MacManus MP, Matthews JP, *et al.* Early FDG-PET imaging after radical radiotherapy for non-small-cell lung cancer: inflammatory changes in normal tissues correlate with tumor response and do not confound therapeutic response evaluation. *Int J Radiat Oncol Biol Phys* 2004; **60**: 412–18.

63. Wieder HA, Brucher BL, Zimmermann F, *et al.* Time course of tumor metabolic activity during chemoradiotherapy of esophageal squamous cell carcinoma and response to treatment. *J Clin Oncol* 2004; **22**: 900–8.

64. Bredella MA, Caputo GR, Steinbach LS. Value of FDG positron emission tomography in conjunction with MR imaging for evaluating therapy response in patients with musculoskeletal sarcomas. *AJR Am J Roentgenol* 2002; **179**: 1145–50.

65. Kattan MW, Leung DH, Brennan MF. Postoperative nomogram for 12-year sarcoma-specific death. *J Clin Oncol* 2002; **20**: 791–6.

66. Fleming JB, Cantor SB, Varma DG, *et al.* Utility of chest computed tomography for staging in patients with T1 extremity soft tissue sarcomas. *Cancer* 2001; **92**: 863–8.

67. Einarsdottir H, Wejde J, Bauer HC. Pre-operative radiotherapy in soft tissue tumors. Assessment of response by static post-contrast MR imaging compared to histopathology. *Acta Radiol* 2001; **42**: 1–5.

68. DeLaney TF, Spiro IJ, Suit HD, *et al*. Neoadjuvant chemotherapy and radiotherapy for large extremity soft-tissue sarcomas. *Int J Radiat Oncol Biol Phys* 2003; **56**: 1117–27.

69. Pisters PW, Patel SR, Varma DG, *et al*. Preoperative chemotherapy for stage IIIB extremity soft tissue sarcoma: long-term results from a single institution. *J Clin Oncol* 1997; **15**: 3481–7.

70. Pezzi CM, Pollock RE, Evans HL, *et al*. Preoperative chemotherapy for soft-tissue sarcomas of the extremities. *Ann Surg* 1990; **211**: 476–81.

71. Meric F, Hess KR, Varma DG, *et al*. Radiographic response to neoadjuvant chemotherapy is a predictor of local control and survival in soft tissue sarcomas. *Cancer* 2002; **95**: 1120–6.

72. Evilevitch V, Weber WA, Tap WD, *et al*. Reduction of glucose metabolic activity is more accurate than change in size at predicting histopathologic response to neoadjuvant therapy in high-grade soft-tissue sarcomas. *Clin Cancer Res* 2008; **14**: 715–20.

73. Schuetze SM, Rubin BP, Vernon C, *et al*. Use of positron emission tomography in localized extremity soft tissue sarcoma treated with neoadjuvant chemotherapy. *Cancer* 2005; **103**: 339–48.

Chapter 18

Endocrine tumours

Yong Du and Jamshed Bomanji

Introduction

The endocrine system includes not only the discrete endocrine glands but also the diffuse endocrine systems of the gut, respiratory tract, heart, and endothelium[1]. Endocrine tumours are rare, and range from well-differentiated indolent tumours to poorly-differentiated aggressive malignancies[2]. Thyroid carcinoma is the most common endocrine gland malignancy, accounting for <0.5% of all new malignancies and <0.5% of all cancer deaths in the UK[3,4]. Pituitary, thyroid, and ovarian tumours are discussed more extensively in other chapters, this chapter deals with other endocrine tumours.

18.1 Apudomas

Pearse first described that several apparently disparate cell series in the body—initially adrenomedullary chromaffin cells, enterochromaffin cells, the corticotroph, the melanotroph, the pancreatic islet B cell, and the thyroid C cell share—common cytochemical and ultrastructural properties including amine precursor uptake and decarboxylase (APUD) activity within the cells. A generic name—APUD cells—was later proposed for these cells and its list has since expanded. The structural and chemical similarity of APUD cells to neurons suggested a neural crest origin and these cells are distributed throughout the body, where they are all prone to both hyperplasia and neoplasia[5].

18.1.1 Gastroenteropancreatic (GEP) endocrine tumours

18.1.1.1 Clinical background

GEP tumours are rare and produce excessive amounts of varied hormones. Laboratory tests are more specific in diagnosing excessive secretion of particular hormones[6-8]. Patients may present with characteristic symptoms suggesting the possible existence of particular tumour type. Insulinoma is probably the most common tumour (incidence 1 per million per year) and usually present with hypoglycaemic symptoms.

Other functioning tumours include gastrinomas, glucagonomas, VIPomas, and somatostatinomas. Gastrinomas produce a large amount of gastrin which stimulates the secretion of excessive gastric acid leading to ulcers and diarrhoea (Zollinger–Ellison syndrome). Glucagonomas produce excessive glucagon and lead to hyperglycaemia, which causes frequent urination, increased thirst, increased hunger, and a rash that spreads on the face, abdomen, or lower extremities. VIPomas produce vasoactive intestinal peptide (VIP), a hormone that plays a role in intestinal water transport and causes chronic, watery diarrhoea, low serum potassium, low gastric hydrochloric acid, flushing, fatigue, and nausea. Somatostatinomas produce somatostatin, a hormone that inhibits the secretion of several other hormones such as growth hormone, insulin, and gastrin. Thus it can produce type II diabetes, gallstones, steatorrhoea, diarrhoea, weight loss, and lower the gastric hydrochloric acid. Functioning tumours also include PPomas (watery diarrhoea syndrome or absence of clinical symptoms), GRFoma (acromegaly due to ectopic secretion of GH-releasing factor) and ACTHoma (ectopic ACTH, Cushing's syndrome). These are all relatively rare, and overlap with non-pancreatic gut-derived neuroendocrine tumours with and without the carcinoid syndrome[9,10].

Non-functioning tumours make up the majority of islet cell tumours[8]. They produce none of the hormones and thus present with no characteristic clinical syndromes as already mentioned. As a result, they are typically diagnosed at more advanced stages of disease. Approximately 90% of insulinomas are benign, but the percentage is considerably less for gastrinomas. Between 8% insulinomas and 20–25% glucagonomas, and gastrinomas are associated with multiple endocrine neoplasia type-1 (MEN-1) syndrome, where they are multicentric, and all have a capacity for metastatic spread. The prognosis and survival of patients with GEP tumours are related to pathological features, including tumour differentiation, Ki-67 index, tumour size, invasion, and the presence of metastases[9,10].

18.1.1.2 Diagnosis and staging

Diagnosis is usually established following clinical suspicion, serum tests, and imaging[2, 9–12]. Serum tests include gut hormone profile and other relevant endocrine tests, in particular plasma chromogranin A, a useful marker in all these tumours. Computed tomography (CT) or magnetic resonance imaging (MRI) and endoscopic ultrasound (EUS) play an important role in locating the primary tumour and detecting metastases[9–12]. Scintigraphy with radiolabelled somatostatin analogue ^{111}In-octreotide has a sensitivity of 82–95% for detecting islet-cell tumours and their metastases (80% of gastrinomas, glucagonomas and VIPomas, and 60% of insulinomas)[12,13]. The recent introduction of Ga-68 labelled octreotate positron emission tomography (PET)/CT imaging will further improve the diagnostic accuracy[13,14] (Fig. 18.1). Scintigraphy with ^{111}In-octreotide also provides the ability for targeted therapy with ^{90}Y or [177]Lu. In addition, following scintigraphy, a hand-held detection probe may be used intraoperatively to locate occult disease[12].

18.1.1.3 Therapeutic assessment and follow-up

The primary treatment for GEP tumours is surgical removal of all resectable primary and secondary lesions and biochemical follow-up is far more sensitive than imaging. Gut neuroendocrine tumours often pursue an indolent course over many years, and symptomatic palliation of the sequelae of their endocrine products forms an important part of management. Most inoperable or metastatic neuroendocrine tumours express a high density of somatostatin receptors. Various radiolabelled (^{111}In, ^{90}Y, and ^{177}Lu) somatostatin analogues have been used to deliver tumour-targeted radiotherapy. Prior to radionuclide therapy, all patients should have pre-treatment scintigraphy to confirm tumour avidity of the therapeutic radiopharmaceutical[9,12]. Partial remission or

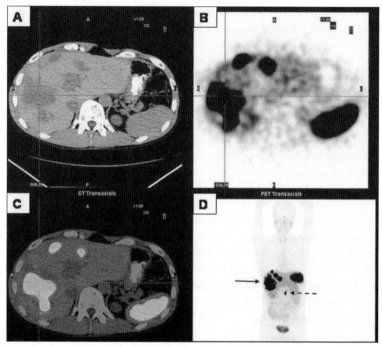

Fig. 18.1 A 35-year-old male patient with known metastatic pancreatic neuroendocrine tumour. PET/CT scan illustrates Ga-68-octreotate avid multiple liver metastases (arrow) and a pre-aortic node (dash arrow). (A), (B), and (C) are CT, PET, and PET/CT fused axial tomographic images respectively.

disease stabilization has been reported in 70–80%, of patients but complete remission rates remain low (<10%).

18.1.2 Carcinoid tumours

18.1.2.1 Clinical background

Carcinoid tumours arise from the argentaffin cells. They may be found in any age group. About 85% of carcinoid tumours develop in the gastrointestinal tract, 10% in the lung, and the rest in various organs such as thymus, kidney, ovary, and prostate[15,16]. Carcinoid tumours are usually classified on the basis of their topographical location as foregut (arising from thymus, lung, stomach, duodenum, and pancreas), midgut (jejunum, ileum, and ascending colon), and hindgut tumours (arising from distal colon and rectum). The most common sites are the appendix, the small bowel, and the rectum. Carcinoids constitute about 34% of all tumours in the small intestine but only 1% of all neoplasms in the stomach, colon, or rectum. Liver is the most common metastatic site and the metastases have one of the longest doubling times of any malignant human tumour. Despite enormous hepatomegaly, patients may remain well for a long time[9,10,17].

Bronchial carcinoids are the most common 'benign' bronchial tumour. They arise endobronchially and frequently in the major bronchi. They usually present with haemoptysis or bronchial obstruction, and resection (lobectomy, pneumonectomy) is usually curative[18]. Approximately 5% of bronchial carcinoids show nodal metastases and atypical carcinoids show more aggressive behaviour and could metastasize to mediastinal lymph nodes (30–50% cases), with a 5-year survival rate of 40–60%[18,19].

Several factors should be considered when evaluating carcinoid tumours for metastatic behaviour. These include the location of the primary tumour (approx 70% of colonic carcinoids give rise to metastases, compared to 30–60% of ileal tumours and only 2–5% of appendical carcinoids), the size of the primary tumour (70% of tumours >2cm and 6% <1cm develop metastases). In addition, the depth of tumour penetration into the bowl wall and the histological growth pattern of the tumour are also important factors[16,20,21].

18.1.2.2 Diagnosis and staging

The diagnosis of a carcinoid tumour may be suspected by clinical symptoms suggestive of carcinoid syndrome or by the presence of other symptoms such as abdominal pain[16,21]. Urinary 5-HIAA has been reported to have a sensitivity of around 70% and a specificity of 100% in patients with carcinoid syndrome. Plasma chromogranin A is the most sensitive marker (100%) but its specificity is lower than urinary 5-HIAA[5,21,22,23] since almost all neuroendocrine tumours show increased levels of chromogranin A.

Imaging plays a crucial role in detecting and characterizing carcinoid tumour[5,21,23]. Scintigraphy using radiolabelled somatostatin analogues such as ^{111}In-octreotide has demonstrated high sensitivity and specificity in the detection of carcinoid tumour[12,22,24]. The recent advent of intergrated ^{68}Ga-OCTREOTATE and ^{18}F fluorodeoxyglucose (FDG) PET/CT could potentially improve the detection accuracy further[7,8,12].

18.1.2.3 Therapeutic assessment and follow-up

Surgical treatment should be considered in every patient with a carcinoid tumour and operable disease should be resected[16,21,23,25]. Although the majority of patients with midgut carcinoid tumours presenting with a carcinoid syndrome have liver metastases and cannot be cured surgically, excision of discrete hepatic metastases of this slowly growing tumour is perceived to be clinically beneficial[26–28].

Whilst external beam radiotherapy has been mostly reserved for treating painful bone metastases, radionuclide therapy is becoming of increasing importance[21,27]. If the relevant tracer scanning is positive, radionuclide targeted therapy such as ^{131}I-MIBG or ^{90}Y-octreotide may replace chemotherapy as initial systemic therapy for all but the most aggressive tumours[29]. For faster-growing disease, aggressive and atypical carcinoids, the combination of cisplatin and etoposide is favoured, as for the more malignant islet cell tumours[21].

Somatostatin analogues effectively control symptoms in 40–80% patients with the carcinoid syndrome, with a reduction of biochemical markers in up to 40%. Stabilization of tumour growth has been observed in 24–57% of patients with documented tumour progression prior to somatostatin therapy[21,25,30]. However, partial and complete tumour response has been observed in <10% of patients. The problem of tachyphylaxis to somatostatin analogues occurs in the great majority of patients and hinders the duration of therapeutic response (median 12 months).

18.1.3 **Phaeochromocytomas**

18.1.3.1 Clinical background

Phaeochromocytomas are catecholamine-secreting tumours arising from the adrenomedullary chromaffin cells. About 10%, arise from extra-adrenal chromaffin tissue located next to sympathetic ganglia are known as paragangliomas[31–33].

Phaeochromocytomas are rare, with a prevalence of 1:6500–1:10 000, and are reported in <0.1% of hypertensive patients[34]. Sporadic phaeochromocytomas are often single and unilateral, whereas familial phaeochromocytomas (about 10%) are often multi-centric, bilateral, have an earlier onset, and a lower risk of being malignant. About 10% of phaeochromocytomas are malignant, metastasizing to bone, lung, brain or liver[31–33,35].

18.1.3.2 Diagnosis and staging

The diagnosis of phaeochromocytoma is based on the demonstration of increased levels of catecholamine or their metabolites[32,33,35]. The measurement of 24-hour urinary free catecholamine has a high sensitivity for phaeochromocytoma. In a symptomatic patient, sensitivity approaches 100%. Plasma catecholamine levels are of lesser sensitivity than 24-hour urinary catecholamine levels but are useful if measured during a suspect event.

Biochemical evidence of a phaeochromocytoma should be followed by imaging for tumour localization[31,35,36]. CT and MRI scanning can localize small adrenal, extra-adrenal, or metastatic lesions, but despite a high sensitivity (>95%), the specificity remains about 65–75%. Where there is unequivocal biochemical evidence of a catecholamine-secreting tumour, but a negative CT/MRI scan, ^{123}I-MIBG scintigraphy offers better specificity (95–100%) and reasonable sensitivity (78–83%) for tumours with catecholamine uptake. More recently, PET imaging using ^{18}F-fluorodopamine appears to offer superior detection/localization results[35].

18.1.3.3 Therapeutic assessment and follow-up

The treatment of phaeochromocytoma is primarily surgical resection[36–39]. Annual urinary free catecholamines test is recommended in all patients for at least 5 years after surgical excision. In contrast to the 5-year survival rate of 96% for patients with benign lesions, malignant phaeochromocytoma carries a 44% survival rate. ^{131}I-MIBG therapy is promising[39–41] and in advanced disease, ^{131}I-MIBG produces partial response and stabilization of disease in more than 80% patients[39–42] (Fig. 18.2). Similar encouraging results have been achieved with ^{90}Y-octreotide and this radiopharmaceutical holds more potential in the treatment of bulky diseases, owing to the more favourable physical property of ^{90}Y [31,32,35,38].

18.2 **Adrenocortical tumours**

18.2.1 Clinical background

The vast majority (99%) of adrenal gland tumours are adenomas, they are benign non-functioning tumour of the adrenal cortex and usually of no clinical importance. Most functioning cortical adenomas are found in female patients[43,44]. Those occurring in

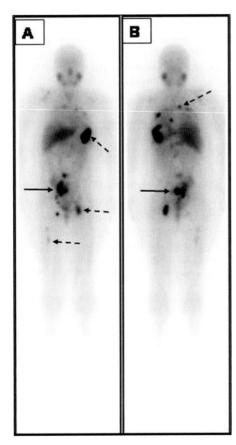

Fig. 18.2 A 34-year-old female patient with known metastatic prapganglioma. Anterior and posterior whole body views (A, B) taken 3 days after the administration of a therapeutic dose (11.1 GBq) of I-131-MIBG demonstrate MIBG avid pelvic retroperitoneal tumour (arrow) and multiple bone metastases (dash arrows).

pre-pubertal patients tend to present with virilization, whereas those in post-pubertal patients present with Cushing's syndrome[45]. Adrenocortical carcinoma is a rare malignancy, with an annual incidence of 4–12 cases per million population[43]. It can be functioning or non-functioning. The left adrenal has been documented as the more common site and the disease is rarely bilateral[43,46,47].

18.2.2 Diagnosis and staging

Non-specific abdominal symptoms such as fullness, indigestion, nausea, vomiting, and pain are usually the most common clinical presenting features[43,44]. Between one-quarter and one-third of patients with primary adrenal carcinoma have clinical evidence of endocrine dysfunction at presentation, most commonly Cushing's syndrome, often supplemented by virilism. A slightly higher fraction of the patients show evidence of abnormal hormone secretion, i.e. subclinical dysfunction. Feminizing tumours due to over-secretion of oestrogens are rare (10%), as are aldosterone-secreting tumours (2%). As for suspected cortical adenomas, diagnostic tests include the demonstration of excessive and non-suppressible levels of adrenal steroids[43].

Imaging is an essential adjunct to clinical and biochemical findings in the diagnosis of adrenal tumours[12,43,44]. Both CT and MRI have capability to detect adrenal tumours <5mm and indeed, small adrenal tumours are sometimes being detected on imaging of the abdomen by CT or MRI for an ostensibly unrelated reason—the so-called 'incidentaloma'. FDG-PET/CT has been shown to detect metastases and recurrence of adrenocortical tumours with impressive sensitivity of 96%, specificity of 99%, and accuracy of 98%.

18.2.3 Therapeutic assessment and follow-up

The treatment of an adrenal tumour depends on the size and location of the tumour[43,44,46,47]. Various algorithms have been proposed to differentiate tumours that require surgical removal from those that can be simply monitored, most attempting to exclude a hypersecretory state biochemically and assess the probability of adrenal malignancy on imaging criteria. In general, small (<3cm) lesions with 'benign' imaging characteristics can be simply observed and rescanned at intervals[43,46,47].

18.3 Summary

- Endocrine tumours represent a diverse group of tumours.
- Diagnosis is suggested by clinical presentation and usually confirmed by biochemical tests but a variety of imaging techniques may be used to localize and stage disease including CT, MRI, EUS, scintigraphy, and PET/CT with tracers including Ga-68 labelled octreotate and ^{18}F-fluorodopamine.

References

1. Morris J. Structure and development of the endocrine system. In: Sheaves R, Jenkins PJ, Wass JAH (eds). *Clinical endocrine oncology*, pp. 11–24. London: Blackwell Science, 1997.

2. Tomassetti P, Migliori M, Lalli S, *et al*. Epidemiology, clinical features and diagnosis of gastroenteropancreatic endocrine tumours. *Annals of Oncology* 2001; **12**: S95–9.

3. Nicholson A. Epidemiology of endocrine tumours. In: Sheaves R, Jenkins PJ, Wass JAH (eds). *Clinical endocrine oncology*, pp. 25–9. London: Blackwell Science, 1997.

4. Office for National Statistics. *Cancer Statistics registrations: Registrations of cancer diagnosed in 2004.England*. Series MB1 No.35. London: National Statistics, 2007.

5. Gueorguiev M, Grossman AB, Plowman PN. Endocrine cancer. In: Price P, Sikola K, Illidge T (eds). *Treatment of cancer*, 5th edn, pp. 438–67. United Kingdom: Hodder Education, 2008.

6. Dixon E, Pasieka JL. Functioning and nonfunctioning neuroendocrine tumors of the pancreas. *Curr Opin Oncol* 2007; **19**: 30–5.

7. Posner MR, Mayer RJ. The Use of Serologic Tumor-Markers in Gastrointestinal Malignancies. *Hematol Oncol Clin North Am* 1994; **8**: 533–53.

8. Mizuno N, Naruse S, Kitagawa M, *et al*. Insulinoma with subsequent association of Zollinger-Ellison syndrome. *Internal Medicine* 2001; **40**: 386–90.

9. Plockinger U, Rindi G, Arnold R, *et al*. Guidelines for the diagnosis and treatment of neuroendocrine gastrointestinal tumours - A consensus statement on behalf of the European Neuroendocrine Tumour Society (ENETS). *Neuroendocrinology* 2004; **80**: 394–424.

10. Plockinger U, Wiedenmann B. Neuroendocrine tumours of the gastrointestinal tract. *Z Gastroenterol* 2004; **42**: 517–26.

11. Howman-Giles R, Shaw PJ, Uren RF, *et al*. Neuroblastoma and other neuroendocrine tumors. *Semin Nucl Med* 2007; **37**: 286–302.

12. Tamm EP, Kim EE, Ng CS. Imaging of neurcendocrine tumors. *Hematol Oncol Clin North Am* 2007; **21**: 409–32.

13. Amthauer H, Ruf J, Bohmig M, *et al*. Diagnosis of neuroendocrine tumours by retrospective image fusion: is there a benefit? *Eur J Nucl Med Mol Imaging* 2004; **31**: 342–8.

14. Kayani I, Bomanji J, Groves A, *et al*. Functional imaging of neuroendocrine tumors with combined PET/CT using Ga-68-DOTATATE (Dota-DPhe-1, Tyr-3-octretotate) and F-18-FDG. *Cancer* 2008; **112**: 2447–55.

15. Newton JN, Swerdlow AJ, dos Santos Silva IM, *et al*. The epidemiology of carcinoid tumours in England and Scotland. *Br J Cancer* 1994; **70**: 939–42.

16. McStay MK, Caplin ME. Carcinoid tumour. *Minerva Med* 2002; **93**: 389–401.

17. Ramage JK, Davies AH, Ardill J, *et al*. Guidelines for the management of gastroenteropancreatic neuroendocrine (including carcinoid) tumours. *Gut* 2005; **54** (Suppl. 4): iv1–16.

18. Ruggieri M, Scocchera F, Genderini M, *et al*. Therapeutic approach of carcinoid tumours of the lung. *Eur Rev Med Pharmacol Sci* 2000; **4**: 43–6.

19. Tastepe AI, Kurul IC, Demircan S, *et al*. Long-term survival following bronchotomy for polypoid bronchial carcinoid tumours. *Eur J Cardiothorac Surg* 1998; **14**: 575–7.

20. Krysiak R, Okopien B, Herman ZS. Current concepts on diagnosis and treatment of carcinoid. *Przegl Lek* 2007; **64**: 103–10.

21. Modlin IM, Kidd M, Lye KD. Biology and management of gastric carcinoid tumours: a review. *Eur J Surg* 2002; **168**: 669–83.

22. Burgess A. Diagnosing, treating and managing carcinoid tumours. *Nurs Times* 2005; **101**: 32–4.

23. Modlin IM, Tang LH. Diagnostic, clinical, and therapeutic aspects of gastric carcinoids. *Chir Gastroenterol* 1997; **13**: 260–7.

24. Caplin ME, Buscombe JR, Hilson AJ, *et al*. Carcinoid tumour. *Lancet* 1998; **352**: 799–805.

25. Granberg D, Sundin A, Janson ET, *et al*. Octreoscan in patients with bronchial carcinoid tumours. *Clin Endocrinol (Oxf)* 2003; **59**: 793–9.

26. Burkitt MD, Pritchard DM. Review article: Pathogenesis and management of gastric carcinoid tumours. *Aliment Pharmacol Ther* 2006; **24**: 1305–20.

27. O'Donnell ME, Carson J, Garstin WI. Surgical treatment of malignant carcinoid tumours of the appendix. *Int J Clin Pract* 2007; **61**: 431–7.

28. Taal BG, Smits M. Developments in diagnosis and treatment of metastatic midgut carcinoid tumors. A review. *Minerva Gastroenterol Dietol* 2005; **51**: 335–44.

29. Kerstrom G, Hellman P, Hessman O. Midgut carcinoid tumours: surgical treatment and prognosis. *Best Pract Res Clin Gastroenterol* 2005; **19**: 717–28.

30. Oberg K, Eriksson B. Nuclear medicine in the detection, staging and treatment of gastrointestinal carcinoid tumours. *Best Pract Res Clin Endocrinol Metab* 2005; **19**: 265–76.

31. Roumeliotis A, Barkas K, Amygdalos G. Carcinoid: modern aspects on its therapy. *Tech Coloproctol* 2004; **8**(Suppl. 1): s164–6.

32. Karagiannis A, Mikhailidis DP, Athyros VG, *et al*. Pheochromocytoma: an update on genetics and management. *Endocr Relat Cancer* 2007; **14**: 935–56.

33. Mittendorf EA, Evans DB, Lee JE, *et al.* Pheochromocytoma: advances in genetics, diagnosis, localization, and treatment. *Hematol Oncol Clin North Am* 2007; **21**: 509–25.

34. Reisch N, Peczkowska M, Januszewicz A, *et al.* Pheochromocytoma: presentation, diagnosis and treatment. *J Hypertens* 2006; **24**: 2331–9.

35. Pimenta E, Calhoun DA. Resistant hypertension and aldosteronism. *Curr Hypertens Rep* 2007; **9**: 353–9.

36. Chrisoulidou A, Kaltsas G, Ilias I, *et al.* The diagnosis and management of malignant phaeochromocytoma and paraganglioma. *Endocr Relat Cancer* 2007; **14**: 569–85.

37. Kasturi S, Kutikov A, Guzzo TJ, *et al.* Modern management of pheochromocytoma. *Nat Clin Pract Urol* 2007; **4**: 630–3.

38. Kuruba R, Gallagher SF. Current management of adrenal tumors. *Curr Opin Oncol* 2008; **20**: 34–46.

39. Scholz T, Eisenhofer G, Pacak K, *et al.* Clinical review: Current treatment of malignant pheochromocytoma. *J Clin Endocrinol Metab* 2007; **92**: 1217–25.

40. Bomanji J, Britton KE, Ur E, *et al.* Treatment of Malignant Pheochromocytoma, Paraganglioma and Carcinoid-Tumors with I-131 Metaiodobenzylguanidine. *Nucl Med Commun* 1993; **14**: 856–61.

41. Bomanji JB, Wong W, Gaze MN, *et al.* Treatment of neuroendocrine tumours in adults with I-131-MIBG therapy. *Clin Oncol* 2003; **15**: 193–8.

42. Bomanji JB. Radionuclide therapy. *Clin Med* 2006; **6**: 249–53.

43. Mukherjee JJ, Kaltsas GA, Islam N, *et al.* Treatment of metastatic carcinoid tumours, phaeochromocytoma, paraganglioma and medullary carcinoma of the thyroid with I-131-meta-iodobenzylguanidine (I-131-mIBG). *Clin Endocrinol (Oxf)* 2001; **55**: 47–60.

44. Libe R, Fratticci A, Bertherat J. Adrenocortical cancer: pathophysiology and clinical management. *Endocr Relat Cancer* 2007; **14**: 13–28.

45. Bertherat J, Groussin L, Bertagna X. Mechanisms of disease: adrenocortical tumors–molecular advances and clinical perspectives. *Nat Clin Pract Endocrinol Metab* 2006; **2**: 632–41.

46. Bourdeau I, Lampron A, Costa MH, *et al.* Adrenocorticotropic hormone-independent Cushing's syndrome. *Curr Opin Endocrinol Diabetes Obes* 2007; **14**: 219–25.

47. Rodriguez-Galindo C, Figueiredo BC, Zambetti GP, *et al.* Biology, clinical characteristics, and management of adrenocortical tumors in children. *Pediatr Blood Cancer* 2005; **45**: 265–73.

Chapter 19

Skeletal tumours

Steven James and David Spooner

Introduction

Modern radiological imaging has transformed the ability to accurately locate and define the extent of primary and secondary skeletal tumours. Using information available from such imaging and the recent provision of computed tomography (CT) planning facilities, both the clinical target volume (CTV) and critical normal organs at risk (OAR) can be more reliably defined.

19.1 Imaging modalities

19.1.1 Plain films

Simple radiographs have limited value in defining the extent of primary bone tumours or identifying the precise location of metastases (Fig. 19.1). Bone destruction has to be advance in order to identify lysis on plain radiographs (usually >60% of the volume) and sclerotic metastases tend to be very diffuse (Fig. 19.2). However, plain radiographs may provide sufficient evidence to inform important decisions about surgical stabilization situations of actual or impending pathological fracture prior to radiotherapy.

19.1.2 Bone scintigraphy

Bone scintigraphy alerts clinicians to the presence of systemic or local skeletal disease (Fig. 19.3), but is unreliable, being dependent on increased osteoblastic cell activity within tumours. Therefore, precise localization and definition of tumour extent is difficult to determine. Purely lytic lesions with advanced bone destruction may not be apparent on bone scintigraphy. This technique has poor sensitivity and specificity. Occasionally generalized skeletal increased uptake may be identified (superscan).

19.1.3 CT and magnetic resonance imaging (MRI)

Both CT and MRI can more accurately define the extent of areas of bone involvement and especially bone destruction. CT is particularly useful in identifying local soft tissue extent, especially in tissues adjacent to air filled cavities (lungs, paranasal sinuses). MRI is able to characterize the extent of the lesion within the medullary cavity of long bones and also the adjacent soft tissue. Skip metastases within the medullary cavity are not unusual in both Ewing's sarcoma (ES) and osteosarcoma and their presence and extent can be determined by MRI. Areas of malignant involvement are often of low or

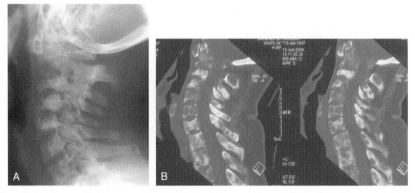

Fig. 19.1 Metastatic breast carcinoma: lateral view of the cervical spine shows patchy sclerosis and lucency (A). Sagittal CT reconstruction of the cervical spine illustrates the mixed sclerotic and lytic metastases (B).

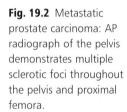
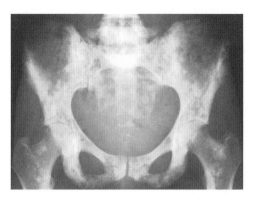

Fig. 19.2 Metastatic prostate carcinoma: AP radiograph of the pelvis demonstrates multiple sclerotic foci throughout the pelvis and proximal femora.

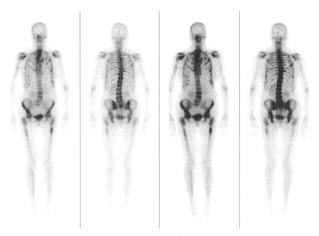

Fig. 19.3 Bone scintigraphy demonstrates multiple areas of increased uptake in keeping with diffuse metastatic disease.

intermediate signal on T1-weighted and of high signal on T2-weighted or STIR sequences on MRI.

19.2 Skeletal metastases

Improved oncology therapies have extended the intermediate to long-term survival of patients with skeletal metastases. As the skeleton is the most prognostic favourable systemic site of metastatic disease more precise delivery of radiotherapy becomes increasingly appropriate.

Availability of bisphosphonates have significantly contributed to the management of painful skeletal metastases and reduced fracture rates and maybe will improve survival. However, local radiotherapy remains effective in improving local bone pain.

19.2.1 Diagnosis

The presence of local metastases are poorly delineated on plains films and often only 'hinted at' by bone scintigraphy. CT and MR images can delineate the presence and extent of local disease accurately (especially in adjacent vertebrae; Fig. 19.4) and therefore optimal management can be discussed and planned. Fig. 19.1 illustrates that CT images of the cervical spine better demonstrate widespread sclerosis than plain films in a patient with breast cancer.

19.2.2 Radiotherapy planning

Plain films may be useful in the radiotherapy planning of patients with poor prognosis, widespread disease and poor performance status. However, they fail to demonstrate the precise extent of local metastasis, which are often optimally seen on axial MRI scans (Fig. 19.5). Both CT and MRI diagnostic images can be successfully fused with CT planning scans to more precisely identify clinical target volume (CTV) and organs at risk (OAR). Plain films are useful for the delineation of the CTV following surgical fixation or endoprosthetic replacement, which usually involves metallic implants with bone allografts very rarely used in this situation. The entirety of the intended CTV is usually apparent on plain films.

The longevity of patients with skeletal metastases brings challenges, e.g. subsequent treatment of adjacent bones, especially vertebral bodies, and possible re-irradiation of sites and sensitive organs at risk (e.g. spinal cord). Both CT and MRI diagnostic studies can inform on CT planning, allowing more accurate localization of abutting treatment target volumes, and thus avoiding overlap.

19.3 Ewing's sarcoma (ES)

ES is a highly aggressive malignant primary bone tumour of childhood and young adults, characterized by the presence of small blue round cells of uncertain origin, which do not produce a tumour matrix. It can occur universally, but most commonly in the proximal metadiaphyseal region of long bones (55%); pelvis (30%), chest wall (5%), and vertebral body (5%) are some of the axial skeleton sites.

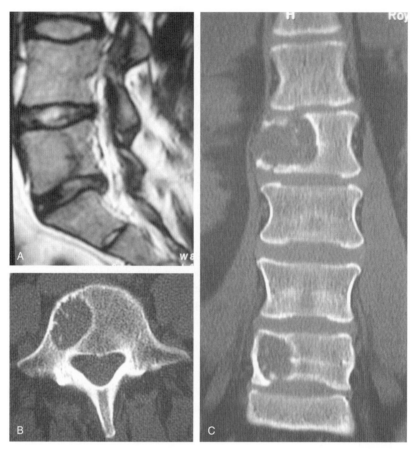

Fig. 19.4 Renal metastasis: sagittal MRI demonstrating focal lesion in the anterior portion of L5 vertebra (A). Axial CT demonstrates a lytic lesion in the anterior portion of the L5 vertebra (B). Coronal reconstruction confirms the presence of multifocal disease (C).

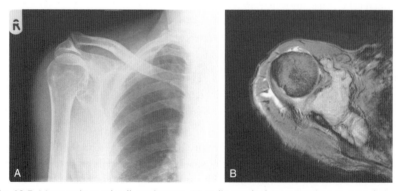

Fig. 19.5 Metastatic renal cell carcinoma: AP radiograph demonstrating an osteolytic lesion in the right glenoid with bony expansion (A). Axial MRI shows the extent of the destructive lesion in the scapula to be more extensive than identified on radiographs (B).

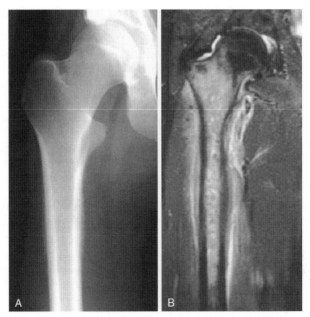

Fig. 19.6 Ewing's sarcoma: AP radiograph of the femur demonstrates an area of sclerosis with periosteal reaction in the proximal diaphysis (A). Coronal MR image demonstrates the true extent of the lesion which is often underestimated on radiographs (B).

19.3.1 **Diagnosis and staging**

19.3.1.1 Plain films

Diagnostic imaging of ES shows an ill-defined bony destructive process with a permeative moth-eaten pattern. A periosteal reaction is often present which typically has an interrupted lamellated pattern. The classic 'onion skin' or 'sun burst' pattern may also be present as well as the 'Codman triangle' and is frequently associated with a large soft tissue component (Fig. 19.6).

19.3.1.2 MRI and CT

MRI will optimally characterize the extent of the intramedullary, periosteal, and local soft tissue components. Typically it demonstrates an intermediate signal on TI-weighted and high signal on T2-weighted sequences (Fig. 19.6). CT staging of the chest to exclude lung metastases (Fig. 19.7) and also bone scintigraphy are required for initial staging.

19.3.2 **Radiotherapy planning**

Radiation therapy plays a major role in both local and systemic therapy of this disease. With the exception of small tumours (<200mL) with 100% cellular necrotic response to neoadjuvant cytotoxic chemotherapy, all primary tumours receive local radiotherapy with or without surgery. When treating pelvic tumours the insertion of a spacer to

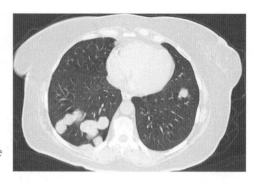

Fig. 19.7 Axial CT chest demonstrates multiple large pulmonary metastases.

move small bowel away from the CTV may be valuable, as shown in Fig. 19.8. Radiotherapy is normally delivered in two phases; the first delineated using CT/MRI axial and sagittal images taken prior to the commencement of systemic therapy. The second phase using similar diagnostic images taken immediately preoperatively, i.e. after neoadjuvant chemotherapy (Fig. 19.9). In patients presenting with metastatic disease, local radiotherapy is delivered to all possible sites as part of the initial definitive treatment.

Diagnostic thoracic CT scans inform on whole lung volume delineation and radiation dosimetry. Together with appropriate MRI, careful PTV definition of other metastatic sites requiring radiation can be achieved.

19.4 **Osteosarcoma (OS)**

OS is the commonest primary malignant bone tumour in children and young adults. It accounts for approximately 20% of all primary bone malignancies of any age. Eighty percent occur in the metaphysis of long tubular bones, with the knee (55%) being the commonest site.

19.4.1 **Diagnosis and staging**

19.4.1.1 **Plain films**

Plain films display considerable variation. Most commonly, a mixed lytic/sclerotic pattern is commonly seen, but purely lytic or dense sclerotic variations occur. Typically there

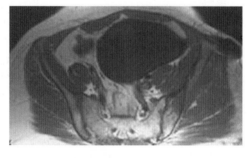

Fig. 19.8 Ewing's sarcoma: axial MR image showing the lesion in the left ilium and pelvic soft tissue spacer in the pelvis.

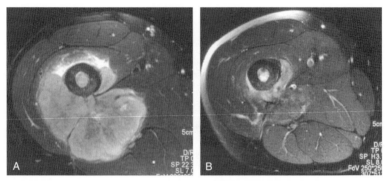

Fig. 19.9 Ewing's sarcoma: pre-chemotherapy axial MRI of the thigh demonstrates a large soft mass (A). Post-chemotherapy axial MRI 10 weeks following the original study demonstrates a marked reduction in the soft tissue component of the tumour (B).

is an indistinct margin and disorganized periosteal reaction; the classic 'Codman triangle' being secondary to periosteal elevation (Fig. 19.10).

19.4.1.2 Bone scintigraphy

Bone scintigraphy is essential for initial staging. Often both soft tissue and skeletal metastases are osteoblastic rich with avid uptake on bone scintigraphy (Fig. 19.11).

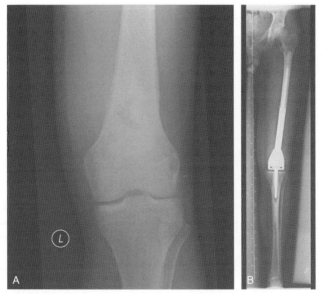

Fig. 19.10 Osteosarcoma: AP radiograph of the distal femur demonstrates an area of patchy sclerosis and periosteal reaction in the distal femur (A). Postoperative view of the limb showing a distal femoral prosthesis (B).

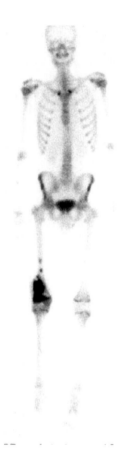

Fig. 19.11 Osteosarcoma:
bone scintigraphy
demonstrating avid
increased uptake in the
distal femoral tumour with
further areas of uptake in
the skip metastases.

19.4.1.3 MRI and CT

MRI defines the local tumour extent within the joint medullary compartment and identifies 'skip' lesions (Fig. 19.12). Adjacent neurovascular involvement is also well visualized by MRI scan, which is important to assess operability. CT chest to identify lung metastases is an integral part of staging.

19.4.2 Radiotherapy planning

The role of radiotherapy in this disease stills needs to be clearly determined. It is of value at inoperable sites, e.g. facial bones, pelvis, and axial skeleton. If possible, high doses (in the order of 70Gy in 35 daily fractions) are used. Optimal PTV localization uses a combination of MRI, CT, and bone scintigraphy for tumour site definition.

Postoperative radiotherapy is used in situations of close or involved surgical margins and attempts to reduce local recurrence or to avoid amputation. Preoperative MRI and postoperative plain films in the presence of an EPR are required (Fig. 19.10).

Local tumour planning is optimally performed using a combination of MRI, CT, and bone scintigraphy imaging.

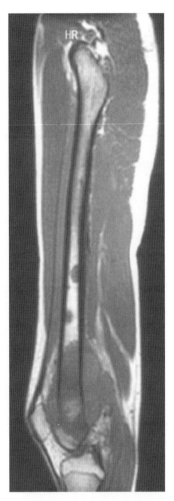

Fig. 19.12 Osteosarcoma: sagittal MRI showing a distal femoral lesion with two proximal skip metastases.

19.5 **Primary lymphoma of bone**

19.5.1 Diagnosis and staging

19.5.1.1 Plain film

Radiological presentation is normally as a lytic destructive lesion with a permeative pattern and associated soft tissue mass which may be apparent on plain films (Fig. 19.13).

19.5.1.2 MRI and CT

MRI and CT are the images of choice to localize this rare tumour. MRI most effectively demonstrates both intra- and extratumour extent (Fig. 19.14). The appearances are variable and lesions may show increased or decreased signal intensity on T2-weighted sequences and low signal on T1-weighted imaging. The characteristic feature is the relative preservation of the bony cortex in the presence of a large soft tissue mass.

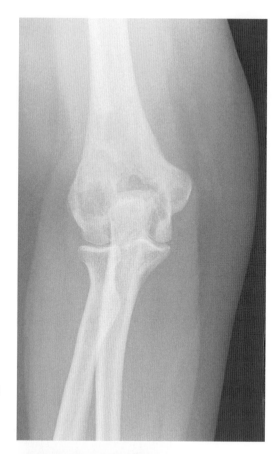

Fig. 19.13 Lymphoma: AP view of the elbow joint demonstrating ill defined lucency in the distal humerus.

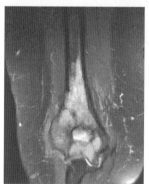

Fig. 19.14 Lymphoma: coronal MRI of the distal humerus showing the extent of the tumour infiltration.

19.5.2 Radiotherapy planning

Although low doses of radiotherapy are required (30Gy in 15 daily fractions) there is a relatively high risk of subsequent avascular necrosis and fracture and careful localization is required using the diagnostic information from CT and MR. The CTV should encompass the entire marrow cavity of the bone but should avoid

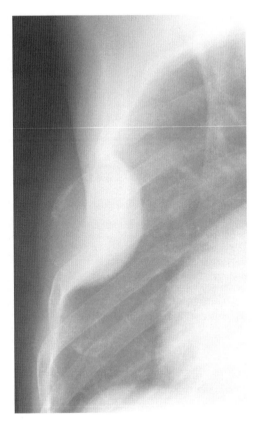

Fig. 19.15 Plasmacytoma: oblique view of the ribs showing an expansile lytic lesion.

articular surfaces and despite the low dose a corridor for lymph drainage should be preserved.

19.6 **Plasmacytoma**

19.6.1 **Diagnosis and staging**

Typically plasmacytoma will be seen on plain X-ray as a lytic lesion (Fig. 19.15) and in long bones significant cortical destruction may result in pathological fracture as shown in Fig. 19.16. Frequently there is a significant soft tissue component for which CT and MRI are essential for evaluation.

19.6.2 **Radiotherapy planning**

Local radiation is used in the treatment of unresectable isolated plasmacytoma. As for primary lymphoma of bone there is a significant risk of pathological fracture, and initial plain films and MRI are important to assess the need for appropriate pre-radiotherapy structural fixation or endoprosthetic replacement (Fig. 19.16).

Because of the soft tissue extension, plain films are inadequate for accurate volume definition. The GTV and CTV will be defined using CT planning and relating this to

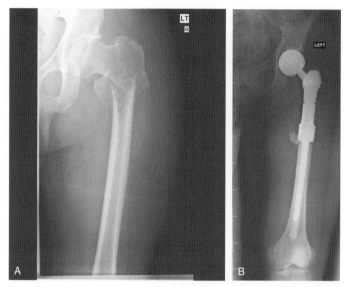

Fig. 19.16 Plasmacytoma: AP radiograph of the femur demonstrates a pathological fracture through a lytic lesion (A). Postoperative view following resection and prosthesis implantation (B).

the diagnostic imaging. The CTV will represent a 5–10mm volumetric expansion from the GTV constrained to tissue planes such as the skin surface.

19.7 **Summary**

- Modern three-dimensional imaging with CT and MRI has revolutionized the visualization of local skeletal tumours.
- More careful and precise radiotherapy can be delivered thereby increasing the therapeutic ratio, with increased tumour control and reduced damage to adjacent healthy organs at risk.

Chapter 20

Paediatrics

Paul Humphries, Francesca Peters, and
Mark Gaze

Introduction

There are various definitions of what constitutes 'paediatric' or 'adolescent' patients, and the terms 'children', 'teenagers', and 'young people' are sometimes used loosely. In its guidance *Improving Outcomes in Children and Young People with Cancer*, the National Institute for Health and Clinical Excellence regards those aged less than 15 years as children, and those aged from 15–24 as young people. The Children's Cancer and Leukaemia Group reports patients aged up to 15 years separately from those older than 15 years, so in this chapter 15 years will be taken as the cut-off point.

Paediatric cancer is a diverse and heterogeneous group of diseases. Table 20.1 sets out the principal categories of malignant disease, and their relative proportion, in children. Although there are cancer types which usually occur in those under 15, and other types which almost always occur in individuals aged over 15 years, there are exceptional cases when cancers occur in the 'wrong' age group, and there are other cancer types which commonly affect both children and older patients.

Paediatric malignancy is uncommon, with 0.5% of all cancers seen in children less than 15 years of age[1]. This corresponds to an annual incidence of about 1600 cases per year in Britain and Ireland.

20.1 The role of imaging in paediatric oncology

Imaging has a number of roles in children suspected of having, or proven to have, some form of cancer. These include:

♦ Assessment of a suspicious lesion, with the aim of providing a differential diagnosis and guiding a biopsy procedure.

♦ Staging the local extent of disease and identifying nodal or distant metastases.

♦ Assessment of response to therapy.

♦ Target volume definition for radiotherapy.

♦ Management of complications and late effects.

There are many challenges to overcome when imaging children, particularly in the setting of malignant disease. The inherent heterogeneity of the population of 'paediatric' patients in terms of age, body size, and understanding and tolerance of imaging procedures, demands a flexible and age-appropriate approach.

Table 20.1 Approximate relative frequency of paediatric cancer types

Leukaemia	32%
Acute lymphoblastic leukaemia	26%
Other leukaemias	6%
Central nervous system tumours	23%
Low grade astrocytoma	7%
Medulloblastoma/PNET	4%
Other central nervous system tumours	12%
Lymphoma	10%
Hodgkin's lymphoma	5%
Non-Hodgkin's lymphoma	5%
Neuroblastoma	6%
Soft tissue sarcomas	6%
Renal tumours	6%
Retinoblastoma	2%
Germ cell tumours	2%
Liver tumours	1%
Other tumour types	12%

PNET, primitive neuroectodermal tumour.

Simply being in hospital can be bewildering and frightening for any child. It is worse if the child is unwell or in pain, or has had prior experience of distressing procedures. It is important to engage with both the child and their parents to facilitate a successful examination. Older children can cooperate with imaging investigations when the purpose and practicalities of the procedure are simply explained. In younger children, the input of a hospital play specialist and the use of distraction techniques (e.g. the use of toys, books, or videos) are particularly useful. Sometimes adopting a non-standard scanning position, e.g. with the child being cuddled by a parent or carer, may facilitate ultrasound (US) examinations. In younger children, especially if the scan time is long as with MRI, or when it is not advisable for a parent to remain in the room during the procedure, the use of sedation or general anaesthesia is required.

In general terms, the use of ionizing radiation investigations should be kept to a minimum. This is because of the greater radiosensitivity of children and their expected longer lifespan in which radiation effects, especially carcinogenesis, have a longer time to manifest themselves. To this end there is a greater emphasis on non-ionizing techniques, with US and magnetic resonance imaging (MRI) being utilized where possible. Where ionizing techniques (such as computed tomography (CT) or positron emission tomography (PET)) are needed, radiation dose reduction strategies are employed in order to minimize exposure.

US enables real-time evaluation and is particularly helpful with abdominal masses in assessing their relationship with solid organs and vessels. MRI provides excellent anatomical detail without the use of ionizing radiation, and although central nervous system (CNS) imaging is relatively straightforward, MRI of body tumours remains a challenge in paediatric practice.

Particular difficulties include:

- Relatively long scan times (compared with multislice CT), leading to motion artefact.
- Relatively poor signal-to-noise ratio of the images when patients are small in size, necessitating innovative use of 'adult' coils, e.g. using knee coils or flex coils to image abdominal tumours in infants.
- Issues related to patients tolerating the MRI examination.

Logistic difficulties may occur in relation to radiotherapy planning and delivery as patients are often imaged in a number of separate hospitals. For example, a tumour may be imaged at presentation to a district general hospital, and further imaging may be performed at the paediatric oncology centre, whereas radiotherapy may be planned and administered at a third separate hospital. It is important for the clinical oncologist to have all relevant imaging to enable accurate target volume definition. For different cancers, treatment may be planned on the extent of disease at diagnosis or following initial chemotherapy, or on the presurgical tumour or the postoperative residual mass. Digital imaging sent in DICOM format on a disc is preferable to hardcopy images as it can be uploaded into radiotherapy planning computers, and fused with other images. It is essential to have adequate administrative staff to locate and retrieve the required images from other hospitals in order to avoid unnecessary re-imaging of children simply because previous imaging is not to hand.

20.2 **CNS tumours**

20.2.1 **Clinical background**

As a group, CNS tumours are the second most common paediatric malignancy after leukaemia. Clinical presentation includes:

- Symptoms of raised intracranial pressure, including headaches and vomiting, which is often due to the development of obstructive hydrocephalus,
- Focal neurological signs including cranial nerve palsies or a hemiparesis,
- Epileptic manifestations of various sorts including complex partial seizures and grand mal convulsions are an uncommon presentation,
- Infants may present with increasing head circumference, lethargy, and nausea and vomiting
- Pituitary, suprasellar, and hypothalamic tumours may present with a variety of symptoms including visual loss, appetite disturbance, precocious or delayed puberty, growth failure, or other endocrine dysfunction

20.2.2 **Diagnosis and staging**

The first step in the differential diagnosis of a CNS tumour is to define its anatomical location. Anatomically, CNS tumours can be considered as infra- or supratentorial. Supratentorial tumours are more common between 1–3 years, infratentorial (posterior fossa) tumours more common between 4–10 years, with an equal distribution over 10 years of age. Primary spinal cord tumours are very rare[2].

Both CT and MRI can be utilized in the investigation of a child with a suspected CNS tumour. CT, by virtue of its wider availability and shorter scanning times, is often used as the first or screening investigation. It may confirm the presence of a tumour and associated features such as obstructive hydrocephalus. CT is relatively more sensitive for the detection of calcification, which may be seen in craniopharyngiomas. Subsequent MRI is required if an abnormality is shown. MRI has the advantage of defining the extent of tumour more accurately, and is very sensitive to the presence of blood products. MRI has replaced myelography in assessment of the spine for metastatic disease from primary intracranial tumours. While spinal metastases are most common in medulloblastoma and other primitive neuroectodermal tumours, germ cell tumours, and ependymoma, MRI of the spine should be performed in all patients with brain tumours as spinal metastatic disease, although less common, can occur in almost all brain tumour types including both high-grade and low-grade gliomas.

While imaging including CT, diffusion-weighted MR and MR spectroscopy may give a strong indication of the type of tumour, in most cases surgery or at least a biopsy is essential to define its histological type.

Exceptions to this general rule include:

◆ Diffuse intrinsic pontine gliomas which have characteristic MR appearances and where biopsy may be hazardous (Fig. 20.1);

◆ Bifocal midline masses in the pineal and suprasellar regions with normal blood and cerebrospinal fluid (CSF) tumour markers which are diagnostic of germinoma

◆ A midline mass associated with significantly elevated levels of the tumour markers αFP (alpha-fetoprotein) and/or βHCG (beta-human chorionic gonadotrophin) in blood or CSF, diagnostic of a secreting intracranial germ cell tumour.

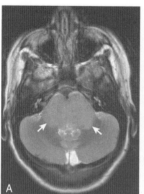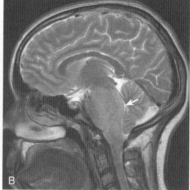

Fig. 20.1 (A) Axial T2-weighted image of a brainstem glioma, showing marked swelling and signal change of the pons, with abnormal signal extending into both cerebellar peduncles (short arrows) (B) Sagittal T2-weighted image of a brainstem glioma causing expansion of the pons and medulla, with marked effacement of the IV ventricle (short arrow).

For the majority of primary tumours, complete surgical resection is attempted when it is believed that this can be achieved without undue morbidity. Otherwise limited surgery such as cyst aspiration or biopsy only is indicated because of the morbidity which would be associated with radical surgery, and the effectiveness of non-surgical treatment. Where a lesion is difficult to access, MRI or CT-guided biopsy may be helpful.

Following surgery for a brain tumour, a postoperative MRI scan with gadolinium should be performed to assess the extent of residual disease. This is particularly important as a surgeon's intraoperative judgement about the completeness of removal may be wrong. It is important to image the spine at this point in time if it was not done preoperatively in those tumour types where there is any risk of metastasis. This includes gliomas of all types as well as intracranial germ cell tumours, ependymomas, and medulloblastoma/primitive neuroectodermal tumours (PNETs). It is important to perform postoperative MR within 48 hours, as beyond that time it can be more difficult to distinguish between residual or metastatic disease and surgical artefact. Risk stratification depends on the extent of postoperative residual disease in medulloblastoma, and this affects clinical trial eligibility and the radiotherapy dose prescribed.

20.2.3 Imaging for radiotherapy planning

Patients will have a CT scan performed, usually without intravenous contrast, in the treatment position in their immobilization shell in the radiotherapy department. This will be of head only when localized cranial radiotherapy is to be given, or of the head and whole spine if craniospinal radiotherapy is necessary (Fig. 20.2). Image fusion of pre- and/or postoperative MRI scans will be performed to help with target volume definition. Contrast administration may be helpful if there is an incompletely resected tumour and MR imaging for fusion is not available. For localized tumours, the gross tumour volume (GTV) is usually the area of gadolinium enhancing tumour without surrounding oedema. The clinical target volume (CTV) is the GTV plus a defined margin depending on tumour type as below, or extended to the meninges. The margin for the planning target volume (PTV) will depend on the results of departmental audits of movement within the shell, but will usually be of the order of 3–5mm.

20.2.4 Therapeutic assessment and follow-up

A baseline post-treatment MRI scan with gadolinium enhancement should be performed about 6 weeks after completion of treatment. This may reasonably be brain-only for tumours without metastatic potential such as craniopharyngioma, but should be of the whole CNS in tumour types which do have potential for seeding through the CSF pathways such as medulloblastoma/PNET and germ cell tumours. Routine follow-up imaging is performed at 3-6-monthly intervals, usually until 5 years have elapsed, unless protocol dictates otherwise. Interval scans may be required if new symptoms develop. A normal scan performed previously to investigate new symptoms should not be allowed to provide undue reassurance if symptoms or signs continue to develop subsequently. A second scan after an interval of 4–6 weeks may be needed as sometimes the first symptoms of a recurrence or second tumour may precede imaging changes. If there is a clinical suggestion of the development of raised

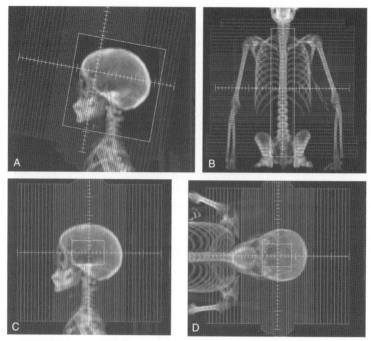

Fig. 20.2 Radiotherapy images. Medulloblastoma/PNET, germ cell tumours, and other central nervous system tumours with leptomeningeal metastases require whole CNS radiotherapy. (A) Planning DRR shows the lateral head field covering the brain and cervical spine. Multileaf collimation is now used to shield the facial structures, rather than cast lead alloy blocks used previously. The clinical target volume covers the meninges and its reflections and a margin is added to define the PTV. Care is taken to ensure adequate coverage of the cribriform plate area anteriorly which means that the eyes cannot be fully shielded. (B) Planning DRR shows the field covering the whole spine. Care is taken to ensure a precise match with the cranial fields, and to ensure adequate coverage of the spinal theca inferiorly. (C) Planning DRR of the lateral phase II field covering the suprasellar intracranial germ cell tumour. (d) Planning DRR of the phase II anterosuperior field.

intracranial pressure, an uncontrasted CT scan may be adequate as an emergency investigation to confirm or exclude the development of obstructive hydrocephalus.

20.3 Renal tumours

20.3.1 Clinical background

Wilms' tumour or nephroblastoma is the most common renal tumour in childhood, accounting for approximately 6% of all childhood cancers. The peak incidence is at 2 years of age, with 75% of affected children being under 4 years of age. There is an equal sex distribution. It typically presents as an asymptomatic abdominal mass or with pain and fever. Bilateral tumours are seen in approximately 10% of cases, with two-thirds of these being synchronous.

There are several associated conditions that predispose to the development of Wilms' tumour including:

♦ Beckwith–Wiederman.

♦ Denys–Drash.

♦ Perlman's.

♦ WAGR syndromes.

Nephroblastomatosis is the persistence of multiple immature nephrogenic rests within the kidney. These should normally involute after 36 weeks of gestation. It is seen in up to 40% of unilateral, and in nearly all cases of multicentric or bilateral, Wilms' tumour. It is thought to be a precursor to the development of Wilms' tumour. In the UK, children with an associated condition having risk of developing Wilms' tumour of 5% or more are screened using US every 3 months until the age of 7 years.

Rarer histologies of renal tumours in childhood include clear cell sarcoma of the kidney, malignant rhabdoid tumour, mesoblastic nephroma, and renal cell carcinoma[3].

20.3.2 Diagnosis and staging

At US examination, Wilms' tumour typically appears as a mass with increased echogenicity, with or without cystic areas. US is particularly useful in evaluating the renal vein and IVC for tumour extension. The contralateral kidney should be examined for a synchronous lesion or nephroblastomatosis. On cross-sectional imaging it is seen to arise from the kidney, classically with a 'claw' of normal renal tissue seen stretched around the periphery of the tumour. Wilms' tumour classically displaces, rather than encases, vessels in contrast to neuroblastoma (Fig. 20.3). MRI may have a role in differentiating hyperplastic nephroblastomatosis and Wilms' tumour from sclerotic (regressive) nephroblastomatosis.

When the presence of a renal tumour has been demonstrated by imaging, a percutaneous needle biopsy is usually performed to confirm the diagnosis and characterize the pathological tumour type.

Staging for distant metastases will be performed before treatment. Detection of pulmonary nodules has historically been based on plain chest radiography. This should include both PA and lateral views. It is well recognized that when CT is used to stage the chest, there are cases that have nodules on CT that cannot be detected on

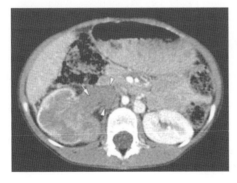

Fig. 20.3 Contrast-enhanced CT of right Wilms' tumour, with right renal vein (short arrow) and IVC tumour thrombosis (arrowheads)—stage 2 or 3 determined by complete/incomplete surgical resection respectively.

chest X-ray. These patients are treated according to their primary tumour stage, rather than as stage IV pulmonary disease[4].

Preoperative chemotherapy is utilized to reduce both tumour size and chance of tumour rupture at surgery. Pathology of the resected tumour is very important for two reasons: to determine the local disease stage and to assign the patient to a pathological risk group. Tumours completely excised and confined to the kidney are stage I. Tumours which have extended beyond the kidney but have been completely excised are stage II. Tumours incompletely excised, and therefore with either microscopic or macroscopic residual disease, or with lymph node involvement are stage III. Stage IV has haematogenous metastatic disease, usually in the lung, less commonly in the liver. 'Stage V' is used to designate bilateral disease. The pathological risk groups are low, intermediate, or high, and together with the stage determine the details of postoperative therapy.

20.3.3 Imaging for radiotherapy planning

Radiotherapy to the flank or abdomen and pelvis is indicated in Wilm's tumour in the case of stage III intermediate or stage II or III high-risk disease (Fig. 20.4), and to the thorax in patients with lung metastases which have not resolved completely with

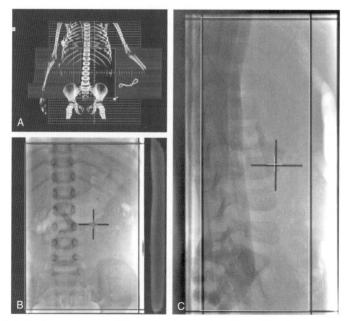

Fig. 20.4 Radiotherapy images. This patient has undergone surgery for an extensive stage III left-sided Wilms' tumour extending into the pelvis. Target volume definition was based on the extent of the tumour and kidney at diagnosis, and extends medially across the midline to cover the full width of the vertebral bodies and para-aortic lymph node region. (A) Anterior planning DRR to show the extent of the field as shaped with multileaf collimators. (B) Anterior machine isocentre check to ensure accuracy of field placement compared with planning image. (C) Lateral isocentre check.

preoperative chemotherapy. The use of abdominal radiotherapy in stage IV and stage V disease is dependent on the local extent of disease.

When radiotherapy is required for the treatment of pulmonary metastases, the whole of both lungs is treated, regardless of the number and extent of metastases. If there is a need to treat both the lungs and the whole or part of the abdomen, it is best to do this together to avoid the possibility of overdose or underdose at junctions.

In the current era, even though treatment techniques are usually still simple anterior and posterior parallel opposed fields, CT planning is used. This allows fusion with earlier diagnostic MR or CT images to allow accurate target volume definition based on the preoperative tumour extent, for example. Shaped fields can be put on at virtual simulation, dosimetry can be optimized, and dose volume histograms of normal tissues can be calculated.

20.3.4 Therapeutic assessment and follow-up

Early detection of local recurrence or distant metastases is the purpose of imaging at follow-up. Postero-anterior and lateral CXR should be obtained every 9 weeks during treatment, every 2 months for the first year and every 3 months for the second year after completion of treatment, with Stage IV patients continuing with 3-monthly chest X-rays fo a further year. Abdominal US at the end of treatment with further US every 6 months for 2 years is recommended to assess for local relapse.

20.4 Neuroblastoma

20.4.1 Clinical background

Neuroblastoma arises from neural crest cells in the sympathetic chain. The most common primary site is in the adrenal medulla or elsewhere in the retroperitoneum, about 60%. Less commonly it arises in the posterior mediastinum (20%), or rarely in the neck, pelvis, or with no identifiable primary tumour. Neuroblastoma is most common in the first year of life and 90% are less than 5 years of age at diagnosis, although rarely it presents in teenagers and young adults. The disease shows marked heterogeneity, with age at presentation, stage of disease and tumour biology affecting outcome.

The clinical presentation depends on the site of the primary disease, locoregional extent, and any metastatic spread (Fig. 20.5). The most common presentation is with an abdominal mass. Often the tumour grows through the intervertebral foraminae, forming a dumbbell tumour which may lead to spinal cord compression or radiculopathy. Metastatic disease may present as bone pain, symptoms of marrow infiltration, fever, and malaise. Infantile metastatic neuroblastoma can present with multiple skin lesions, the so-called 'blueberry muffin' appearance. Asymptomatic presentation is not uncommon. Adrenal masses may be found on antenatal ultrasonography or during investigation of other problems, and thoracic neuroblastoma may be detected incidentally on chest radiography.

20.4.2 Diagnosis and staging

US typically reveals a heterogeneous solid mass, separate from and often displacing the ipsilateral kidney. Further staging investigations include bone marrow trephines,

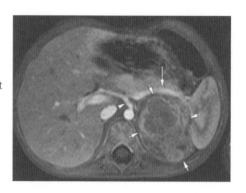

Fig. 20.5 Post-gadolinium T1-weighted axial MRI of left suprarenal neuroblastoma (short arrows) with no involvement of coeliac axis (arrowhead) or splenic artery (long arrow)—stage L1 (INRGSS).

cross-sectional imaging (either CT or MRI, depending on local availability and experience) and I^{123} labelled metaiodobenzylguanidine (MIBG) scintigraphy to evaluate the primary tumour and metastases. The classical imaging appearance of abdominal NBL is that of a large soft tissue mass encasing vascular structures (Fig. 20.6), with calcification seen in approximately 80% on CT. MRI better delineates extradural intraspinal extension of tumour and bone marrow involvement than CT, with the added advantage of lack of ionizing radiation, and is becoming more widely utilized[5].

The International Neuroblastoma Staging System (INSS) was until recently the accepted worldwide staging system for neuroblastoma[6,7]. Now it is being replaced by the International Neuroblastoma Risk Group (INRG) staging system (Table 20.2). The key distinguishing feature of the INRG is that it is based on objective radiological staging, suitable for use at diagnosis, rather than a post-surgical system, in which an individual tumour may be stage 1 or stage 3 depending on the enthusiasm of the surgeon. Disease extent is determined by Image Defined Risk Factors (IDRF) (Table 20.3) at diagnosis[8,9].

Metastatic disease is now defined as any disease spread that is not in continuity with the primary tumour, including non-contiguous lymph node spread (Fig. 20.7). In addition, the new stage Ms (corresponding to INSS stage 4S) now has an upper age limit of 18 months, following statistical analyses of previous NBL trials, showing that benefit of young age extends beyond infancy[10]. Biopsy of the primary tumour is undertaken at diagnosis to evaluate the histology and cell ploidy of the tumour and determine if MycN amplification is present. Approximately 20% of cases will demonstrate MycN

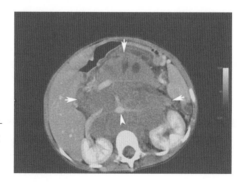

Fig. 20.6 Contrast-enhanced CT of neuroblastoma (short arrows) encasing and displacing the aorta (arrowhead), renal vessels, coeliac artery and its branches—stage L2 (INRGSS).

Table 20.2 INRGSS—International neuroblastoma risk group staging system for neuroblastoma

Stage L1	Locoregional tumour not involving vital structures as defined by the list of image defined risk factors
Stage L2	Locoregional tumour with presence of one or more image defined risk factors
Stage M	Distant metastatic disease (except stage Ms)
Stage Ms	Metastatic disease confined to skin and/or liver and/or bone marrow in children under the age of 18 months

Table 20.3 IDRF—image defined risk factors for neuroblastoma

Neck	Tumour encasing carotid and/or vertebral artery and/or internal jugular vein
	Tumour extending to base of skull
Cervico-thoracic junction	Tumour encasing brachial plexus roots
	Tumour encasing subclavian vessels and/or vertebral and/or carotid artery
	Tumour compressing the trachea
Thorax	Tumour encasing the aorta and/or major branches
	Tumour compressing the trachea and/or principal bronchi
	Lower mediastinal tumour, infiltrating the costo-vertebral junction between T9 and T12
	Significant pleural effusion with or without presence of malignant cells
Thoraco-abdominal	Tumour encasing the aorta and/or vena cava
Abdomen/pelvis	Tumour infiltrating the porta hepatis
	Tumour infiltrating branches of the superior mesenteric artery at the mesenteric root
	Tumour encasing the origin of the coeliac axis, and/or of the superior mesenteric artery
	Tumour invading one or both renal pedicles
	Tumour encasing the aorta and/or vena cava
	Tumour encasing the iliac vessels
	Pelvic tumour crossing the sciatic notch
	Ascites with or without presence of malignant cells
Dumbbell tumours	Symptoms of cord compression, whatever the location
Involvement/infiltration of adjacent organs/structures	Pericardium, diaphragm, kidney, liver, duodeno-pancreatic block, mesentery and others

amplification, which is associated with metastatic disease and a poorer prognosis[11]. A combination of INRGSS, age of the patient (younger or older than 18 months), MycN status and histology define the Risk Group for each case, which determines the treatment received.

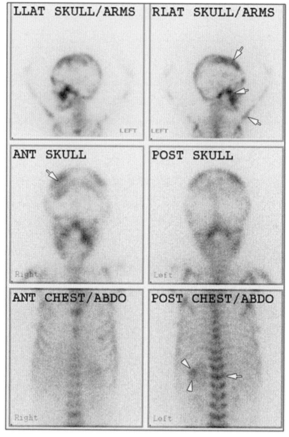

Fig. 20.7 MIBG study of metastatic neuroblastoma (arrow heads) with multifocal bone uptake (short arrows).

20.4.3 Imaging for radiotherapy planning

The treatment of neuroblastoma often involves complex multimodality therapy including surgery, chemotherapy, radiotherapy[12], and biological treatments[13], but the precise treatment schedule is very dependent on risk-group assignment. Radiotherapy is indicated to the primary tumour site in all patients with high-risk disease, that is to say children over 18 months of age with stage M disease, and in patients with MycN amplified disease stage L2 or M regardless of age (Fig. 20.8). Selected patients with intermediate-risk disease, those MycN non-amplified stage L2 aged over 18 months with undifferentiated histology, should also receive radiotherapy to the primary site. Patients with low risk disease, principally those with L1, L2, or Ms disease under 18 months of age without MycN amplification are managed with much less intensive treatment, surgery or chemotherapy alone or in combination, or sometimes observation alone in the hope of spontaneous regression.

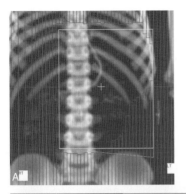

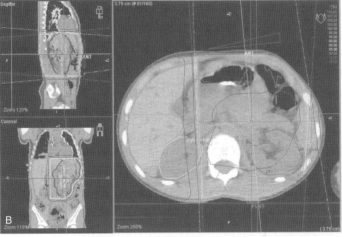

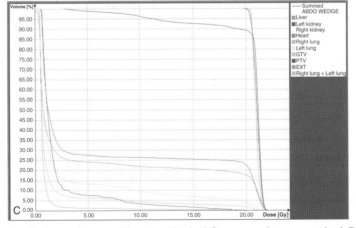

Fig. 20.8 Radiotherapy images. This patient had a left suprarenal tumour excised. Target volume definition was based on the post-chemotherapy, pre-surgical extent of the tumour. (A) Planning DRR to show anterior field. (B) Isodose plans in axial, coronal, and sagittal planes through the isocentre to show dose distribution to the target volume and organs at risk including the left kidney, right kidney, and liver. (C) Dose volume histograms demonstrating coverage of PTV and acceptable doses to organs at risk. See colour section.

Target volume definition for radiotherapy in the local control of the primary tumour in patients with high-risk neuroblastoma and intermediate-risk disease requiring irradiation is based on the postchemotherapy, presurgery, extent of the tumour. Patients will be assessed by contrast-enhanced CT or MRI following induction chemotherapy, and a radiotherapy planning CT scan may be performed at this time. Subsequently patients will undergo resection of their tumour if it is deemed operable and often high-dose chemotherapy, so an interval of 3 months may elapse before they are ready for radiotherapy. A planning scan done at this time may be fused with the earlier scan. The initial scan is used to define the virtual GTV, based on the extent of the primary tumour and any contiguous nodal spread. A 1–2-cm margin is added to define the CTV. This may be modified to include whole vertebrae to avoid the development of a scoliosis. This means that the upper and lower field borders should lie in an intervertebral space, and that the full width of the backbone should be encompassed. Further modification to allow for the fact that uninvolved organs such as liver may have moved into the space previously occupied by tumour may be required. To minimize irradiation of critical normal structures such as the contralateral kidney the CTV may be reduced again. A further margin, usually 1cm, is added to allow for uncertainty and errors in set-up and the likely movement of the child during treatment. The radiotherapy planning scan is used to define organs at risk including the kidneys, liver, and lungs to enable dose volume histograms to be calculated.

The art of target volume definition in paediatric radiotherapy is to achieve the best balance between full coverage of the tumour and avoidance of organs at risk. Sometimes it is necessary to compromise on the recommended protocol treatment of the tumour with regard to total dose, volume or both to reduce the risk of unacceptable normal tissue damage.

20.4.4 Therapeutic assessment and follow-up

In addition to standard cross-sectional imaging, ^{123}I-MIBG scintigraphy is important to assess the response to therapy of metastatic disease. Semi-quantitative scoring systems have been devised for this purpose and are being evaluated. Criteria to assess response to therapy are as detailed by the INSS (Table 20.4).

20.5 Lymphoma

20.5.1 Clinical background

Lymphoma accounts for approximately 10% of all childhood cancers. Approximately half is Hodgkin lymphoma (HL) and half non-Hodgkin lymphoma (NHL)[14]. Radiotherapy is very important in the management of HL, but the treatment of NHL in childhood is an almost exclusively with chemotherapy. The rest of this section therefore relates only to HL.

The most typical clinical presentation is of painless lymphadenopathy. Alternative presentations include incidental detection of mediastinal lymphadenopathy on a chest radiograph performed for evaluation of respiratory symptoms or superior vena cava obstruction. Systemic symptoms such as fever, night sweats, and weight loss may also be present.

Table 20.4 International Neuroblastoma Staging System response criteria

Response	Primary tumour	Metastatic sites
CR (complete response)	No tumour	No tumour, normal catecholamines
VGPR (very good partial response)	Decreased by 90–99%	No tumour, normal catecholamines
PR (partial response)	Decreased by > 50 %	All sites decreased by >50%
		Bone/bone marrow sites decreased by >50%
		No more than 1 positive bone marrow site
MR (mixed response)	No new lesions	
	>50% reduction any measurable lesion with <50% reduction in any other	
	<25% increase in any lesion	
NR (no response)	No new lesions	
	<50% reduction but <25% increase in any existing lesion	
PD (progressive disease)	Any new lesion	
	Increase in any measurable lesion by >25%	
	Previously negative bone marrow now positive	

20.5.2 Diagnosis and staging

Initial imaging investigations usually include a CXR and US of both the neck and abdomen, including high-resolution US imaging of the liver and spleen to assess for small focal lesions; however, cross-sectional imaging has a central role in staging, as the anatomical extent of disease at diagnosis has a profound impact on outcome. Imaging of the neck, abdomen, and pelvis can be performed with either CT or MRI, depending on local experience; however the chest should be imaged using CT, as current MRI techniques are not sufficiently sensitive to detect small pulmonary nodules. HL is staged according to Cotswolds revision of the Ann Arbor classification (Table 20.5)[15].

Histological diagnosis is made by biopsy of abnormal nodal tissue identified by staging investigations. Tissue can be obtained via surgical excision of a node or by percutaneous, image-guided core biopsy; the strategy employed depends on local expertise of both histopathologists and radiologists.

[18]F-fluorodeoxyglucose positron emission tomography (FDG PET) enables an assessment of the metabolic activity, as a marker of disease activity, of involved nodal groups and organs to be made, in addition to the purely anatomical evaluation obtained with CT or MRI[16]. Whole body FDG PET/CT is now a standard investigation at both diagnosis and follow-up in paediatric and adolescent HL (Fig. 20.9).

20.5.3 Therapeutic assessment and follow-up

Patients are reassessed after two cycles of chemotherapy and again at end of treatment with CT or MRI of the neck, abdomen and pelvis, with CT of the thorax if pulmonary

Table 20.5 Cotswolds revision of the Ann Arbor staging system for lymphoma

Stage I	Single lymph node region involvement, including isolated splenic involvement
Stage II	Two or more lymph node regions involved on the same side of the diaphragm
Stage III	Lymph node groups or lymph structures involved on both sides of the diaphragm
Stage IV	Discontinuous extra-nodal involvement: Liver lesions Pulmonary lesions: nodule >1cm or >three nodules <1cm size Bone or bone marrow involvement CNS involvement
A	Absence of 'B' symptoms
B	Presence of at least one of: ◆ Unexplained weight loss of >10% in 6 months ◆ Drenching night sweats ◆ Unexplained persistent or recurrent fever >38°C
E	Involvement of a single extra-nodal site in continuity with nodal disease Except liver or bone marrow involvement—always implies S IV disease

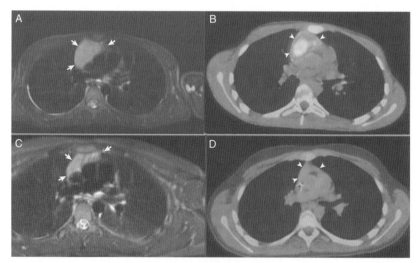

Fig. 20.9 Anterior mediastinal mass. (A) Staging axial MR image of anterior mediastinal mass (short arrows) with corresponding fused PET/CT (B) showing FDG avidity (arrowheads). Restaging following two cycles of chemotherapy. (C) MR image showing reduction in size, but persistant mediastinal disease. (D) Fused PET/CT image showing an excellent metabolic response to chemotherapy, with no residual FDG avidity. See colour section.

Table 20.6 Imaging assessment of response to therapy in childhood and adolescent lymphoma

Local complete remission (local CR)	Residual tumour volume ≤5% reference volume at initial staging
	Residual tumour volume ≤2mL
Local complete remission unconfirmed (local CRu)	No local CR and:
	◆ Residual tumour volume ≤25% reference volume
	◆ Residual tumour ≤2mL
Local partial remission (local PR)	No local CR or local CRu and:
	◆ Residual tumour volume ≤50% reference volume
	◆ Residual tumour volume is ≤5mL
Local no change (local NC)	No local CR or local CRu or local PR and:
	◆ No local progression
Local progression (local PRO)	Residual tumour volume >125% of reference volume or significantly increases compared with best previous response

disease was present at diagnosis, to assess anatomical response to chemotherapy (Table 20.6). The overall response is defined by both the local anatomical response and clinical response.

A PET scan is also performed after two cycles of chemotherapy to assess metabolic response. It is recognized that both false positive and false negative PET findings can be seen if the PET scan is performed too soon after completion of the chemotherapy cycle and hence at least a 2-week gap between the end of chemotherapy and the PET study being performed is recommended. Ongoing clinical trials utilize PET response to two cycles of chemotherapy to determine if radiotherapy may be omitted. The presence of any persistently FDG PET avid nodes or organs after two cycles of chemotherapy denotes an inadequate response and therefore radiotherapy will be administered to all involved fields, as defined by the initial staging investigations.

In the first year following end of treatment, in addition to clinical examination, it is recommended that abdominal US be performed as a surveillance tool, initially four times a year, decreasing in frequency in the third year following end of treatment.

20.5.4 Imaging for radiotherapy planning

Radiotherapy is given to patients with HL who fail to respond adequately to two courses of chemotherapy. A positive PET scan, or persistently enlarged nodes even if PET negative, at this time point is an indication for radiotherapy on completion of chemotherapy. The duration of chemotherapy is based on initial stage rather than response to treatment.

Current radiotherapy is based on CT planning (Fig. 20.10). A planning CT scan is performed for target volume definition, optimization of the plan, and dosimetry of normal tissues. If it is possible to have therapy radiographers present at the reassessment PET/CT scan to place skin markers, and use a flat couch top with the patient in the treatment position, it is possible to use the CT component of the PET/CT scan

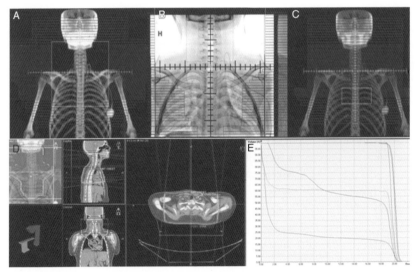

Fig. 20.10 Radiotherapy images. (A) Planning DRR to show complete anterior field covering neck, supraclavicular, and superior mediastinal nodal areas. (B) Simulator check film confirming correct field placement. (C) Planning DRR of anterior boost field used to achieve dose homogeneity. (D) Isodose plans showing dose distribution in axial, coronal, and sagittal planes. (E) Dose volume histograms confirming good coverage of target volumes and acceptable doses to organs at risk. See colour section.

for treatment planning rather than perform a repeat CT scan for planning purposes in the treatment department.

All the lymph node areas identified by cross-sectional imaging and PET as being involved at the time of diagnosis are treated, irrespective of response. The nodal groups are identified on CT. The whole length of lymph node chains, e.g. down the mediastinum are treated, but if there has been a good shrinkage of an initial bulky mass it is sufficient to use the residual width as the GTV, and not necessary to treat the whole width at diagnosis.

20.6 **Primary bone tumours: osteosarcoma and Ewing's sarcoma**

20.6.1 **Clinical background**

Osteosarcoma (OS) is the commonest malignant paediatric primary bone tumour, characterized histologically by the presence of malignant mesenchymal cells that produce immature bone or osteoid[17]. It is rare in young children, the peak incidence is in adolescents between the ages of 15–19 years. It becomes rarer again in adult life, although it is recognized as a complication of Paget disease of bone in the elderly. Males are affected more frequently.

There are many histological subtypes; however the commonest, high-grade central osteosarcoma (also known as classic or conventional OS) accounts for >90% of cases.

Whilst it can affect any bone, the majority of cases arise in the appendicular skeleton, most commonly around the knee (up to 75% cases) or proximal humerus. Presentation is typically delayed, patients complaining of localized pain and swelling often attributed to trivial injury. Referred pain felt in the knee may mask the presentation of a proximal femoral lesion.

The Ewing family of tumours are a rare group of paediatric small round blue cell tumours arising from primitive neural elements, which includes classic Ewing's sarcoma (ES) of bone, soft tissue ES and peripheral primitive neuroectodermal tumours (pPNET). Care must be taken to avoid confusion with central nervous system PNETs which are a quite distinct disease entity. ES is the second most common primary bone tumour in adolescents. It is more common than OS in young children. Cases continue to be seen into adult life. Pain is the presenting symptom in most cases, which typically persists through the night and, as in OS, is often attributed to trivial injury or growing pains. Additional symptoms include swelling and constitutional signs such as fever.

Patients with bone tumours should be managed at designated supraregional bone tumour units. Patients should be referred to such a centre for diagnosis when the suspicion is raised, rather than being imaged and biopsied close to home in general orthopaedic units.

20.6.2 Diagnosis and staging

Plain films are the initial investigation in most cases of suspected primary bone tumour. Appearances of OS are variable, with conventional OS typically having a mixed sclerotic/lytic appearance involving the metaphysis of a long bone, often accompanied by an aggressive periosteal reaction and soft tissue mass. Extension into the diaphysis and/or epiphysis is common, occasionally in association with a pathological fracture[18].

In ES, pelvic bones, long bones, and ribs are most commonly affected. Tumours involving long bones typically have an aggressive permeative, lytic appearance within the diaphysis often accompanied by a soft tissue mass (Fig. 20.11); however up to a quarter of lesions are sclerotic at presentation.

For both OS and ES, MRI of the whole bone is used to evaluate local extent owing to its multiplanar capabilities and superior soft tissue resolution, with emphasis on defining intra- and extraosseous tumour extent, and involved tissue compartments that will ultimately influence the surgical approach (Fig. 20.12). MRI has also proven useful in the detection of skip lesions (defined as secondary tumour foci occurring simultaneously within the same bone) seen in up to 25% of OS cases, contralateral lesions, and relationship of tumour to nearby neurovascular structures[19].

Histological confirmation requires bone biopsy, which will be performed at the designated bone tumour treatment centre. The approach taken should be discussed with the bone tumour surgeon to avoid contamination of unaffected soft tissue compartments and to ensure resection of the biopsy tract at primary surgery.

Further staging includes CT chest and technetium-99m (^{99m}Tc)-phosphonate bone scan, reflecting the propensity of both tumours to metastasise to lung and/or bone. Between 10–20% of OS patients have metastases at presentation, 80% of which involve lung.

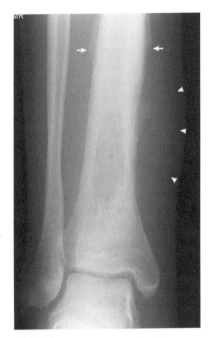

Fig. 20.11 AP radiograph of distal right tibial Ewing's sarcoma showing a lytic lesion with associated aggressive, lamellated periosteal reaction (short arrows) and a soft tissue mass (arrowheads).

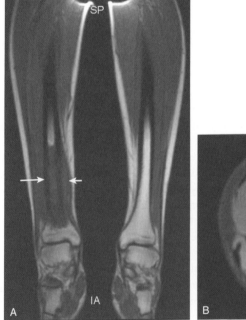
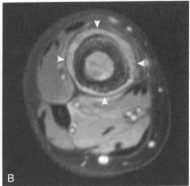

Fig. 20.12 Ewing's sarcoma. (A) Coronal T1-weighted MR image of the right distal femur, with intramedullary tumour, periosteal reaction (long arrow), and an extraosseous soft tissue mass (short arrow). (B) Axial STIR MR image demonstrating the extent of the extra-osseous tumour mass (arrowheads).

Twenty-five percent of ES patients have metastatic disease at presentation, involving the lung, bone or bone marrow.

Whilst not part of routine staging, FDG PET has proven to be both sensitive and specific in detecting bone metastases; however, it has yet to become part of an international staging system for either OS or ES, owing to limited availability. There is also increasing evidence that whole body MRI combined with FDG PET improves the detection of bone and bone marrow metastases in children and adolescents compared with either imaging modality alone or standard skeletal scintigraphy, owing to earlier detection of intramedullary tumour deposits before osteoblastic responses occur which result in uptake on a conventional bone scan[20]. However, owing to availability, costs, and a limited amount of evidence at present this combination is unlikely to be incorporated into staging protocols in the near future.

Treatment of patients with ES is influenced by disease stage. Currently there is no single widely accepted staging system for ES. Whilst each system differs slightly, their universal aim is the identification of prognostic factors influencing both local recurrence rates and metastatic disease[21–23]. Adverse prognostic factors include primary site, metastases, and age at presentation (>15 years), tumour volume or diameter >8cm, elevated lactate dehydrogenase (LDH) levels and poor histological response to induction chemotherapy[24].

20.6.3 Imaging for radiotherapy planning

Current treatment strategies rely on neoadjuvant chemotherapy with surgery for local disease control and all respectable metastases. Radiotherapy has only a limited role in the management of extremity OS, being reserved for inoperable disease or following incomplete resection. Radical radiotherapy may be used as the sole local control modality in axial OS which is felt to be inoperable. Treatment planning is based on the extent of disease as determined by MRI.

Ewing's tumours are radiosensitive. Preoperative radiotherapy is considered in borderline cases based on their response to induction chemotherapy assessed using a variety of imaging modalities including CT, whole body MRI, FDG/PET, and thallium studies. Radiotherapy may be used alone in cases where only intralesional surgery would be possible or where metastatic disease is present.

Prior to radiotherapy planning, careful consideration needs to be given to the positioning of the area to be treated to allow for adequate treatment with maximum sparing of uninvolved normal tissues. Limbs should be immobilized in custom-made shells, and, with the body part fixed in the shell a planning CT scan should be undertaken. Target volumes are planned based on the initial diagnostic MRI. The GTV is the tumour extent demonstrated by imaging. The CTV includes an additional longitudinal margin of up to 3cm in long bones, leaving an unirradiated corridor of skin and subcutaneous tissue in the limb to prevent the development of lymphoedema. Any surgical scars or drainage sites should be included in the radiation field to ensure all potential sites of microscopic disease are treated.

20.6.4 Therapeutic assessment and follow-up

Local response to treatment is best monitored with regional MRI. Metastatic disease can be evaluated with an array of imaging techniques dependent on the site, the frequency, and combination of which will differ according to trial protocol and the individual patient but include CT chest, total body MRI, FDG PET, and isotope bone scans.

Studies report between 30–40% of patients experience recurrent disease either locally, at a distance from the primary site or a combination of the two. Recurrence is associated with a poor prognosis, worse still if disease recurs within 2 years of initial diagnosis. Current guidelines recommend follow-up for at least 15 years.

20.7 Soft tissue sarcomas: rhabdomyosarcoma and other types

20.7.1 Clinical background

Rhabdomyosarcoma (RMS) is the commonest childhood soft tissue sarcoma. It is a highly malignant tumour arising from primitive mesenchymal cells prior to their differentiation into striated muscle. Histologically there are two main types. About 75% are embryonal rhabdomyosarcoma (eRMS). Alveolar rhabdomyosarcoma (aRMS) carries a worse prognosis and is diagnosed on the basis of characteristic morphology and a high level of myogenin positivity on immunohistochemistry[25]. There are many other types of soft tissue sarcoma encountered in children and young people. They tend to be grouped together as non-RMS soft tissue sarcoma. As far as imaging goes, RMS and non-RMS soft tissue sarcomas can be considered together, as imaging is more dependent on anatomical site than histological type.

Clinical presentation is largely dependent on the site and extent of the primary disease and the presence/absence of metastases. RMS can arise almost anywhere within the body, the more commonly affected sites involve the head and neck (40%), the genitourinary system (30%), and the extremities (16%)[26].

Within the head and neck, a distinction is drawn between those tumours confined to the orbit which carry a very good prognosis, and other sites which are divided into parameningeal and non-parameningeal primary sites. Parameningeal tumours are sited near the skull base, and there is a tendency for intracranial spread to occur through the neural and vascular foramina. Such sites include the nasopharynx, nasal cavity, and paranasal sinuses, middle ear and mastoid, infratemporal fossa, and pterygopalatine fossa. Non-parameningeal sites include the oral cavity, cheek, and larynx.

Genitourinary primary sites are divided into bladder (Fig. 20.13) and prostate primary sites, which are less favourable, and non-bladder/prostate sites including the vulva, vagina, and cervix in girls and paratesticular tissues in boys which carry a more favourable prognosis.

Age and site at presentation differ for the subtypes, eRMS typically presenting in the younger children with orbital or other head and neck or genitourinary primaries whilst aRMS tends to affect older children and adolescents involving the extremities.

20.7.2 Diagnosis and staging

Initial diagnostic investigations will be guided by the site of primary tumour and its associated symptoms and signs. Genitourinary RMS is typically imaged with US in the first instance followed by CT or MRI to assess extent and nodal involvement whilst

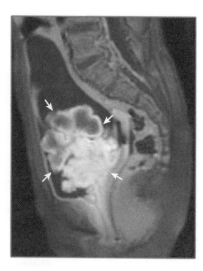

Fig. 20.13 Post-gadolinium sagittal T1-weighted MR image of a partly cystic, partly solid bladder rhabdomyosarcoma.

head/neck and extremity primaries are best imaged with MRI owing to its superior soft tissue resolution.

Approximately 20% of patients present with metastases at diagnosis. Evaluation for metastatic disease includes CT chest and ^{99m}Tc-diphosphonate bone scan reflecting the propensity of RMS to metastasize to lung and bone. Bone marrow aspirates and trephines are also essential to diagnose bone marrow involvement. More focused staging investigations will depend on the knowledge of spread from specific primary sites, e.g. CSF sampling required in cases of primary CNS disease. Currently there is no established role for PET/CT in the staging of RMS, however it has proven useful in quantifying disease activity in non-RMS soft tissue tumours. The main staging system for risk stratification is the IRS (Intergroup Rhadomyosarcoma Study) system, which defines four categories based on the extent of spread at diagnosis and volume of residual disease following initial surgery.

◆ Group I: primary complete resection with clear margins.

◆ Group II: complete resection but positive margins on histology.

◆ Group III: macroscopic residual tumour or biopsy only.

◆ Group IV: distant metastases.

Full risk stratification takes into account the size of the tumour (5.0cm or less in maximum diameter, or greater than 5.0cm), age, histology, site, and lymph node involvement as well as IRS group.

20.7.3 Imaging for radiotherapy planning

Radiotherapy is indicated for the majority of patients with RMS (Fig. 20.14). Exceptions include very young children, IRS group I, or IRS group II or III where there is a secondary complete resection. The target volume definition is usually based on the size of the primary tumour at diagnosis. Exceptions to this include tumours which extend into a body cavity without direct invasion, and shrink back to the tissue of

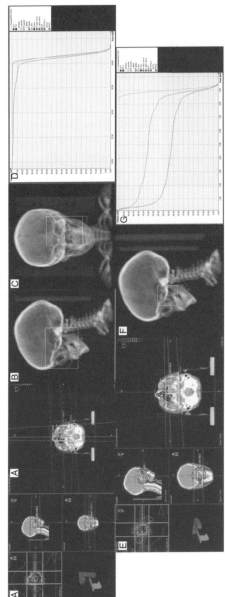

Fig. 20.14 Radiotherapy images. This patient had a parameningeal (nasopharyngeal) rhabdomyosarcoma, treated by a two phase technique. (A) Isodose distribution in axial, coronal, and sagittal planes showing coverage of the phase 1 PTV. (B) Planning DRR of the phase 1 lateral field. (C) Planning DRR of the phase 1 anterior field. (D) Dose volume histograms for phase 1. (E) Plan in three planes for the smaller phase 2 volume avoiding further dose to the eyes. (F) planning DRR of phase 2 field. (G) Dose volume histograms for phase 2. See colour section.

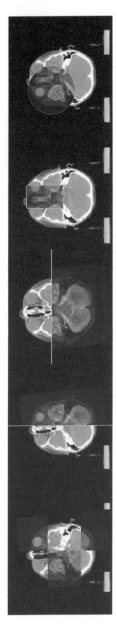

Fig. 20.15 Radiotherapy CT/MR fusion planning. Images to show MRI/CT fusion for radiotherapy planning. The planning CT scan images have been fused with the initial (pre-chemotherapy) diagnostic MRI scans. The target volumes have been drawn on the MRI and the planning is done on the CT images. See colour section.

origin with chemotherapy. For example, a chest wall tumour may extend significantly into the pleural cavity. Following a good response to chemotherapy it is still necessary to irradiate all of the chest wall initially involved, but not the lung which occupies the intrathoracic space previously occupied by tumour. The pretreatment T1 postcontrast MRI is usually the optimum imaging study for defining the GTV. These images can be fused with the planning CT scan performed with the patient immobilized as necessary in the treatment position (Fig. 20.15). The CTV is usually the GTV plus 1.0cm, but adjustments need to be made for areas of possible subclinical extension (such as the full thickness of the skull base in parameningeal cases) or if there are natural barriers to spread, and to include scars, drain sites, and biopsy tracts.

20.7.4 Therapeutic assessment and follow-up

Response to therapy in RMS is usually with the same imaging modality as was used at diagnosis. If there is a definite residual mass after therapy, FDG PET/CT imaging may be useful to identify persistent metabolic activity, or an image-guided biopsy may be undertaken to differentiate between residual active disease and fibrosis or scarring. Often there is a residual abnormality on imaging but without mass effect in which case PET will probably be unhelpful. Response Evaluation Criteria in Solid Tumours (RECIST) are sometimes used in clinical trial settings to define response, but are not part of normal practice in most centres outside trials.

20.8 Summary

- Malignant disease in children is uncommon.
- Childhood tumours are a pathologically heterogeneous group.
- Children with a suspected malignancy should be assessed at a designated paediatric oncology centre.
- An age-appropriate approach is required for both imaging and radiotherapy.
- Close multidisciplinary team working is vital for success

References

1. Parkin DM, Kramarova E, Draper GJ, *et al* (eds). *International Incidence of childhood cancer, Vol 2. IARC Scientific publications No. 144.* Lyon: IARC Press, 1998.
2. Kleihues P, Louis DN, Scheithauer BW, *et al.* The WHO classification of tumours of the central nervous system. *J Neuropathol Exp Neurol* 2002; **61**: 215–25.
3. Vujanic GM, Sandstedt B, Harms D, *et al.* Revised International Society of Paediatric Oncology (SIOP) working classification of renal tumours of childhood. *Med Pediatr Oncol* 2002; **38**: 79–82.
4. Grundy P, Perlman E, Rosen NS, *et al.* Current issues in Wilms tumor management. *Curr Probl Cancer* 2005; **29**: 221–60.
5. Rha SE, Byun JY, Jung SE, *et al.* Neurogenic tumors in the abdomen: tumor types and imaging characteristics. *Radiographics* 2003; **23**: 29–43.
6. Brodeur GM, Seeger RC, Barrett A, *et al.* International criteria for diagnosis, staging, and response to treatment in patients with neuroblastoma. *J Clin Oncol* 1988; **6**: 1874–81.

7. Brodeur GM, Pritchard J, Berthold F, *et al.* Revisions of the international criteria for neuroblastoma diagnosis, staging, and response to treatment. *J Clin Oncol* 1993; **11**: 1466–77.

8. Cohn SL, London WB, Monclair T, *et al.* Update on the development of the international neuroblastoma risk group (INRG) classification schema. *J Clin Oncol* (Meeting Abstracts) 2007; **25**: 9503.

9. Maris JM, Hogarty MD, Bagatell R, *et al.* 'Neuroblastoma'. *Lancet* 2007; **369**: 2106–20.

10. London WB, Castleberry RP, Matthay KK, *et al.* Evidence for an age cut-off greater than 365 days for neuroblastoma risk group stratification in the Children's Oncology Group. *J Clin Oncol* 2005; **20**: 6459–65.

11. Rubie H, Hartmann O, Michon J, *et al. N-myc* amplification is a major prognostic factor in localized neuroblastoma: Results of the French NBL 90 Study. *J Clin Oncol* 1997; **15**: 1171–82.

12. Marcus KC, Tarbell NJ. The changing role of radiation therapy in the treatment of neuroblastoma. *Semin Radiat Oncol* 1997; **7**: 195–203.

13. Matthay KK. Neuroblastoma: Biology and therapy. *Oncology* 1997; **11**: 1857–66.

14. Weinstein HJ, Tarbell NJ. Leukaemias and lymphomas of childhood. In: DeVita VT, Hellman S, Rosenberg SA (eds). *Cancer: Principles and Practice of Oncology*, pp. 2235–56. Philadelphia, PA: Lippencott Williams & Wilkins, 2001.

15. Mauch P, Armitage J, Volker D, *et al. Weiss Hodgkin's Disease*, pp.223–8. Philadelphia, PA: Lippincott Williams & Wilkins, 1999.

16. Young H, Baum R, Cremerius U, *et al.* Measurement of clinical and subclinical tumour response using [18F]-fluorodeoxyglucose and positron emission tomography: review and 1999 EORTC recommendations. European Organisation for Research and Treatment of Cancer (EORTC) PET Study Group. *Eur J Cancer* 1999; **35**: 1773–82.

17. Unni KK. *Dahlin's bone tumours: general aspects and data on 11,087 cases*, 5th edn. Philadelphia, PA: Lippincott-Raven, 1996.

18. Resnik D, Kyriakos M, Greenaway GD. Tumours and tumour-like lesions of bone: imaging appearances and pathology of specific lesions. In: Resnick D (ed). *Diagnosis of bone and Joint Disorders*, 4th edn, pp. 3800–15. Philadelphia, PA: Saunders Co, 2002.

19. Saifuddin A. The accuracy of imaging in the local staging of appendicular osteosarcoma. *Skeletal Radiol* 2002; **31**: 191–201.

20. Daldrup-Link H, Franzius C, Link T, *et al.* Whole-Body MRI Imaging for detection of Bone metastases in children and young adults: Comparison with skeletal scintgraphy and FDG PET. *AJR Am J Roentgenol* 2001; **177**: 229–36.

21. Paulussen M, Craft AW. Ewing Tumours: Management and Prognosis. *Supplement SIOP* 2006: 50–2.

22. Saeter G, Oliveira J, Bergh J. ESMO minimum clinical recommendations for diagnosis, treatment and follow-up for Ewing's sarcoma of bone. *Ann Oncol* 2005; **16** (Suppl.1): i73–4.

23. Bernstein M, Kovar H, Paulussen M, *et al.* Ewing's sarcoma family of tumours: current management. *Oncologist* 2006; **11**: 503–19.

24. Cotterill SJ, Ahrens S, Paulussen M, *et al.* Prognostic factors in Ewing's tumour of bone: analysis of 975 patients from the European intergroup cooperative Ewing's sarcoma study group. *J Clin Oncol* 2000; **18**: 3108–14.

25. McDowell HP. Update on childhood rhabdomyosarcoma. *Arch Dis Child* 2003; **88**: 354–7.

26. Dagher R, Helman L. Rhabdomyosarcoma: An Overview. *Oncologist* 1999; **4**: 34–44.

Chapter 21

Imaging for common complications

Charlotte Whittaker and Vicky Goh

Introduction

Patients with cancer are prone to multiple complications which can be a significant cause of morbidity and mortality. Imaging plays a critical role in the diagnostic pathway. It is beyond the scope of this chapter to present a detailed review but the imaging appearances of the most commonly encountered complications in clinical practice are outlined.

21.1 Venous thromboembolism (VTE)

Malignancy is a major risk factor for VTE[1] with the highest incidence occurring in metastatic pancreatic, stomach, bladder, uterine, renal, and lung cancer. The risk of recurrent thrombosis is also significantly higher in cancer patients than non-cancer patients. Other contributory risk factors include therapy, surgery, and immobility[2]. Cancer-associated VTE is serious and potentially life threatening, being the second leading cause of mortality in cancer patients following the disease itself[2].

21.1.1 Guidelines for imaging suspected VTE

Prior to the introduction of multidetector computed tomography (CT), the majority of cases of suspected pulmonary embolism (PE) were investigated with ventilation perfusion lung scans (Fig. 21.1), with conventional pulmonary angiography considered the 'gold standard'. Following the Prospective Investigation of Pulmonary Embolism Diagnosis (PIOPED II)[3] the following recommendations have been adopted by the British Thoracic Society (BTS)[4]:

21.1.1.1 Clinical assessment

To determine the clinical probability of PE, PIOPED II, and BTS recommend an objective clinical assessment scoring index to allow for the inexperience of junior doctors whose ability to make an accurate estimate of the likelihood of PE may be less than that of their senior colleagues[5].

The BTS guidelines require that: *the patient has clinical signs and symptoms compatible with PE, i.e. breathlessness and/or tachypnoea with or without pleuritic chest pain and/or haemoptysis.*

Two other factors are considered:

1) The absence of an alternative reasonable clinical explanation

2) The presence of a major risk factor (Table 21.1)

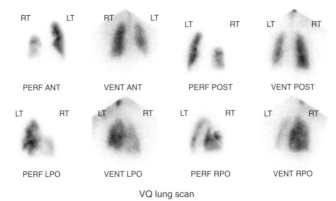

RT   LT   RT   LT   LT   RT   LT   RT

PERF ANT   VENT ANT   PERF POST   VENT POST

LT   RT   LT   RT   LT   RT   LT   RT

PERF LPO   VENT LPO   PERF RPO   VENT RPO

VQ lung scan

Fig. 21.1 Ventilation/ perfusion scan showing multiple unmatched perfusion defects giving a high probability of pulmonary embolus.

High probability is assigned where 1) and 2) are true. Intermediate probability is assigned where only 1) or 2) is true. Low probability is assigned where neither 1) nor 2) are true. PIOPED II used the validated Wells score to assign a clinical probability[1].

21.1.1.2 D-dimer

While the sensitivity ranges from 87–98%, there is poor specificity and raised levels are commonly seen in patients with cancer in the absence of VTE[6]. The overall negative predictive value has been shown to be much higher in patients with low clinical probability[7]. Therefore, D-dimer assays are only recommended in patients with low or intermediate clinical probability. They are not recommended in patients with high pre-test probability.

Table 21.1 Major risk factors for VTE as defined by the British Thoracic Society

Surgery	Major abdominal/pelvic surgery
	Hip/knee replacement
	Postoperative intensive care
Obstetrics	Late pregnancy
	Caesarian section
	Puerperium
Lower limb problems	Fracture
	Varicose veins
Malignancy	Abdominal/pelvic
	Advanced/metastatic
Reduced mobility	Hospitalization
	Institutional care
Miscellaneous	Previous proven VTE

The BTS guidelines conclude that: *a negative D-dimer test reliably excludes PE in patients with low or intermediate clinical probability (for details of specific assays please refer to the original guidelines).*

21.1.1.3 Ventilation/perfusion scanning

The initial PIOPED study determined that PE can only be diagnosed or excluded reliably with scintigraphy in a minority of patients[8]. In all patients with either an indeterminate lung scan or discordant clinical and scintigraphic probabilities, further imaging is mandatory. However, a normal scan will reliably exclude PE. Interpretation is only reliable when a current high quality erect chest radiograph is available and indeterminate scans are often seen in patients with an abnormal chest radiograph. Ventilation/perfusion scanning may also be a helpful option for patients with renal impairment.

The BTS recommends that: *ventilation/perfusion scans should only be used as the initial imaging assessment when the facilities are available, the chest radiograph is normal and further imaging is always performed following an inconclusive result[5].*

21.1.1.4 Computed tomographic pulmonary angiography (CTPA)

This is the initial imaging investigation recommended by both BTS and PIOPED II for all patients except those with low or intermediate clinical probability and a negative D-dimer[3,4] (Fig. 21.2). This method has higher specificity for diagnosis of PE, detection of alternative pathology, wider availability, and very short scanning time. Potential disadvantages include the use of iodinated contrast and the reduced sensitivity for subsegmental thrombus when compared to pulmonary angiography. However, with defined protocols, thin section collimation, and the use of imaging work stations and computer-aided detection, interpretation is likely to be improved when compared to earlier published results[9].

The BTS concludes that: *patients with a good quality negative CTPA do not require further investigation for PE.*

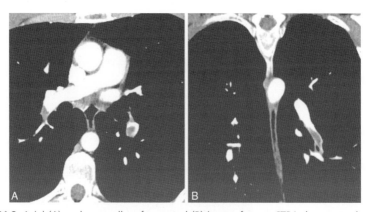

Fig. 21.2 Axial (A) and coronally reformatted (B) image from a CTPA demonstrating filling defects in the right and left main pulmonary arteries, and in the left lower lobe pulmonary artery consistent with thrombus.

21.1.1.5 Magnetic resonance (MR) angiography

Whilst appearing promising on initial studies, it is not currently widely used, with limited access and concern about low sensitivity for subsegmental clot[10,11]. It is also less useful in detecting alternative or concurrent pulmonary disease when compared to CTPA.

21.1.1.6 Echocardiography

Both transoesophageal and transthoracic echocardiography can be diagnostic in massive PE, but are rarely definitive in other situations. It may be useful in critically ill patients as it can be performed at the bedside, but is not recommended for patients who are clinically stable enough to tolerate CTPA[4].

21.1.1.7 Ultrasonography

Compression ultrasonography (US) is the imaging procedure of choice in patients with suspected DVT, with 95% sensitivity and 98% specificity for thrombus in the proximal deep veins (Fig. 21.3)[12]. The principal criterion for diagnosis is the inability to completely compress the vein lumen, with supportive signs including distention of the involved vein and absence of flow on Doppler evaluation. Accuracy rates for the detection of thrombus isolated to the deep calf veins are lower (73% sensitivity in one meta-analysis)[13] and the evaluation of deep calf veins is more technically challenging, in addition to being more time consuming.

Approximately 10–20% of patients with symptomatic DVT have thrombus confined to the deep calf veins, of which 20–30% will subsequently propagate to the proximal venous system[12]. Therefore, in patients with a high pre-test probability for acute DVT, serial US testing is recommended, with at least one additional follow-up compression US study over a 1-week interval. Compression US may also be useful in the investigation of suspected PE, as 70% of patients with proven PE have proximal DVT[4]. In patients with coexisting clinical DVT, BTS recommend compression US as the initial imaging test. Serial bilateral studies may also be helpful in patients with renal impairment, severe contrast allergy, or pregnant patients[3].

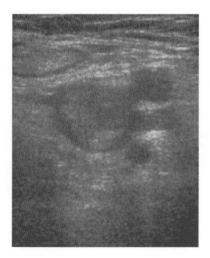

Fig. 21.3 Transverse US image showing common femoral vein distended and filled with echogenic thrombus.

21.1.1.8 Venography

Conventional venography for the initial investigation of suspected DVT is no longer recommended. MR venography is performed by a number of centres and has been shown to have a high sensitivity for the detection of iliofemoral DVT. A number of sequences can be used. Time-of-flight techniques do not require the use of IV contrast. Contrast-enhanced imaging has the advantage of reduced imaging time and high spatial resolution three-dimensional imaging is achievable[14].

CT venography (CTV), performed following CTPA was undertaken in all analyzed patients in the PIOPED II study[3]. There is a reported 93% accuracy in identifying DVT when compared to compression US[15]. This method has the advantage of increasing the rate of detection of VTE with a single contrast injection required for both the CTPA and CTV, but disadvantages include an increased radiation dose, particularly when the pelvic veins are imaged.

21.2 Superior vena cava obstruction (SVCO)

SVCO can occur either from external compression due to a mediastinal mass, or from intraluminal thrombus, usually associated with an intravascular device. Malignant causes account for approximately 65% of cases of SVCO, the most common associated malignancies being (in descending order of frequency) non-small cell lung cancer, small cell lung cancer, lymphoma, and metastases. The resultant clinical syndrome involves oedema of the affected areas, which can rarely cause airway or neurological compromise due to involvement of the upper respiratory tract or cerebral oedema respectively. Symptoms usually progress initially over a few weeks, then may improve somewhat as a collateral network develops.

Contrast-enhanced CT of the chest is the most useful initial imaging modality (Fig. 21.4). CT phlebography, in which there is cannulation of veins within both antecubital fossae has been shown to be a useful technique for demonstration of the site of the occlusion and associated collateral vessels[16]. Conventional venography is usually reserved for planning subsequent intervention, such as placement of a stent. MR venography may be helpful in patients with a severe contrast allergy, while positron emission tomography (PET) can influence the design of the radiotherapy field[17,18].

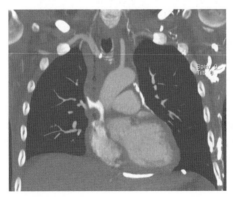

Fig. 21.4 Coronal contrast-enhanced CT image showing extensive thrombus in the superior vena cava and right brachiocephalic vein.

Percutaneous intravascular stenting is usually reserved for patients with severe symptoms requiring urgent intervention such as respiratory or neurologic compromise, or for patients with disease resistant to chemoradiation such as mesothelioma. It is also helpful in cases due to catheter associated thrombus[19,20]. Stent placement is associated with more rapid improvement in symptom than chemoradiation and oedema usually resolves within 48–72 hours. The rate of relapse after stent placement has been reported to be between 9–20%, with a complication rate of 3–7%[20]. Potential complications of stent placement include stent migration, pulmonary embolus, haematoma at the puncture site, and perforation.

21.3 The acute abdomen

A number of conditions related to the malignancy itself or as a complication of treatment can present with acute abdominal pain and gastrointestinal symptoms in patients with cancer. Surgical oncological referrals for patients presenting with an acute abdomen whilst undergoing chemotherapy include acute appendicitis, paralytic ileus, neutropenic colitis, intestinal perforation, acute intestinal obstruction, obstructed hernia, and intussusception in descending order of frequency[21]. Clinical evaluation, particularly in the immunocompromised patient, can be difficult as symptoms and signs may not develop until late in the course of the illness and are often non-specific.

An erect chest radiograph and supine abdominal film are helpful as an initial evaluation, particularly assessing for pneumoperitoneum or bowel obstruction. However, abdominal CT is usually the most valuable non-invasive and rapidly available imaging modality. The imaging appearances of some of the most common causes for an acute abdomen in this population are briefly discussed in the rest of this section.

21.3.1 Colitis

There are several causes for the development of colitis in oncology patients, the most common being neutropenic colitis or typhlitis, pseudomembranous colitis due to *Clostridium difficile*, ischaemia, infections related to immunodeficiency such as cytomegalovirus, and the direct effects of treatment including radiotherapy and certain chemotherapeutic regimens[22,23].

The supine abdominal radiograph is the most important single radiograph and may be helpful as an initial assessment of the extent of colitis as well as detecting the presence of toxic megacolon. Extensive colitis is likely when there is a complete absence of faecal residue. Intraluminal gas usually accumulates where there are areas of severe disease and can help to delineate mucosal abnormalities. However, in the absence of gas, these abnormalities can be underestimated. Plain film findings include thumb printing, thickened haustra, dilatation of small and or large bowel, mucosal abnormalities, or a 'gasless abdomen'.

Abdominal CT is a more sensitive method for the detection of colitis, is not associated with the potential risks of endoscopy and biopsy, and the results are more rapidly available than those from stool assays. A number of findings are common to all of the causes of colitis described here, although certain appearances may help to refine the diagnosis somewhat.

The hallmark appearances of colitis on CT consist of bowel wall thickening to >3mm. Other findings include mucosal enhancement, wall nodularity, the presence

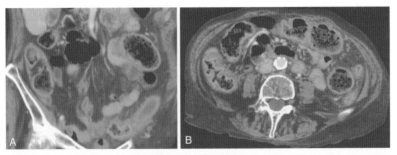

Fig. 21.5 Coronal (A) and axial (B) images from a CT abdomen examination in a patient with pseudomembranous colitis demonstrating diffusely abnormal colon with wall thickening and abnormally enhancing mucosa.

of air within the bowel wall (pneumatosis intestinalis), bowel dilatation, mesenteric stranding, and ascites.

21.3.1.1 Pseudomembranous colitis

Pseudomembranous colitis is limited to the colon, with no small bowel involvement seen; it almost always involves the rectum and left hemicolon, with a pancolitis often demonstrated[24] (Fig. 21.5). Mean bowel wall thickening was greatest and wall nodularity significantly more common in pseudomembranous colitis than other causes in a review of 76 neutropenic patients with radiologic bowel abnormalities. Abnormal CT appearances were seen in 50% of a series of 152 scanned hospitalized patients with *C. difficile* colitis[24].

21.3.1.2 Neutropenic enterocolitis

Neutropenic enterocolitis or typhlitis is a poorly understood entity, but is thought to result from compromise of bowel wall integrity, with subsequent bacterial or fungal invasion. It was the most common final diagnosis in neutropenic patients with radiologic bowel abnormalities[23]. The caecum is the most common site of disease, although any segment of the small or large bowel may be involved (Fig. 21.6). Pneumatosis intestinalis, the combined involvement of small and large bowel and/or disease isolated to the right hemicolon may be helpful pointers to this disease.

21.3.1.3 Ischaemic colitis

Ischaemic colitis is classically a disease of the elderly with arteriosclerotic disease. However, other precipitating causes include sudden hypotensive episodes, distal colonic obstruction, and vascular occlusion related to neoplasia[25]. A segmental pattern of colitis is most commonly reported, which can be left- (Fig. 21.7) or right-sided, although a pancolitis can also be seen. Intramural air is a relatively specific, but insensitive finding and may be associated with portal venous gas.

21.3.2 Obstruction

There are multiple possible causes of intestinal obstruction in patients with cancer. Small bowel obstruction is most commonly caused by adhesions and peritoneal carcinomatosis, but rarer causes include metastases to the bowel wall, reported with breast cancer, melanoma, and osteosarcoma among other tumours[26].

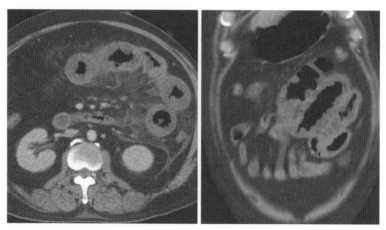

Fig. 21.6 Axial (A) and coronal (B) CT image showing marked small bowel wall thickening with associated mesenteric stranding in a patient with neutropenic colitis. The ascending and descending colon are decompressed.

On the supine abdominal radiograph, mechanical small bowel obstruction usually causes distention of small bowel with gas and fluid, with associated collapse of the large bowel. Small bowel loops can be discriminated from large bowel due to their central position, multiple loops, and the presence of valvulae conniventes which traverse the entire diameter of the bowel as opposed to colonic haustra. Multiple fluid levels may be seen on an erect radiograph, although this is not usually required. The 'string of beads' sign, due to bubbles of gas trapped beween valvulae conniventes, is seen only when very dilated small bowel is almost entirely fluid filled.

Appearances of large bowel obstruction are dependent on the site of obstruction and the competence of the ileo-caecal valve. Small bowel distention is seen when this valve is incompetent, although the combination of small and large bowel dilatation can also be seen in paralytic ileus. The presence of air in the rectum, which may be more visible on a left lateral radiograph can help to confirm an ileus and exclude a distal obstruction. Large bowel can be identified by its peripheral position within the abdomen and the presence of a haustral margin.

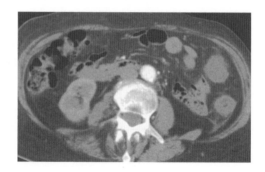

Fig. 21.7 Axial CT image showing a thick-walled descending colon with mesenteric stranding in ischaemic colitis. The ascending colon contains faeces and appears unremarkable.

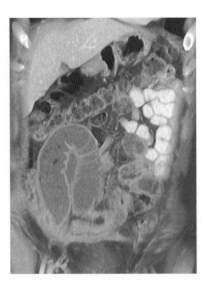

Fig. 21.8 Coronal CT image showing closed loop small bowel obstruction due to peritoneal metastases secondary to ovarian carcinoma.

Abdominal CT is useful in evaluating the site of obstruction and determining the cause. Specific forms of obstruction such as a closed loop or an intussusception may also be demonstrated (Fig. 21.8).

21.3.3 **Pneumoperitoneum**

The presence of free intraperitoneal gas almost always indicates perforation of a viscus. An erect chest radiograph is the usually the initial imaging performed and can detect as little as 1mL of free gas. However, the patient is required to remain erect for 10min prior to the radiograph and this may not be possible depending on the clinical condition. A horizontal ray lateral decubitus radiograph may also be helpful, but often only a supine portable abdominal film can be obtained. Signs of pneumoperitoneum on a supine radiograph may be present in 60% of cases and include Rigler's sign (gas on both sides of the bowel wall), gas outlining the falciform ligament, the football sign (gas outlining the peritoneal cavity), and the inverted V sign (gas outlining the medial umbilical folds)[27]. Localized gas in the right upper quadrant is most frequently seen, but is prone to frequent errors in interpretation. Abdominal CT is the most sensitive imaging modality for the detection of free air (Fig. 21.9), with 100% sensitivity on one series[28]. It may also help to localize the source of perforation.

21.4 **Metastatic epidural spinal cord compression (MESCC)**

MESCC occurs when an epidural metastatic lesion causes true displacement of the spinal cord from its normal position in the spinal canal. It is a relatively common complication of malignancy, occurring in 5–10% of cancer patients and in up to 40% of patients with pre-existing known spinal skeletal metastases[29-31]. If left untreated, virtually 100% of patients with MESCC would become paraplegic and this is therefore considered a true medical emergency requiring immediate intervention[32]. Whilst therapy is primarily palliative, up to one-third of patients may survive beyond 1 year and preservation of quality of life is essential.

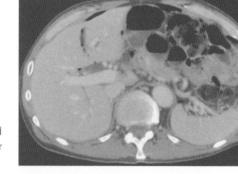

Fig. 21.9 Axial CT image showing free intraperitoneal air. Locules of air are present around the falciform ligament and anteriorly within the upper abdomen.

As multiple studies have demonstrated a correlation between neurological function at the time of diagnosis and prognosis from MESCC, diagnosis before the development of neurological deficit is particularly important. MR imaging (MRI) is considered the gold standard imaging modality (Fig. 21.10), with improved sensitivity as compared to the previously regarded myelography, with superior depiction of paravertebral tumour extension and identification of additional metastatic lesions[33,34].

It is non-invasive and provides excellent depiction of soft tissues, tumour margins, and neural elements. Most imaging protocols include sagittal T1- and T2-weighted sequences followed by relevant axial scans of the same sequences through identified regions of interest. Osteolytic metastases display low signal on T1-weighted and high or intermediate signal intensity on T2-weighted scans. Highly sclerotic metastases such as seen in breast or prostate cancer show low signal intensity on all sequences[35].

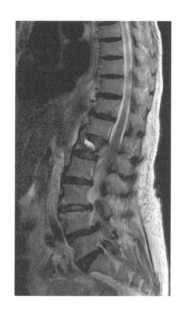

Fig. 21.10 T2-weighted sagittal MRI of the same patient demonstrating there is significant compression of the conus medullaris by the heterogeneous high signal soft tissue mass.

21.5 **Sepsis**

Fever is a common symptom among patients with cancer and may be caused by a variety of factors. A prospective study of 477 episodes of fever in cancer patients found that infectious causes represented 47%[36]. The most common sites of infection are the respiratory tract, followed by the urinary tract, gastrointestinal system, and soft tissues[36,37]. Febrile patients are usually initially assessed with a thorough history and clinical examination, chest radiography and routine cultures. If chest radiography shows an opacity, then broncholaveolar lavage may be performed[38]. In patients with persistent fever, but no evidence of respiratory tract infection including chest CT, CT of the abdomen and paranasal sinuses, MRI of the head and liver and transoesophageal echocardiography may be considered[38].

21.5.1 **Respiratory tract infections**

Bacteria are the most frequent cause of pneumonia in immunocompromised patients. The radiographic features of lobar or segmental consolidation usually do not differ from those in the general population, although there may be an increased delay in their appearance (Fig. 21.11).

Fungal infections are important pathogens, particularly *Candida* and *Aspergillus fumigatus*. *Candida pneumonia* often occurs in association with other pathogens and in the presence of systemic disease with mucous membrane involvement. The radiographic findings vary from diffuse bilateral non-segmental opacities of varying sizes to a miliary pattern or unilateral or bilateral lobar or segmental consolidation[39]. Cavitation is not thought to be a feature. *Aspergillus* in the immunocompromised patient may be suggested by ground glass opacification, consolidation, poorly defined nodules, and cavitation[38].

Pneumocystis jiroveci (formerly *Pneumocystis carinii*) is an important pathogen. The radiologic appearances are similar to those seen in patients with AIDS, although the clinical course may be more fulminant, with a higher mortality. Radiographic features include diffuse or perihilar reticular and ill-defined ground glass opacities, which may progress within a few days to homogeneous opacification in the untreated patient[39].

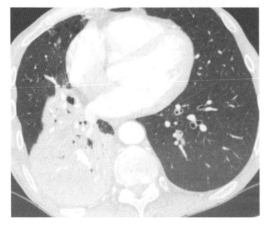

Fig. 21.11 Axial CT image demonstrating presence of air bronchograms indicating consolidation within the right lower lobe.

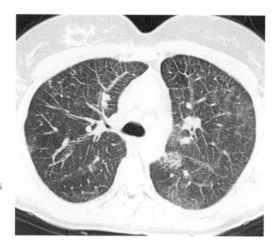

Fig. 21.12 Axial CT image showing extensive nodular interlobular septal thickening with superimposed ground glass opacification consistent with lymphangitis carcinomatosa.

High-resolution thin-section CT is significantly more sensitive for the detection of pulmonary disease and several studies have demonstrated the value of CT in the evaluation of febrile neutropenic patients with a normal chest radiograph[40].

21.6 Lymphangitis carcinomatosis

Lymphangitis carcinomatosis is caused by infiltration of tumour cells into the lymphatic vessels and results histologically in thickening of the interlobular septa and of the bronchovascular interstitium. The most common tumours causing this pattern of disease arise from bronchus, breast, pancreas, stomach, colon, and prostate[41]. Approximately 25% of cases are due to infiltration of hilar lymph nodes causing peripheral lymphatic obstruction, whilst the remainder result from direct haematogenous spread to the lung interstitium[42].

The chest radiographic findings are positive in approximately 50% of cases of pathologically proven lymphangitis and include Kerley A lines, peripheral septal thickening (Kerley B lines), and fine reticulonodular opacification, which may be accompanied by hilar enlargement[43]. In patients with carcinoma of the bronchus the findings may be unilateral, but usually the appearances are diffuse and bilateral, often with associated pleural effusions[41]. The appearances may be very similar to those of pulmonary oedema, particularly in the absence of lymphadenopathy and clinical correlation in association with previous radiographs is helpful in their differentiation.

CT is significantly more sensitive than radiography, particularly thin-section high-resolution CT. Common findings include thickening and irregularity of the fissures, thickening of the bronchovascular bundles and interlobular septa and often associated patchy air space shadowing[42–44]. The nodularity of the septal thickening is not seen in pulmonary oedema and may be a helpful distinguishing feature (Fig. 21.12).

21.7 Radiation induced injury

21.7.1 Radiation-induced lung injury

The effects of radiation therapy are commonly seen on chest radiographs and CT. Although lung injury is usually confined to the radiation field, several studies and reports have demonstrated that damage may occur within the non-irradiated lung possibly related to a hypersensitivity reaction[45,46].

The pattern of radiation injury is described in two distinct phases. The initial phase is a pneumonitis, which develops 1–6 months after therapy, although CT changes have been described as early as 1 week[47]. This phase is characterized by loss of type 1 pneumocytes, increased capillary permeability, interstitial oedema, alveolar capillary congestion, and inflammatory cell accumulation in the alveolar space[48]. Radiographic changes show hazy opacities with obscured vascular margins which are usually confined to radiation portals[49]. Changes may be apparent earlier on CT than on chest radiographs and consist of ground glass opacities or consolidation[47]. Ventilation and perfusion studies may show perfusion defects in areas of lung which appear normal on chest radiographs and CT[49].

The second phase of lung injury is fibrosis, which has a variable time course and a poorly understood mechanism of pathogenesis. More homogeneous linear or angled opacities may be seen on chest radiographs, with accompanying volume loss, which can distort adjacent structures. Traction bronchiectasis may be a dominant feature on CT. Again the appearances are usually geographically rather than anatomically distributed (Fig. 21.13). If there are progressive changes beyond 18 months, an alternative diagnosis should be sought[48].

Other rarer manifestations of lung injury include hyperlucency, pleural effusions, and spontaneous pneuomthorax. Second primary tumours may arise within the radiation field, particularly when radiation therapy is given in childhood. Infection and tumour recurrence should be considered as differential diagnoses in radiation induced lung injury. Infection is not usually confined to the radiation field, although secondary infection can occur in an area of radiation injury.

Tumour recurrence may be detected by the development of focal masses or cavitation on CT. FDG PET scanning can be helpful in distinguishing fibrosis from recurrent tumour, however false positives are likely to occur if this is performed <4–5 months post-completion of radiation therapy.

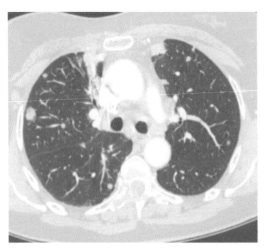

Fig. 21.13 Axial CT image showing volume loss in the right upper lobe anteriorly secondary to fibrosis in the radiation field of a patient with breast cancer. Unfortunately multiple pulmonary metastases have also developed.

21.8 **Insufficiency fractures**

Osteoporosis is increased in many cancer patients, in particular breast and prostate cancer patients receiving hormone manipulation therapy[50,51]; a 78% increase of relative risk for clinical vertebral fractures was noted amongst breast cancer survivors with a breast cancer diagnosis before the age of 55 compared to controls with no cancer history[52].

Bone mineral density (BMD) is assessed by dual-energy X-ray absorptiometry with measurements taken at the posterior-anterior spine, total hip, and total body. A T-score is calculated using a young adult reference group: T-score = (individual BMD − mean of young adult reference BMD population]/standard deviation of young reference BMD population. Osteoporosis is defined as a t-score $<−2.5$.

21.8.1 **Vertebral compression fractures**

When a cancer patient develops an acute vertebral compression fracture then distinction between metastasis or osteoporosis is important (Fig. 21.14). Radiographs are often unhelpful in this situation and bone scintigraphy will show increased activity in either circumstance. A number of studies have shown that MRI may be helpful. Several distinguishing features have been demonstrated, although no single feature should be taken in isolation given the overlap in metastatic and benign disease[53–55].

MRI features suggestive of metastatic compression fractures include:

- A convex posterior border of the vertebral body.
- Abnormal signal intensity of the pedicle or posterior element.
- An epidural mass, particularly when it is encasing the theca.
- A focal paraspinal mass.
- Other spinal metastases.

MR features suggestive of acute osteoporotic compression fractures include:

- A low signal intensity band on T1- and T2-weighted images.
- Spared normal bone marrow signal intensity of the vertebral body.
- Retropulsion of a posterior bone fragment.
- Multiple compression fractures.

21.8.2 **Pelvic insufficiency fractures**

Pelvic insufficiency fractures are a common complication of pelvic radiotherapy. A prospective study with MRI of patients with advanced cervical carcinoma found an incidence of 89%, although only 56% of patients reported pain[56]. Postmenopausal patients appear to be at the highest risk. These fractures have characteristic imaging appearances and it is very important for prognosis and future treatment that they are not misinterpreted as bony metastatic disease.

The most common sites for the development of fractures are within the sacrum and ilium. These are often bilateral and symmetric. Pubic fractures have been reported in association. Fractures may be visualized on radiographs, although these are insensitive. Bone scintigraphy classically shows a bilateral symmetrical pattern of increased uptake within the sacrum/ilium, giving rise to the 'Honda sign' (Fig. 21.15). Areas of increased uptake outside the radiation field are concerning for metastatic disease[57]. CT can

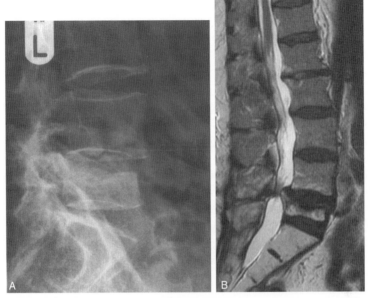

Fig. 21.14 Lateral radiograph (A) and sagittal T2-weighted MRI (B) in a patient post-radiotherapy for rectal cancer. The bone marrow within the radiation field has developed abnormal high signal intensity. There is a subsequent compression fracture of L5, with retropulsion of fragment into the spinal canal, causing narrowing of the theca.

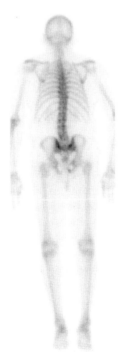

Fig. 21.15 Whole body ^{99m}Tc-MDP bone scintigraphy showing bilateral symmetrical increased uptake in the sacro-iliac regions and fractures of the right superior and inferior pubic rami.

confirm the presence of fractures by demonstrating focal cortical disruption, a fracture line, and/or callus formation in the absence of osteolytic lesions or a soft tissue mass[56].

They are demonstrated on MR as focal and often multiple areas of marrow oedema, with low signal on T1-weighted images and high signal on STIR sequences.

21.9 **Summary**

- Complications either as a result of malignancy or as a consequence of treatment are common.
- Complications may mimic malignancy.
- Imaging plays a critical role in the diagnostic pathway. Final diagnosis may require the use of several imaging modalities. Comprehensive clinical information is essential to aid the radiologist with narrowing the differential diagnosis.

References

1. Wells PS, Ginsberg JS, Anderson DR, *et al.* Use of a clinical model of safe management of patients with suspected pulmonary embolism. *Ann Intern Med* 1998; **129**: 997–1005.
2. Pruemer J. Prevalence, causes and impact of cancer-associated thrombosis. *Am J Health Syst Pharm* 2005; **62**: S4–6.
3. Stein PD, Woodard PK, Weg JG, *et al.* Diagnostic pathways in acute pulmonary embolism: recommendations of the PIOPED II investigators. *Radiology* 2007; **242**: 15–21.
4. British Thoracic Society Standards of Care Committee Pulmonary Embolism Guideline Development Group. British thoracic society guidelines for the management of suspected acute pulmonary embolism. *Thorax* 2003; **58**: 470–84.
5. Rosen M, Sands D, Morris J, *et al.* Does a physician's ability to accurately assess the likelihood of pulmonary embolism increase with training? *Acad Med* 2000; **75**: 1199–205.
6. Kline JA, Johns KL, Colucciello SA *et al.* New diagnostic tests for pulmonary embolism. *Ann Emerg Med* 2000; **35**: 168–80.
7. Kearon C, Ginsberg JS, Douketis J, *et al.* An evaluation of d-dimer in the diagnosis of pulmonary embolism. *Ann Intern Med* 2006; **144**: 812–21.
8. The PIOPED Investigators. Value of the ventilation/perfusion scan in acute pulmonary embolism. Results of the prospective investigation of pulmonary embolism diagnosis (PIOPED). *JAMA* 1990; **263**: 2753–9.
9. Remy-Jardin M, Tillie-Leblond I, Szapiro D, *et al.* CT angiography of pulmonary embolism in patients with underlying respiratory disease: impact of multi-slice CT (MSCT) on image quality and negative predictive value. *Eur Radiol* 2002; **12**: 1971–8.
10. Meany JF, Weg JG, Chenevert TL, *et al.* Diagnosis of pulmonary embolism with magnetic resonance agiography. *N Engl J Med* 1997; **336**: 1422–7.
11. Gupta A, Frazer CK, Ferguson JM, *et al.* Acute pulmonary embolism: diagnosis with MR angiography. *Radiology* 1999; **210**: 353–9.
12. Fraser JD, Anderson DR. Deep venous thrombosis: recent advances and optimal investigation with US. *Radiology* 1999; **211**: 9–24.
13. Kearon C, Julian JA, Newman TE, *et al.* Noninvasive diagnosis of deep venous thrombosis: McMaster diagnostic imaging guidelines initiative. *Ann Intern Med* 1998; **128**: 663–77.
14. Fraser DGW, Moody AR, Davidson IR, *et al.* Deep venous thrombosis: diagnosis by using venous enhanced subtracted peak arterial MR venography versus conventional venography. *Radiology* 2003; **226**: 812–20.

15. Duwe KM, Shiau M, Budorick NE, *et al.* Evaluation of the lower extremity veins in patients with suspected pulmonary embolism: a retrospective comparison of helical CT venography and sonography. *AJR Am J Roentgenol* 2000; **175**: 1525–31.

16. Qanadli SD, El Hajjam M, Bruckert F, *et al.* Helical CT phlebography of the superior vena cava: diagnosis and evaluation of venous obstruction. *AJR Am J Roentgenol* 1999; **172**: 1327–33.

17. Khimji T, Zeiss J. MRI versus CT and US in the evaluation of a patient presenting with superior vena cava syndrome: case report. *Clin Imaging* 1992; **16**: 269–71.

18. Wilson LD, Detterbeck FC, Yahalom J. Superior vena cava syndrome with malignant causes. *N Engl J Med* 2007; **356**: 1862–9.

19. Fine DG, Shepherd RF, Welch TJ. Thrombolytic therapy for superior vena cava syndrome. *Lancet* 1989; **1**: 1200–1.

20. Kee ST, Kinoshita L, Razavi MK, *et al.* Superior vena cava syndrome: treatment with catheter-directed thrombolysis and endovascular stent placement. *Radiology* 1998; **206**: 187–93.

21. Pandey M, Mathew A, Geetha N, *et al.* Acute abdomen in patients receiving chemotherapy. *Indian J Cancer* 2001; **38**: 68–71.

22. Kaur H, Lover EM, David CL, *et al.* Radiologic findings in taxane induced colitis. *Eur J Radiol* 2008; **66**: 75–78.

23. Kirkpatrick ID, Greenberg HM. Gastrointestinal complications in the neutropenic patient: characterization and differentiation with abdominal CT. *Radiology* 2003; **226**: 668–74.

24. Ash L, Baker ME, O'Malley CM, Jr., *et al.* Colonic abnormalities on CT in adult hospitalized patients with Clostridium difficile colitis: prevalence and significance of findings. *AJR Am J Roentgenol* 2006; **186**: 1393–400.

25. Balthazar EJ, Yen BC, Gordon RB. Ischaemic colitis: CT evaluation of 54 cases. *Radiology* 1999; **211**: 381–8.

26. Idelevich E, Kashtan H, Mavor E, *et al.* Small bowel obstruction caused by secondary tumours. *Surg Oncol* 2006; **15**: 29–32.

27. Levine MS, Scheiner JD, Rubesin SE, *et al.* Diagnosis of pneumoperitoneum on supine abdominal radiographs. *AJR Am J Roentgenol* 1991; **156**: 731–5.

28. Stapakis JC, Thickman D. Diagnosis of pneumoperitoneum: abdominal CT vs upright chest film. *J Comput Assist Tomogr* 1992; **16**: 713–16.

29. Barron KD, Hirano A, Arakis S, *et al.* Experiences with metastatic neoplasms involving the spinal cord. *Neurology* 1959; **9**: 91–106.

30. Schaberg J, Gainor BJ. A profile of metastatic carcinoma of the spine. *Spine* 1985; **10**: 19–20.

31. Gerstzen P, Welch W. Current surgical management of metastatic spinal disease. *Oncology (Williston Park)* 2000; **14**: 1013–24.

32. Kwok Y, Tibbs PA, Patchell RA. Clinical approach to metastatic epidural spinal cord compression. *Haematol Oncol North Am* 2006; **20**: 1297–305.

33. Carmody RF, Yang PJ, Seeley GW, *et al.* Spinal cord compression due to metastatic disease: diagnosis with MR imaging versus myelography. *Radiology* 1989; **173**: 225–9.

34. Smoker WR, Godersky JC, Knutzon RK, *et al.* The role of MR imaging in evaluating metastatic spinal disease. *AJR Am J Roentgenol* 1987; **149**: 1241–8.

35. Petren-Mallmin M. Clinical and experimental imaging of breast cancer metastases in the spine. *Acta Radiol Suppl* 1994; **391**: 1–23.

36. Toussaint E, Bahel-Ball E, Vekemans M, *et al.* Causes of fever in cancer patients (prospective study over 477 episodes). *Support Care Cancer* 2006; **14**: 763–9.

37. Gencer S, Salepci T, Ozer S. Evaluation of infectious etiology and prognostic risk factors of febrile episodes in neutropenic cancer patients. *J Infect* 2003; **47**: 65–72.

38. Heussel CP, Kauczor HU, Heussel G, *et al.* Early detection of pneumonia in febrile neutro-penic patients: use of thin-section CT. *AJR Am J Roentgenol* 1997; **169**: 1347–53.

39. Hansell DM, Armstrong P, Lynch DA, *et al.* The immunocompromised patient. In: Hansell DM, Armstrong P, Lynch DA, *et al.* (eds). *Imaging diseases of the chest,* pp. 277–360. London: Elsevier Mosby, 2005.

40. Wendel F, Jenett M, Geib A, *et al.* Low dose CT in neutropenic patients with fever of unknown origin. *Rofo* 2005; **177**: 1424–9.

41. Hansell DM, Armstrong P, Lynch DA, *et al.* Neoplasms of the lungs, airways and pleura. In: Hansell DM, Armstrong P, Lynch DA, *et al.* (eds). *Imaging diseases of the chest,* pp.870–1. London: Elsevier Mosby, 2005.

42. Stein MG, Mayo J, Muller N, *et al.* Pulmonary lymphangitic spread of carcinoma: appearance on CT scans. *Radiology* 1987; **162**: 371–5.

43. Johkoh T, Ikezoe J, Tomiyama N, *et al.* CT findings in lymphangitic carcinomatosis of the lung: correlation with histologic findings and pulmonary function tests. *AJR Am J Roentgenol* 1992; **158**: 1217–22.

44. Munk PL, Muller NL, Miller RR, *et al.* Pulmonary lymphangitic carcinomatosis: CT and pathologic findings. *Radiology* 1988; **166**: 705–9.

45. Martin C, Romero S, Sanchez-Paya J, *et al.* Bilateral lymphocytic alveolitis: a common reaction after unilateral thoracic irradiation. *Eur Resp J* 1999; **13**: 727–32.

46. Bourke SJ, Dalphin JC, Boyd G, *et al.* Hypersensitivity pneumonitis: current concepts. *Eur Resp J* 2001; **32**: 81S–92S.

47. Ikezoe J, Takashima S, Morimoto S, *et al.* CT appearances of acute radiation-induced injury in the lung. *AJR Am J Roentgenol* 1988; **150**: 765–70.

48. Hansell DM, Armstrong P, Lynch DA, *et al.* Drug and radiation induced lung disease. In: Hansell DM, Armstrong P, Lynch DA, *et al.* (eds). *Imaging diseases of the chest,* pp. 516–25. London: Elsevier Mosby, 2005.

49. Bell J, McGivern D, Bullimore J, *et al.* Diagnostic imaging of post-irradiation changes in the chest. *Clin Radiol* 1988; **39**: 109–19.

50. Chen Z, Maricic M, Pettinger M, *et al.* Osteoporosis and rate of bone loss among postmenopausal survivors of breast cancer. *Cancer* 2005; **104**: 1520–30.

51. Malcolm JB, Derweesh IH, Kincade MC, *et al.* Osteoporosis and fractures after androgen deprivation initiation for prostate cancer. *Can J Urol* 2007; **14**: 3551–9.

52. Chen Z, Maricic M, Bassford TL, *et al.* Fracture risk among breast cancer survivors: results from the Women's Health Initiative Observational Study. *Arch Intern Med* 2005; **165**: 552–8.

53. Jung H, Jee W, McCauley T, *et al.* Discrimination of metastatic from acute osteoporotic compression spinal fractures with MR imaging. *Radiographics* 2003; **23**: 179–87.

54. Rupp RE, Ebraheim NA, Coombs RJ. Magnetic resonance imaging differentiation of compression spine fractures or vertebral lesions caused by osteoporosis or tumor. *Spine* 1995; **20**: 2499–503.

55. Fu TS, Chen LH, Liao JC, *et al.* Magnetic resonance imaging characteristics of benign and malignant vertebral fractures. *Chang Gung Med J* 2004; **27**: 808–15.

56. Blomlie V, Rofstad EK, Talle K, *et al.* Incidence of radiation-induced insufficiency fractures of the female pelvis: evaluation with MR imaging. *AJR Am J Roentgenol* 1996; **167**: 1205–19.

57. Abe H, Nakamura M, Takahashi S, *et al.* Radiation-induced insufficiency fractures of the pelvis: evaluation with 99mTc-methylene diphosphonate scintigraphy. *AJR Am J Roentgenol* 1992; **158**: 599–602.

Chapter 22

Radiation protection issues when imaging patients for radiotherapy

Jane Shekhdar and Edwin Aird

Introduction

This chapter discusses radiation protection matters for patients who require imaging with ionizing radiation as part of their radiotherapy management. Although non-ionizing radiation, e.g. ultrasound and magnetic resonance imaging (MRI) will also be used for these patients, these imaging modalities are not discussed here because these radiations are considered 'safe' compared with ionizing radiations. This chapter will include some fundamental scientific aspects of radiation and its effect on the human body, guidance on dosimetry, as well as the regulations themselves.

For the patient the most important regulations are the Ionising Radiation (Medical Exposures) Regulations (IR(ME)R)[1], which are described in section 22.3.1. The imaging performed throughout the radiotherapy (RT) patient pathway for diagnosis, staging, planning, and verification will add to the radiation burden to normal tissue for the RT patient. These doses to normal tissue are likely to be very small compared to those from the 'therapy', except in extreme circumstances.

22.1 The effects of ionizing radiation on the body

The International Commission on Radiological Protection (ICRP) periodically reviews the possible risks of radiation on the human body. The effect on tissue is dependant on the dose level. At high doses a significant number of cells within an organ are killed and a predicted effect will occur, known as a deterministic effect. In radiotherapy it is the killing of the tumour that is the vital deterministic effect. Linked to this (and very relevant to the verification imaging discussed in later sections) is the sparing of critical structures from this deterministic damage.

For a deterministic effect to occur the dose must be above a threshold level, and the severity of the effect increases with dose. The effects of large radiation doses become apparent within a few days. The effects of lower doses are not immediate; they may occur 6–20 months later and still be quite severe in nature. The values for various organs are shown in Appendix 2, Table 1.

At lower doses fewer cells are killed and any harm caused is thought to depend on the probability that a damaged cell is misrepaired and continues to proliferate. It is believed that this can occur at any dose level, but the chance of it occurring increases with dose. The risk model used for these effects is known as the linear-no-threshold (LNT) model.

With this model there is no threshold and no dose is 'safe'. Another feature of this model is that further repair is not possible, and the effect of multiple exposures therefore becomes additive. This is the stochastic effect of radiation and the hazard is the induction of cancers and heritable effects. The risk factors for *stochastic effects* have been estimated from epidemiological studies, such as those individuals exposed to atomic bomb radiations[2]. The data has indicated that certain organs of the body are more likely to develop cancers than others, also that there is a considerable latent period between the time of the exposure and the clinical presentation of the cancer. For leukaemia the latent period is 5–14 years, for solid tumours from 5 years to at least 40 years. Typically the risk factor for cancer induction is taken as 5% per Sievert (Sv)[4].

The risk factors are also age dependent. For children or a fetus exposed *in utero* there is an enhanced risk: this may be due in part to increased sensitivity of the developing organs and in part to the longer time to express this risk. If the fetus is irradiated with a high dose between the 8th–15th week of gestation there is also an increased risk of mental retardation. The risk factor for this is thought to be 25 IQ points per Sv, hence not significant for doses below 100mSv.

Heritable effects from ionizing radiation in humans have not been clearly demonstrated, although mutations have been seen in other species. It is thought that the significant level of spontaneous genetic abnormalities may mask the small number of genetic effects produced by low levels of radiation.

22.2 Dose and dose indicators used in imaging

Diagnostic doses are generally several orders of magnitude lower, typically of the order of 10mGy (quantities defined below), compared to tumorcidal doses of 60–70Gy (fractionated).

Factors affecting patient dose are discussed in detail elsewhere[3] and can be summarized under the headings of:

- Site of patient irradiated.
- Size of the patient at this site.
- Equipment factors (e.g. kV, mAs).
- Technique.
- Image quality required.

These are the factors that affect the dose to the patient. It is important to understand the meaning of dose and the different ways this can be expressed when referring to patient dose. As a fundamental concept the absorbed dose (commonly known as the dose) is the energy absorbed by the tissues per unit mass. The unit of dose is the gray (= 1 joule per kg). Although used in radiotherapy for the target dose this is regarded in the protection field as a very large dose which produces deterministic effects not normally found during diagnostic examinations. The milligray (mGy) and the microgray (μGy) are more commonly used in imaging.

There are further complications to the concept of patient dose:

- In the radiation protection field there is the possibility of the use of radiations other than X-rays and gamma rays. For these other radiations (e.g. alpha particle or neutrons) an absorbed dose of D_T gray, to a specific tissue, will have a different biological effect than D_T gray of X-rays to that tissue. In order to allow for these differences the unit Sievert (Sv) is introduced. This dose unit takes into account the biological effect of different radiations. The equivalent dose to a specific tissue (H_T) is given by the sum of the dose to the tissue (D_T) multiplied by the radiation weighting factor:

$$H_T = \Sigma_R w_R D_T$$

where w_R is the weighting factor for the type of radiation.

Fortunately the value of w_R is normalized to photon radiation, the value of w_R is 1 for photons (also electrons and positrons). Thus equivalent dose to tissues H_T (Sv) for all imaging procedures has the same numerical value as the absorbed dose D_T (Gy).

◆ For the purpose of radiation protection and the setting of dose limits for workers and members of the public, the ICRP introduced the concept of effective dose (E) (which can be used to express risk) also with the unit of Sv. The effective dose is the dose to the whole body that would incur the same risk as a partial exposure of the body, when specific tissues receive an equivalent dose of H_T:

$$E = \Sigma_T w_T H_T$$

where w_T is the weighting factor for the specific tissue. The sum is performed over all organs and tissues of the body considered to be sensitive to the induction of stochastic effects. The value given to w_T reflects the radiation sensitivity of the tissue, it is however, averaged over both sexes and all ages. The value of effective dose calculated using these average weighting factors therefore does not represent the characteristics of a particular individual.

◆ The values for w_T, the named organs, and the calculation of E has changed with time as more evidence has been gathered. The organs and factors used in the 1990 ICRP publication[4] and currently by ICRP[5] are given in Appendix 2, Table 2.

◆ It has become common practice to use effective dose when considering radiation risks from diagnostic radiology where doses are relatively low and only stochastic effects are being considered. All the values of E given in this chapter are calculated using ICRP 60 weighting factors. The uncertainties of the value of E are large (± 40%) even for a reference patient and will be much greater for the individual[6]. Bearing in mind the above limitations of the averaging process in calculating E, the use of E does allow for comparisons of dose between different X-ray examinations, provided that a similar patient sample is considered.

The effective doses for some typical examinations are shown in Table 22.1. Further values are given in Appendix 2 Table 6.

22.3 Radiation protection legislation

The ICRP[4] has recommended that the principles of radiation protection for practices involving ionizing radiation be: justification, optimization, and dose limitation.

These recommendations have been incorporated into Euratom directives, Basic Safety Standard (BSS)[7] directive, (96/29/Euratom and Medical Exposures (ME) Directive (97/43/Euratom)[8].

Table 22.1 Effective dose and risk of fatal cancer induction

Examination: pre-treatment imaging	Typical E	Risk of cancer* induction
CT	10mSv	0.05%
Bone scan	4mSv	0.02%
Diagnostic PET (400 MBq FDG)	11mSv	0.05%

*detriment adjusted nominal risk coefficient for cancer (adults) ICRP 60.

The BSS was implemented in the UK by legislation 'The Ionising Radiations Regulations 1999' (IRR99)[9]. These regulations are supported by a further document from the HSE the 'Approved Code of Practice and Guidance'[10]. Compliance with these regulations is enforced by the HSE. These regulations apply to workers and members of the public and will not be considered here.

The ME directive was implemented in the UK by the Department of Health legislation 'Ionising Radiation (Medical Exposure) Regulations' 2000 (IR(ME)R)[1]. Compliance with these regulations is enforced by the Care Quality Commission. Further guidance, of a more practical nature, for both these regulations is given in the Medical and Dental Guidance Notes[11].

22.3.1 Ionising radiation medical exposure regulations (IR(ME)R)

The IR(ME)R lay down measures to protect patients and other persons undergoing medical exposures from exposure to unnecessary radiation. The ICRP principles of justification and optimization are incorporated into the regulations; dose limits, however, are not applicable to patient procedures, but the benefit to the patient (or society through research, see Appendix 1) must outweigh any detriment from exposure to radiation for the exposure to be justified.

Applied to radiotherapy the scope of the IR(ME)R is to justify and optimize:

◆ The exposure of patients as part of their own medical diagnosis or treatment.

◆ The exposure of patients or other persons voluntarily participating in medical or biomedical, diagnostic, or therapeutic research programmes.

22.3.1.1 Duty holders

Regulation 2 of this legislation defines the roles of duty holders as:

◆ The employer, the referrer, the practitioner, the operator, and the MPE.

22.3.1.1.1 **The employer** The definition of the employer in this legislation is 'any natural or legal person who, in the course of trade, business or other undertaking, carries out, or engages others to carry out, medical exposures or practical aspects at a given radiological installation'.

The employer as a duty holder under IR(ME)R is responsible for providing a framework for radiation protection for patients. This frame work is based on a minimum set of written procedures the 'Employers Procedures' (EPs) (these are set out in schedule 1 of the legislation), written protocols and quality assurance programmes (Reg. 4).

A procedure must be in place to identify individuals who are entitled to act as referrers, practitioners, or operators and the scope of practices for duty holders must be clearly identified and documented.

The employer has a responsibility to ensure that all entitled practitioners and operators are adequately trained to perform their tasks in their defined scope of practice. A list of topics that training must cover is given in schedule 2 of the regulations, but training at local level on specific equipment, procedures, and protocols is also required. The training underpins the entitlement of the individual to act as a practitioner or operator for the range of practices for which they have been deemed competent. The employer must keep a record of all training and make it available for inspection.

The employer must also establish recommendations concerning referral criteria, including radiation doses, for medical exposures and make these available to the referrer.

22.3.1.1.2 **The referrer** The referrer must be a registered medical practitioner, dental practitioner or healthcare professional who under the employer's written procedures, is entitled to refer for medical exposures. The referrer does so under a protocol that conforms to the employer's procedures and the referral criteria. The employer must specify the scope of practice for which an individual can refer.

22.3.1.1.3 **The IR(ME)R practitioner** The primary responsibility of the IR(ME)R practitioner is to ensure that the requested medical exposure is justified and authorized in accordance with the employers written procedures.

Local employers procedures must indicate who may act as an IR(ME)R practitioner. To justify a procedure the IR(ME)R practitioner must use the clinical data supplied by the referrer to assess the benefit of the examination or therapy. The practitioner must have adequate training and be competent to weigh up the potential detriment of the exposure against the potential benefits for that individual (or society in the case of a research exposure, see Appendix 1).

22.3.1.1.4 **The operator** The operator is any person who carries out any practical aspect of the medical exposure. The primary responsibility of the operator is to optimize those aspects of the exposure for which they are responsible, in accordance with the employer's written procedures.

The range of work for an operator is extensive, and the employer must document for the individual the scope for which they are entitled to act as an operator. The employer must ensure operators are suitably trained and document the training. An operator often authorizes an exposure, where it has been previously justified by an IR(ME)R practitioner.

22.3.1.1.5 **Medical physics expert (MPE) (Reg. 9 (1))** The MPE is defined as a state-registered clinical scientist with appropriate experience in the clinical speciality. The expertise of an MPE is required to some extent for all medical exposures, the level of involvement being commensurate with the level of radiation risk. For radiotherapy there is a legal requirement on the employer that an MPE shall be full-time contracted to the radiation employer and available at all times.

The involvement will include advice and measurement of patient dose, advice on equipment purchase and use, measurement of equipment performance both at the commissioning stage and routinely. This involvement aids the justification and optimization required by the legislation. Input from an MPE is also required for research projects that require exposure to ionizing radiation (see Appendix 1).

Consideration of the above duty holders as relevant to imaging in radiotherapy is given in section 22.4. A member staff may have the role of more than one duty holder if the Employers Procedures entitle them to do so. For example the oncologist may be the referrer, IR(ME)R practitioner and operator.

22.3.1.2 Diagnostic reference levels

Patient diagnostic examinations are not subject to dose limits but the IR(ME)R legislation requires that diagnostic reference levels (DRLs) be set for diagnostic examinations. The values are for the relevant dose indicator for a specific examination for a standard size patient. National DRLs are in place in terms of entrance skin dose (ESD) (mGy) for individual radiographs and dose area product (DAP) (Gy·cm^2) for more complex examinations. For CT exams the DRL is given in terms of CT dose index (CTDI$_{vol}$) or dose length product (DLP).

The dose given for X-ray examinations to paediatrics is very dependant on the size of the child, but some typical dose values are given in the Appendix 2, Table 3.

The DRL for NM and PET scans is the ARSAC recommended level of activity (MBq) for that specific examination. DRL values and typical doses are given in the Appendix 2, Table 4.

For planning scans and simulator images there is no such guidance at present, but it is being discussed and guidance is likely to come. Meanwhile a principle such as 'as low as reasonably practicable' (ALARP) is applied to these exposures.

22.3.1.3 Issues concerning pregnancy status (Reg. 7(7))

It is recognized that diagnostic dose levels are very much lower than those given to the patient during radiotherapy, but checking for pregnancy will, be made first at the diagnostic stage for each individual patient. At diagnostic dose levels the only adverse effect of radiation on the fetus which is likely to pose a risk is that of cancer induction. The implementation of official recommendations (HPA 2009[12]) is discussed in the next paragraph. The procedure will apply to 12–55-year-old women (RCR 2007[13] has discussed the problems associated with asking teenage girls about pregnancy).

It is possible, though rare, that the practitioner may proceed with radiotherapy even if the patient is found to be pregnant, in which case the MPE will be asked to make a very careful estimate of risk to the unborn fetus.

In the diagnostic department (X-ray, nuclear medicine, or positron emission tomography (PET) or PET/computed tomography (CT)), the referrer ascertains the pregnancy status and the operator confirms this before carrying out the exposure. If the patient is pregnant, the examination may still continue, provided further justification takes place that indicates the exposure is of net benefit. This must be documented.

To avoid any significant risk from irradiating an unknown fetus if the diagnostic procedure is likely to give a dose of 10mGy or more to the uterus the imaging procedure may be carried out during the first 10 days of the woman's menstrual cycle. This has become known as 'the 10-day rule'.

In the radiotherapy department the procedure will include the following:

♦ It is the referrer's responsibility to ensure whether the patient may be pregnant and that the patient is informed about the risks of becoming pregnant (particularly if the patient is going to proceed to radiotherapy treatment).

♦ The IR(ME)R practitioner (consultant oncologist) will re-assess the pregnancy status before prescribing the RT treatment.

♦ The Operator's responsibilities will include, ensuring the patient be asked to sign a certificate declaring they are not pregnant and informing them that they must tell a radiographer before any ionizing radiation procedure that they may be pregnant.

22.3.1.4 Special treatment of infants, children, and young adults

The process of justification and optimization is particularly important for infants and young children since the risk of inducing a cancer is higher. This is due partly to the increased sensitivity to radiation of bone marrow in children and for young girls the developing breast tissue. Exposure protocols used for imaging should be specific to paediatrics, this is particularly important for CT scanning where the use of techniques used for adults can lead to unnecessarily high doses. Some details of the increase of breast cancer induction per mGy are shown in the Appendix 2, Table 5.

22.3.5 Reporting of incidents

Employers are obliged under regulation 4(5) to investigate where an incident has occurred or may have occurred in which a person has been exposed to ionizing radiation to an extent 'much greater than intended'.

If the investigation shows that such an exposure has occurred then the appropriate authority (in England this is CQC; in Wales, National Assembly for Wales: Health and Social Division; and in Scotland, Scottish Ministers: Scottish Executive Health Department) must be notified and the employer must arrange for a detailed investigation of the circumstances of the exposure and an assessment of the dose received. Appendix 2, Table 7 illustrates the existing guidance (second edition of PM77[14]) as to what constitutes a dose 'much greater than intended'. It can be seen that for radiotherapy the only criteria are for the fractional or total dose to the target.

22.3.6 Quality assurance

In order to maintain standards within the imaging departments and the radiotherapy department it is vital to have a quality assurance programme. This will cover all aspects of the work, staffing, and equipment within each department and will ensure that IR(ME)R matters are covered (equipment QA is under IRR99).

Patient dose audit—it is vital that the entire procedure for a particular examination is checked routinely and that the dose given by each procedure is in line with the national guidelines. Employer's procedures must be regularly reviewed, it should be documented how this is done, and which individual is responsible for the review being done.

Senior management must take responsibility for ensuring that procedures are reviewed at a sufficient frequency to take into account the impact of new technology and role development which will impact on ways of working.

22.4 The radiotherapy episode: justification and assessing patient dose

22.4.1 Diagnostic and staging imaging before the commencement of RT

A referral for imaging to diagnostic radiology is deemed to be a request for a professional opinion, which the radiologist as practitioner will justify and authorize if s/he thinks the exposure appropriate.

Exposures which meet referral criteria, as drawn up by the radiology department, may not need individual justification; however, they need to be authorized by the person carrying out the exposure. Where imaging involves nuclear medicine or PET scanning the practitioner must be the ARSAC certificate holder.

22.4.2 Planning and simulator images

It is simplest to consider doses incurred during planning and simulation as included in the radiotherapy prescription. The above exposures are requested by the oncologist (IR(ME)R referrer) in accordance with written and signed protocols drawn up by the lead specialist oncologist (IR(ME)R practitioner). The protocols should be sufficiently flexible to allow for additional planning images and for more than one simulator session but must not be open ended. If exposures additional to those detailed in the protocol are required the exposures must be additionally justified and authorized. The protocols must be regularly reviewed as the number of simulator sessions may decrease as verification imaging becomes standard.

22.4.3 Verification imaging

These are the images taken during radiotherapy, either just before each treatment exposure is made or during the treatment exposure. They may be carried out at each fractionated treatment exposure, or less frequently in line with local protocols. Except for the exposures using the treatment field, all these verification methods give additional dose to the patient. The treatment itself and the concomitant verification images (using portal imaging or CT as defined in the treatment protocol) will be justified by a consultant clinical oncologist.

22.4.4 Justification and dose assessment

This requires that the benefit and detriment of every exposure be considered, taking into account the intention of each exposure and the characteristics of the individual patient. Any exposures performed outside of protocol must be justified separately (and a note made in the patient's record). This consideration is not a simple task. The target volume must be planned optimally with as much information from the scans as possible in order to define the target and critical structures optimally. The radiotherapy delivery must be checked regularly (both inter- and intrafraction), using verification imaging (see section 22.4.3) including the various forms of CT and cone beam CT (CBCT), to ensure that these volumes have been correctly covered or avoided respectively by the high radiation dose region. If this set of tasks is not performed optimally then the clinical oncologist is failing the radically treated patient. There is also a balance to be drawn for each patient between the potential for deterministic damage to critical structures and the risk of radiation-induced cancer. In addition, as delivery techniques become more complicated and treatment is tailored to inter/intra fractional organ movement more verification imaging will be required.

To make a full risk assessment for the individual patient, it is necessary under IR(ME)R to understand all those doses associated with the various images procedures during a radiotherapy episode. For the diagnostic images this may be considered to be straightforward by using effective dose. For a fuller interpretation of all the doses received by the radiotherapy patient, including those doses to organs/critical structures outside the treatment volume, it will be necessary to approach the problem differently. The treatment doses to organs immediately surrounding the target volume can be very high, for example: if the target dose is 70Gy then even at levels of 1–10% the doses to surrounding organs may be 700–7000mGy.

To estimate the risk of inducing a cancer in these organs (or damaging non-tumour tissue) it is necessary to determine individual organ doses (the most heavily irradiated organs for a particular treatment site) from all the imaging and treatment received by

Table 22.2A Prostate patient with the approximate dose per examination

Examination	E (mSv)	Typical max skin dose (mGy)	Iso centre dose (mGy)	Bladder dose (mGy)
Pre-treatment images				
CT (kV)	10	22	11	21
Diagnostic PET (400MBq FDG)	11	NA	NA	68
Simulator fluoroscopy, per min (pelvic area)	2.5	25	7	12
CBCT (kV)	3–15	35	17	33
Verification images				
CBCT (6MV)**	25	100	100	100
Tomotherapy image (3MV)	2.5	10	12	12
In room CT (kV)	10	22	11	21
CBCT (kV)	3–15	35	17	33
Portal imaging 6MV per image/MU	0.34	11	8	9
Portal kV image	0.1	1	0.2	0.4

**see references[15,16]

Table 22.2B Prostate patient. The approximate dose and risk per imaging regime

Protocol: verification imaging only	Typical E (mSv)	% Risk of cancer (r.f.of 5%/mSv)	Critical organ: bladder dose (mGy)	% Risk of bladder cancer (r.f. of 0.4%/Gy)
1) High (3 CBCT(kV) + portal 6MV 36 pairs of 2MU)	94	0.47	1395	0.56
2) CBCT kV (3 full pelvis + 36 half pelvis)	315	1.58	1287 (assumes all bladder in field)	0.51
3) Typical UK (1CTkV portal 6MV 10 pairs of 2MU)	24	0.12	381	0.15
4) Low UK (1CT + portal kV 10 pairs)	11	0.06	25	0.01

Table 22.3A Breast patient with the approximate dose per examination

Examination	Typical E (mSv)	Critical organ	
		Contralateral breast mGy	Lung mGy
Pre-treatment images			
Mammogram	0.3	0	0
Bone scan 500MBq Tc^{99m}	4	0	0
Sentinal node 20–40MBq Tc^{99m}	<1	0	0
CT (kV) full chest	8	12	20
CBCT (kV)	3–12	5–18	9–33
Simulator fluoroscopy for 1min	1.5	5	3
Verification images			
CBCT (6MV)	20	80	80
CT (kV)	8	12	20
Lat Portal imaging 6MV/image/MU	0.6	1.1	1.8
Lat Portal imaging kV /image	0.04	0.15	0.1

the patient and then to attach a stochastic risk factor to that total organ dose. This will have more meaning since effective dose combines together all ages and does not discriminate between the sexes. This is particularly important when considering infants, children and young adults in order to attribute the appropriate risk factor for cancer induction. A few examples of this approach have been given here, but it must be recognized that this is a developing subject.

Table 22.3B Breast patient. Approximate dose and risk per imaging regime

	Typical E (mSv)	% risk of cancer (r.f. 5%/Sv)	Critical organ: contralateral breast (mGy)	% risk of cancer induction in breast (r.f. 1.16 %/Gy)	Critical organ: lung (mGy)	% risk of cancer induction in lung (r.f. 1.74 %/Gy)
1) High (10CT full chest portal 6 MV 25 pairs of 2MU)	140	0.7	230	0.27	383	0.67
2) Typical UK (1CT full chest + 8 portal 6MV pairs of 2MU)	27	0.14	47	0.05	60	0.10
3) Motion tracking (1CT full chest + 25 of 4DCT half length of chest.)	508	2.5	1512	1.75	1270	2.2

Methods for making these exposures include:

- *Megavoltage portal imaging.* This is mainly now done using an electronic portal imaging device (EPID) attached to the gantry of the linear accelerator. Full imaging is achieved using a radiation field larger than the treatment field and often using an orthogonal pair of images. Most linacs also have a facility which allows the actual treatment field to be viewed on every field and every treatment; however, this can usually only be used to verify the shape of the multileaf collimator (MLC).

- *Kilovoltage imaging.* It is now possible to install in the treatment room, either attached to the linac or in the ceiling/floor of the room, a kilovoltage unit that can be used for routine imaging of the radiotherapy patient. When this is attached to the gantry of the linac the X-ray set and imaging plate (digital) are mounted orthogonally to the megavoltage beam (for Varian and Elekta models) and in-line (for Siemens). Other manufacturers install ceiling and floor mounted combinations of X-rays sets and imaging plates.

- *Megavoltage CT.* Tomotherapy[a] units image with megavoltage spiral CT (the energy of the imaging beam is slightly lower than the treatment beam); megavoltage cone beam CT is also available on conventional linacs (Siemens Unit).

- *Kilovoltage CT.* Siemens linacs can be combined in the treatment room with a conventional CT unit and a common couch that can be used both for the CT and the treatment.

---

[a] Tomotherapy is the name of the linac/CT product made by Tomotherapy Inc. (Madison, WI, USA)

- *Kilovoltage cone beam CT (CBCT)*. When a kV set is mounted on the linac gantry (Varian and Elekta) it can be used to take CT images with cone beam; a volume CT is achieved by using the cone beam and rotating the gantry through 360° in 1min.

In order to illustrate the above points a few examples have been taken from the various examinations required for the following tumour sites: prostate, breast, and lymphoma (Tables 22.2–22.4). The list of examinations is included in these tables together with various illustrative doses—effective dose; skin dose; isocentric dose (which gives a typical value of dose in the central region of the examination for organs close to this region,) and a dose to the most critical organ.

The values given in Tables 22.2–22.4 are an indication only. These values will depend on the geometry of the equipment used, the technique factors selected, the volume of the patient irradiated, and the size of the patient. The value of effective dose from a CT scan is also very dependant on the image length scanned, the image quality required, and the pitch of the scan (couch movement per rotation/X-ray beam width). If CT is used in an over sampling mode (pitch 0.1) to remove motion blurring and to define movement related margins (e.g. for four-dimensional CT imaging of the lungs) there is a theoretical possibility that a dose up to 10 times the conventional CT dose may be given; to be more realistic the table uses a factor of five. The medical physics expert in a cancer centre will be able to provide more specific doses for a particular equipment and image technique.

A number of verification imaging regimens have been considered for each treatment site, to indicate the variation of effective and critical organ doses with imaging modality and frequency of imaging. These doses have been multiplied by the relevant risk factor to give a possible induced cancer risk (life time) expressed as a percentage.

A risk factor (r.f.) of 5% per Sv has been taken from ICRP 60 (1990)[4] to estimate the number of cancers induced when adults (age 16–64 years) are irradiated with an

Table 22.4A Lymphoma (upper body)—age 10 years

Examination	E (mSv)	Critical organ		
		Breast dose (mGy)	Red bone marrow dose (mGy)	Lung dose (mGy)
Pre-treatment images				
Bone scan 355MBq Tc^{99m}	5	0	7	0.9
PET	13	5	6	6
PET with CT	17	22	10	18
CT (kV)	4	17	4	12
Simulator fluoroscopy for 1min (AP)	1.5	7	0.5	3.3
Verification images				
AP Portal kV/image	0.04	0.15	0.01	0.1
AP Portal 6MV/image/MU	2	10	0.5	7

Table 22.4B Lymphoma patient (upper body) aged 10. Approximate dose and risk per imaging regime

Protocol	E (mSv)	% risk of fatal cancer (r.f. 10%/Gy)	Critical organ: breast dose (mGy)	% risk of cancer in breast (r.f. 4.3%/Gy)[18]
1) High (1CT + 20 portal pairs 6MV of 1MU +5 PET with CT)	169	1.7	527	2.3
2) CT based (1CT+ 10kV portal pairs)	4.4	0.04	20	0.1

effective dose of E mSv. This value has been chosen since weighting factors used to calculate E are those given in ICRP 60.

Risk factors for inducing a cancer in an individual organ have been taken from ICRP 103 (2007)[5]. These are the most recent values available from the literature. The risk factors used are for irradiated adults, are gender specific, and are for fatal and non fatal cancers.

For lymphoma the values given in Table 22.4 are approximate but have been included because of potential risks to young patients. For example, PET/CT has become an issue with ethical committees for young people involved in clinical trials since multiple scans are given. However, in general this additional imaging dose may be more than offset by the reduction in radiotherapy dose with the use of involved fields instead of mantle fields. The evidence of secondary cancer for these patients is dramatic. Most of the research work on this appears to demonstrate that the secondary cancers induced in breast and lung are in the margins and high-dose regions of these organs.

22.5 Discussion

22.5.1 Prostate

It is interesting to compare the prostate doses with those found from measurements by Roger Harrison[17]. He also included measurements of the radiotherapy doses (scatter and leakage) and demonstrated that the imaging doses did not exceed a few percent of the radiotherapy doses. For a verification regimen that includes ten CT scans (kV) + 36 portals (MV) (an extreme number of images) the effective dose was found to be 125mSv and the dose to the bladder 1115mSv. Note dose from radiotherapy to bladder: 28,800 mSv (NB mSv has used here to allow a small neutron dose), therefore dose to bladder from concomitant imaging is <4%.

22.5.2 Breast

The use of CT for verification images leads to a higher contralateral breast dose than the use of a lateral portal image. The use of organ dose rather than effective dose gives a more detailed description of the cancer risk. This is clearly indicated by the ratio of breast dose to effective dose. For the regimes shown in Table 22.4B, the risk of cancer from the doses to contralateral breast and lung exceeds the nominal risk calculated from the effective dose.

22.5.3 **Lymphoma**

The total imaging doses under the 'high dose' regimen above are significant. The breast doses (approx 0.5Gy) by themselves give a theoretical risk for second cancer of 2.3% (for a 10–15-year-old girl). It is interesting to compare this dose with the various levels used in modern radiotherapy for these patients. The rate of induction of lung and breast cancer in patients treated for Hodgkin's disease, mainly with mantle fields, is now well understood[19,20]. This risk should now be reduced by the use of involved fields[21] where less of each critical structure is irradiated; so potentially reducing the impact of the increased imaging.

22.6 **Summary**

- Imaging in radiotherapy is very extensive and takes place throughout the patient journey, with images being taken for diagnosis, treatment planning, and verification of treatment.
- The control of these imaging processes is governed by the IR(ME)R.
- The doses received by the patient from pre-treatment imaging are relatively small, the highest effective dose being from a PET with CT examination.
- Verification imaging doses are higher, but are still generally only a few percent of the leakage and scatter dose. However, when frequent verification images, particularly CT, are taken the dose can become comparable to this value.
  - The critical organ typically receives a range of dose from scatter and leakage (depending how close it is to the PTV) from 1–90%.
  - A typical imaging dose to this organ will be about 0.1%, although this could increase to 1%.
- Imaging regimens need to be carefully reviewed in every Radiotherapy Department and this may be achieved by[22]:
  - Where possible using imaging techniques that do not involve ionizing radiation.
  - Reducing the field of view of the image to the smallest required.
  - Using image technique factors that are commensurate with the image quality required for treatment decisions to be made.
- It is vital to give special consideration to children and young adults who are exposed to radiation. This group of patients has a longer period of time over which they may express a radiation induced cancer and they may have more exposures to radiation during that period. It will be of great value to these patients, and the scientific community, to keep records of all these exposures for each individual[23].
- When considering risk to the individual patient the use of effective dose and a general risk factor of 5% per Sv for cancer induction may underestimate the risk. This is particularly true when the breast area is irradiated. The evidence for induction of radiation-induced cancer is sparse but suggests that the second cancers appear in the high-dose regions around the treatment area. This is also the volume that receives the verification imaging dose. Generally the increase in dose due to

this area from imaging is relatively low, but in the cases where frequent imaging, particularly (CT), is used these doses can become significant. However, the clinical oncologist has to weigh up all these issues for each patient when balancing the tumour control, morbidity, and second cancer risks.

References

1. Ionising Radiation (Medical Exposures) Regulations 2000 (SI 2000 no. 1059). London: HMSO, 2000.
2. UNSCEAR 2000 United Nations Scientific Committee on the Effects of Atomic Radiation: Sources and effects of ionising radiation. Report to the general assembly. *Vol. II: Effects.* Geneva: UN.
3. Dendy PP, Heaton B. *Physics for Diagnostic Radiology*, 2nd edn. London: IoP, 1999.
4. ICRP 60: Recommendations of the International Commission on Radiological Protection Publications *Annals of the ICRP* 1990; **21**: 1–3.
5. ICRP 103: Recommendations of the International Commission on Radiological Protection. IRCP Publications, 2007.
6. Martin C. Effective dose: how should it be applied to medical exposures? *Brit J Radiol* 2007; **80**: 639–47.
7. Council of the European Union: Council directive on laying down basic safety standards for the protection of the health of workers and the general public against dangers arising from ionising radiation. *Official J Eur Comm* 1996; **39**: L159.
8. Euratom Council Directive 97/43/Euratom on health protection of individuals against the dangers of ionising radiation in relation to medical exposure, and repealing Directive 84/466/Euratom 30th June 1997.
9. Ionising Radiation Regulations 1999 (SI 1999 No 3232) London: HMSO.
10. *Work with Ionising Radiations: Approved Code of Practice and Guidance Approved Code of Practice.* London: HSE, 2000.
11. Institute of Physics and Engineering in Medicine. *Medical and Dental Guidance Notes. A good practice guide on all aspects of ionising radiation protection in the clinical environment.* York: IPEM, 2002.
12. Documents of the Health Protection Agency. *Protection of Pregnant Patients during Diagnostic Medical Exposures to Ionising Radiation.* March 2009.
13. RCR *Advice on exposure to ionising radiation in pregnancy in children.* Ref. BFCR(07)6 RCR London: RCR, 2007.
14. Health and Safety Executive. *Radiation equipment used for medical exposure.* Guidance Note PM77, 2nd edn. London: HSE, 1998.
15. Gayou O, Miften M. Commissioning and clinical implementation of a mega-voltage cone beam CT system for treatment localisation. *Med Phys* 2007; **34**: 3188–92.
16. Amer A, Marchant T, Sykes J, *et al.* Imaging doses from the Elekta Synergy X-ray cone beam CT. *BJR* 2007; **80**: 276–82.
17. Harrison RM, Wilkinson M, Shemilt A, *et al.* Organ doses from prostate radiotherapy and associated concomitant exposures. *Brit J Radiol* 2006; **79**: 487–96.
18. NHSBSP. *Review of Radiation Risks in Breast Screening. Report by a joint working party of the NHSBSP National Coordinating Group for Physics Quality Assurance and the National Radiological Protection Board.* NHSBSP Publication No 54 (Feb 2003). Sheffield: NHS Cancer Screening Programme, 2003.

19. Travis LB, Hill DA, Dores GM, *et al*. Breast cancer following radiotherapy and chemotherapy among young women with Hodgkin disease. *JAMA* 2003; **290**: 465–75.

20. van Leeuwen FE, Klokman WJ, Veer MB, *et al* Long-term risk of second malignancy in survivors of Hodgkin's Disease treated during adolescence or young adulthood. *J Clin Oncol* 2000; **18**: 487–97.

21. Hoskin P, Smith P, Maughan TS, *et al.* Long term results of a randomised trial of involved field radiotherapy versus extended field radiotherapy in stage I and II Hodgkin lymphoma. *Clin Oncol* (R Coll Radiol) 2005; **17**: 47–53.

22. AAPM The management of imaging dose during image-guided radiotherapy: Report of the AAPM Group 75. *Med Phys* 2007; **34**: 4041–63.

23. Royal College of Radiologists. *Guidance on the retention and destruction of NHS medical records concerned with chemotherapy and radiotherapy.* Clinical Oncology publication BFCO (96)3. London: RCR, 1996.

Additional guidance

The Royal College of Radiologists, Society and College of Radiographers, Institute of Physics and Engineering in Medicine. *A Guide to Understanding the Implications of the Ionising Radiation (Medical Exposure) Regulations in Radiotherapy.* London: The Royal College of Radiologists, 2008.

Appendix 1 to Chapter 22

Research and imaging in radiotherapy

All research involving ionizing radiation must comply with:

- IR(ME)R (2000), and Amendment (2006).
- The Medicines for Human Use (Clinical Trials) Regulations 2004.
- The Medicines (Administration of Radioactive Substances) Regulations 1978 (MARS).
- IRR (1999).
- The Radioactive Substances Act (RSA) 1993.

The National Research Ethics service (NRES) has produced guidance to researchers, radiation experts, employers, and Research Ethics Committees (RES) on the procedures for planning, review, and authorization of all medical and biomedical research involving the use of ionizing radiation. 'Approval for research involving ionising radiation version 2; 2008' can be viewed at: http://www.nres.npsa.nhs.uk/applicants/guidance

The medicines for Human Use regulations 2004[1], requires a single ethical opinion as to the benefit of a research project. IR(ME)R, however, requires the exposure to each individual to be justified, the guidance explains the harmonization of these two processes.

A 'research exposure' is deemed to be, any exposure required by the research protocol. It includes all exposures carried out on the participant as determined by the protocol, including those which would otherwise be part of routine clinical care for patients.

The research is lead by the Chief Investigator (CI) who has overall responsibility for the conduct of the research. S/he is responsible for submitting the research protocol on the electronic form given on the Integrated Research Application System (IRAS) website (https://www.myresearchproject.org.uk/Signin.aspx) and obtaining a single favorable ethical opinion from the main REC.

The CI will need to involve other duty holders:

- A Principle Investigator (PI) is required at each research site. The PI must ensure that their specific site can comply with the research protocols, as given in the application form, and that mechanisms are in place such that the requirements of other legislation, given above, can be met. In addition to the ethical approval by the main REC the PI must ensure that the local ethics committee approves the research. For research carried out at a single site the PI may be the same individual as the CI.
- A Clinical Radiation Expert (CRE) completes the clinical assessment section given on the IRAS form for radiation exposures that are part of the research protocol. The CRE will advise the main REC as to whether the exposures are necessary and whether the potential benefits to the individual (or society) outweigh the possible detriment from the radiation exposure. The role of the CRE may be undertaken by

the CI, a radiologist, an oncologist, or a nuclear medicine specialist with expertise in the imaging modality involved in the study. Where the research involves the administration of radioactive substances, the CRE must be an ARSAC[2] certificate holder.

In addition, if the research involves exposures that are additional to those normally carried out by the certificate holder, then the certificate holder must apply for a 'research ARSAC certificate'. The certificate is site, procedure and holder specific and requires input from the Radiation Protection Advisor (RPA).

- A Medical Physics Expert (MPE) is required to inform the CRE of the total research protocol dose and possible radiation detriment to a research participant. If more than 1 centre is involved the assessment must account for variations in dose due to equipment and imaging techniques used. This information will aid the setting of a dose constraint*/dose target** as required by IRMER. [*Radiation dose constraints are established in studies where there is no health benefit to be expected from the exposure. **Target dose levels are established in studies where there is some expected health benefit for participants from the exposure.]

- For research in RT where the study involves changes in therapeutic dose or volume delivery, the CRE will advise on the expected therapeutic outcome compared to the standard protocol. The MPE may, however, give advice on additional exposures associated with the patient treatment which does not follow standard protocols.

- A Radiation Protection Adviser (RPA) is required if the research involves the use of radioactive materials. The RPA must demonstrate that the site can safely handle the radioactive materials, such that doses to staff and other persons are kept as low as reasonably practical (ALARP), and within dose limits (IRR'99). The RPA must also ensure that the register of nuclides and activities held at the site, as required by the Environment Agency (EA), is not breached and that the site has permission to dispose of (by best practical means) the research nuclides and activities.

The main REC application process generally ensures that any additional radiation exposure required by the protocol is ethically acceptable. However there is still a legal requirement for the employer to demonstrate compliance with IR(ME)R for the research, in particular:

- Dose constraints/target dose levels are established and adhered to.
- Exposures are individually justified by a practitioner.
- Individuals participate voluntarily.
- Participants are informed of the risks related to the radiation exposures.

The arrangements for ensuring IR(ME)R compliance at different NHS Trusts will vary.

References

1. The Medicines for Human Use (Clinical Trials) Regulations. Statutory Inst. 2004 No. 1031. Available at: http://www.opsi.gov.uk/si/si2004/20041031.htm
2. ARSAC. *Administration of Radioactive Substances Advisory Committee. Notes for Guidance.* London: DoH 1988.

Appendix 2 to Chapter 22

Table 1 Deterministic effects from a single dose of radiation[1]

Effect	Organ/dose	Time to develop effect	Absorbed dose mGy
Morbidity			
Main phase of skin reddening	Skin (large areas)	1–4 weeks	3000–6000
Skin burns	Skin (large areas)	2–3 weeks	5000–10000
Temporary hair loss	Skin	2–3 weeks	~4000
Cataract (visual impairment)	Eye	Several years	~1500
Mortality			
Gastrointestinal syndrome with conventional medical care	Small intestine	6–9 days	>6000
Pneumonitis	Lung	1–7 months	6000

Table 2 Tissue-weighting factors—International Commission on Radiological Protection[1,2]

	ICRP 60 1990	ICRP 103 2007
Organ	W_T	W_T
Gonads	0.2	0.08
Bone marrow (red)	0.12	0.12
Colon	0.12	0.12
Lung	0.12	0.12
Stomach	0.12	0.12
Bladder	0.05	0.04
Breast	0.05	0.12
Liver	0.05	0.04
Oesophagus (thymus)	0.05	0.04
Thyroid	0.05	0.04
Skin	0.01	0.01
Bone surface	0.01	0.01
Brain	–	0.01
Salivary glands	–	0.01
Remainder 1	0.025	0.12
Remainder 2	0.025	0

Table 3 Paediatric typical effective dose from diagnostic examinations

Examination	Typical E (mSv)
Abdomen AP	0.09
Chest AP	0.01
Pelvis	0.08

Table 4 Effective dose for nuclear medicine studies—adults and paediatric

FDG tumour imaging

	Adult	15 years	10 years	5 years	1 year
E (mSv/MBq)	0.027	0.032	0.047	0.073	0.13
Wt (kg)	70	58	36	20	10
Activity (MBq)	400	368	284	184	108
E (mSv)	11	12	13	13	14

Tc99m bone imaging

	Adult	15 years	10 years	5 years	1 year
E (mSv/MBq)	0.008	0.01	0.015	0.025	0.05
Activity (MBq)	500	460	355	230	135
E (mSv)	4	5	5	6	7

Table 5 Risk of inducing breast cancer/Gy (mean glandular dose to the breast) (NHSBSP report 54)[3]

Age at exposure	Risk % per Gy
5–15	4.3
20–30	1.8
35–50	1.7–1.4
55–70	1.2–0.6

Table 6 Typical effective doses for some diagnostic examinations[4]

Radiological examination (adults)	mSv
Limbs and joints (except hip)	<0.5
Chest (single PA)	0.02
Skull	0.06
Thoracic Spine	0.7
Lumber spine	1.0
Hip	0.4

Table 6 (continued) Typical effective doses for some diagnostic examinations[4]

Radiological examination (adults)	mSv
Pelvis	0.7
Abdomen	0.7
IVU	2.4
Barium swallow	1.5
Barium meal	2.6
Barium follow-through	3
Barium enema	7.2
CT head	2
CT chest	8
CT abdomen or pelvis	10
Lung Ventilation (Xe-133)	0.3
Lung perfusion (Tc-99m)	1
Kidney (Tc-99m)	1
Thyroid (Tc-99m)	1
Bone (Tc-99m)	4
Dynamic cardiac (Tc-99m)	6
PET head (F-18FDG)	5

Table 7 Multiplication factors defining exposures as 'much greater than intended'

Type of diagnostic examination	Multiplying factor applied to intended dose
Interventional radiology, radiographic, and fluoroscopic procedures involving contrast agents, nuclear medicine with intended dose E > 5mSv and CT examinations	3
Mammography, nuclear medicine with intended dose E <5mSv but >0.5mSv, all other radiographic examinations not referred to elsewhere in this table	10
Radiography of extremities, skull, dentition, shoulder, chest, elbow, knee, and nuclear medicine with intended dose E <0.5mSv	20
Type of treatment	**Multiplying factor applied to intended dose**
Beam therapy, brachytherapy	1.1 whole course or 1.2 any fraction
Unsealed radionuclide therapy	1.2 any administration

References

1. ICRP 60: Recommendations of the International Commission on Radiological Protection Publications *Annals of the ICRP* 1990; **21**: 1–3.
2. ICRP103: Recommendations of the International Commission on Radiological Protection. IRCP Publications, 2007.
3. NHSBSP. *Review of Radiation Risks in Breast Screening. Report by a joint working party of the NHSBSP National Coordinating Group for Physics Quality Assurance and the National Radiological Protection Board.* NHSBSP Publication No 54 (Feb 2003). Sheffield: NHS Cancer Screening Programme, 2003.
4. Royal College of Radiologists. *Making best use of clinical radiology services*, 6th edn. RCR London: RCR, 2007.

Index